Springer Series in Synergetics

Editor: Hermann Haken

Synergetics, an interdisciplinary field of research, is concerned with the cooperation of individual parts of a system that produces macroscopic spatial, temporal or functional structures. It deals with deterministic as well as stochastic processes.

1 **Synergetics** An Introduction 3rd Edition
By H. Haken
2 **Synergetics** A Workshop
Editor: H. Haken
3 **Synergetics** Far from Equilibrium
Editors: A. Pacault, C. Vidal
4 **Structural Stability in Physics**
Editors: W. Güttinger, H. Eikemeier
5 **Pattern Formation by Dynamic Systems and Pattern Recognition**
Editor: H. Haken
6 **Dynamics of Synergetic Systems**
Editor: H. Haken
7 **Problems of Biological Physics**
By L. A. Blumenfeld
8 **Stochastic Nonlinear Systems**
in Physics, Chemistry, and Biology
Editors: L. Arnold, R. Lefever
9 **Numerical Methods in the Study of Critical Phenomena**
Editors: J. Della Dora, J. Demongeot, B. Lacolle
10 **The Kinetic Theory of Electromagnetic Processes** By Yu. L. Klimontovich
11 **Chaos and Order in Nature**
Editor: H. Haken
12 **Nonlinear Phenomena in Chemical Dynamics**
Editors: C. Vidal, A. Pacault
13 **Handbook of Stochastic Methods**
for Physics, Chemistry, and the Natural Sciences
2nd Edition By C. W. Gardiner
14 **Concepts and Models of a Quantitative Sociology** The Dynamics of Interacting Populations By W. Weidlich, G. Haag
15 **Noise-Induced Transitions** Theory and Applications in Physics, Chemistry, and Biology
By W. Horsthemke, R. Lefever
16 **Physics of Bioenergetic Processes**
By L. A. Blumenfeld
17 **Evolution of Order and Chaos** in Physics, Chemistry, and Biology Editor H. Haken
18 **The Fokker-Planck Equation**
By H. Risken
19 **Chemical Oscillations, Waves, and Turbulence**
By Y. Kuramoto
20 **Advanced Synergetics**
By H. Haken
21 **Stochastic Phenomena and Chaotic Behaviour in Complex Systems**
Editor: P. Schuster
22 **Synergetics – From Microscopic to Macroscopic Order** Editor: E. Frehland
23 **Synergetics of the Brain**
Editors: E. Başar, H. Flohr, H. Haken, A. J. Mandell
24 **Chaos and Statistical Methods**
Editor: Y. Kuramoto
25 **Dynamics of Hierarchical Systems**
An Evolutionary Approach By J. S. Nicolis
26 **Self-Organization and Management of Social Systems**
Editors: H. Ulrich, G. J. B. Probst
27 **Non-Equilibrium Dynamics in Chemical Systems** Editors: C. Vidal, A. Pacault
28 **Self-Organization.** Autowaves and Structures Far from Equilibrium
Editor: V. I. Krinsky
29 **Temporal Order**
Editors: L. Rensing, N. I. Jaeger
30 **Dynamical Problems in Soliton Systems**
Editor: S. Takeno
31 **Complex Systems – Operational Approaches**
in Neurobiology, Physics, and Computers
Editor: H. Haken
32 **Dimensions and Entropies in Chaotic Systems**
Quantification of Complex Behavior
Editor: G. Mayer-Kress
33 **Selforganization by Nonlinear Irreversible Processes**
Editors: W. Ebeling, H. Ulbricht
34 **Instabilities and Chaos in Quantum Optics**
Editors: F. T. Arecchi, R. G. Harrison
35 **Nonequilibrium Phase Transitions in Semiconductors**
By E. Schöll
36 **Temporal Disorder in Human Oscillatory Systems**
Editors: L. Rensing, U. an der Heiden, M. C. Mackey

Temporal Disorder in Human Oscillatory Systems

Proceedings of an International Symposium
University of Bremen, 8–13 September 1986

Editors: L. Rensing, U. an der Heiden,
M. C. Mackey

With 122 Figures

Springer-Verlag Berlin Heidelberg New York
London Paris Tokyo

Professor Dr. Ludger Rensing
Fachbereich 2/Biologie, Universität Bremen
D-2800 Bremen, Fed. Rep. of Germany

Professor Dr. Uwe an der Heiden
Fakultät für Naturwissenschaften, Universität Witten/Herdecke
D-5810 Witten (Ruhr), Fed. Rep. of Germany

Professor Dr. Michael C. Mackey
Department of Physiology, McGill University
Montreal, Quebec, Canada H3G 1Y6

Series Editor:

Professor Dr. Dr. h. c. Hermann Haken
Institut für Theoretische Physik der Universität Stuttgart, Pfaffenwaldring 57/IV,
D-7000 Stuttgart 80, Fed. Rep. of Germany

ISBN 3-540-17765-5 Springer-Verlag Berlin Heidelberg New York
ISBN 0-387-17765-5 Springer-Verlag New York Berlin Heidelberg

Offset printing: Druckhaus Beltz, 6944 Hemsbach/Bergstr.
Bookbinding: J. Schäffer GmbH & Co. KG, 6718 Grünstadt
2153/3150-543210

Preface

There has been a rapid expansion of interest in alterations of human physiological rhythms over the past few years. Thus, it seemed timely to invite a diverse group of individuals with interests ranging from clinical medicine through basic biology to mathematical modelling to join intellectual forces for a week to consider the various approaches that may be taken, both experimentally and theoretically, to the study of human temporal disorder. The symposium on "Temporal Disorder in Human Oscillatory Systems" was held at the University of Bremen, September 1986. It was devoted to the analysis of human neural and neuromotor systems, heart and respiration, circadian rhythms and the ovarian cycle. These changes were discussed in terms of general principles, mathematical models and cellular mechanisms. The proceedings contain the invited lectures and selected contributions of the symposium.

We gratefully acknowledge the financial support of this symposium by the Stiftung Volkswagenwerk, Universität Bremen, Gesellschaft der Freunde der Universität Bremen, DuPont de Nemours (Deutschland), H. Jürgens (Bremen) and Siemens AG (Bremen).

Bremen, December 1986

Ludger Rensing
Uwe an der Heiden
Michael C. Mackey

Contents

Temporal Disorder –Introductory Remarks

The Editors

1. Introduction

Those studying basic biological, chemical, and physical processes are quite accustomed to the marked periodic or aperiodic variations in certain variables important for system function and integrity (1,2). Like these phenomena, there are a variety of normal physiological processes that occur at regular, or almost regular, intervals. Abnormalities in many of these physiological rhythms are of major clinical importance. In addition, these oscillations demonstrate that there is a rich variety of dynamics that many physiological control systems can exhibit, ranging from rhythms with differing periodicities to irregular "noise-like" phenomena.

In 1963, Reimann (3) drew attention to a broad group of diseases which he collectively referred to as periodic diseases. In all of these diseases oscillations appeared in physiological systems that were not normally oscillatory. As an extension of the concept of periodic diseases, the concept of a dynamical disease has been introduced (4-7). A dynamical disease is defined as a disease that occurs in an intact physiological control system operating in a range of control parameters that leads to abnormal dynamics. The hallmark of a a dynamic disease is a change in the qualitative dynamics of some observable as one or more parameters are changed. These changes in dynamics correspond mathematically to bifurcations in the relevant non-linear equations describing the physiological system.

Clearly, there is a great deal of subjective interpretation concerning the question of whether or not alterations of physiological rhythms constitute disease. Regardless of this issue we may, in some sense, classify changes from normal to abnormal physiological rhythms as "temporal disorder".

2. Routes to temporal disorder

In general, three types of qualitative changes in dynamics have been observed: 1) the appearance of regular or irregular oscillations in a physiological system not normally characterized by rhythmic processes; 2) the development of an altered or new periodicity in an already periodic process; and 3) the disappearance of a rhythmic process (8).

A. Appearance of rhythms

Changes from a stable steady behaviour to an oscillatory state may occur in a variety of normal situations, such as the development of circadian rhythms in newborns, the development of ovarian hormonal cycles before and during puberty (LACKER) or the shift from quiescent to cycling state in populations of cells. Further, the appearance of a regular, or almost regular, rhythm in a normally stable physiological process has long attracted clinical interest.

Examples include the periodic diseases described by Reimann (3) as well as a number of neurological (BUNZ & HAKEN, FREUND, STARK) and psychological phenomena (ENGELMANN, LEWY), and hematological disorders.

B. Appearance of altered or new periodicities

Situations occur in which an oscillation with a new periodicity and waveform replaces a previously oscillatory process. Well known examples come from cardiology (GLASS, GOLDBERGER, GUEVARA), the appearance of abnormal respiratory cycles such as Cheyne-Stokes respiration, and transitions between periodic states that occur during seizure activity (BABLOYANTZ, MAYER-KRESS) or in response to medication.

These transitions are commonly seen in the interaction of two or more oscillatory processes with one another, and are of great importance for understanding the response of organisms to periodicities in their environment (RENSING). Depending on the characteristic frequencies of the two oscillatory processes, as well as their relative amplitudes and coupling, a variety of phase relations between the oscillations may ensue that have widespread potential significance in psychological and psychiatric contexts (EASTMAN, HILDEBRANDT, LEWY). Similarly, the variable integral phase relations resulting from changes in the coupling of two or more internal circadian osillators may be related to the onset of certain types of depression (PFLUG, ENGELMANN). The appearance of ultradian rhythms in the blood pressure of aging individuals (YATES) may be another example of rhythm desynchronization as are the transitions between various oscillatory domains in developing systems (GOLDBETER, VICKER).

C. Loss of rhythmicity

The final situation occurs in which there is the disappearance of a rhythmic process. Examples of this include alterations associated with aging (YATES), a replacement of the normal cardiac rhythm by atrial or ventricular fibrillation (GOLDBERGER, GUEVARA, KEENER), the development of apneic respiratory rhythms, in the ovarian cycle during pregnancy and after menopause, and in circadian oscillators under very high light intensities (EASTMAN, LEWY). The ability to actually eliminate these circadian rhythms by lesions of appropriate pacemaker regions of the mammalian brain (RIETVELD), or by inducing a mutation in the period locus of *Drosophila* (9), is helpful in understanding the genesis of these rhythms.

3. Models for temporal disorder

Ever increasingly mathematical models offer insight into the origin and potential control of various types of oscillatory phenomena. They are useful for the concise description of underlying mechanisms and for investigating how and why various types of oscillations may arise from these mechanisms. In addition, they often provide a coherent framework for drawing connections between a wide class of different types of oscillations and for predicting when transitions between these various types may occur as parameters within the system are varied.

The ultimate hope for many of us working in this field is that this knowledge will aid the development of therapeutic strategies for moving systems from regions of parameter space in which they exhibit pathological behaviour into a region in which they are again classified as healthy.

There are two basic classes of mathematical models for oscillatory processes. One of them includes autonomous oscillators which, independent of any external oscillatory input, spontaneously generate one or more types of oscillatory patterns (GUEVARA, AN DER HEIDEN & MACKEY). In the other class are included systems which are coupled to some external oscillator. In these, the system of particular interest is that which is spontaneously oscillating but interacting with an external oscillatory input. The coupling of two oscillators may lead to extremely complex types of behaviour as investigated in several of these contributions (GOLDBETER, GLASS, KEENER).

The variety of mathematical models that have been proposed and examined within the context of dynamical diseases and temporal disorder is almost as broad and diverse as the phenomena they purport to model. However, there are a number of underlying regularities and whether the model is framed as a finite difference equation (GLASS), as a set of ordinary differential equations (BUNZ & HAKEN, GOLDBETER), or as partial differential equations (GUEVARA, KEENER) there are certain general types of bifurcation pattern that the solutions display as particular control parameters are varied (10,11).

However, it is now clear that these various bifurcation patterns are neither exhaustive nor universal as shown by the bifurcation patterns in time delay differential equations (AN DER HEIDEN & MACKEY). It is safe to say that almost all physiological systems contain significant nonlinearities in their feedback mechanisms, and in many of these time delays are extremely important. These time delays may arise because, for example, of the time required for a cell to mature, of the time for the nerve impulse to travel along the axon and across the synapse, or the time for hormonal signals to travel from their site of production to target organs by diffusion and/or passage through the circulation.

4. Is chaos sometimes the norm?

As the papers of these proceedings illustrate, a wealth of dynamical behaviour ranging from periodic to irregular, noise-like oscillations can readily be observed in physiological systems both experimentally and clinically. Although many of these individual situations are familiar to the cell biologist, biochemist, physiologist, psychologist, and clinician, the universal and fundamental aspects of their rich dynamical fabric does not yet appear to be fully appreciated. The presumed importance of these qualities becomes more evident when it is realized that relatively simple non-linear mathematical models have these same properties, thus implying that dynamic complexity may be the norm rather than the exception in nonlinear systems.

Most normal physiological oscillations also show variability, though sometimes very small, e.g. in inter-event intervals and consecutive amplitudes. The usual interpretation of this irregularity is to attribute it to biological "noise" or "slop". Although in some cases such an interpretation may be reasonable, irregularity may in fact be a reflection of the intrinsic dynamics of the system,and thus would be observed even in the complete absence of biological "noise". Examples in which there is some evidence to indicate that the observed variability may, at least in part, be of deterministic origin include the cell generaton time (12-14), inter-beat variability in the electrocardiogram (15,16), background activity in the electro-encephalogram (MAYER-KRESS), and irregular glucose-induced oscillations in the electrical activity of mouse pancreatic beta-cells (17,18).

Mathematical techniques are under development to analyze the irregularities noted in experimental data with the goal of learning something about the nature of the underlying system (19, MAYER-KRESS). However, confirmation that oberved irregular dynamics are in fact deterministic chaos is problematic. Indeed, in view of the fact that for almost every time series there are an infinite number of possible deterministic systems that will generate a time series with the same statistical properties (20), it would seem that obtaining a unique solution, at least for arbitrarily chosen examples of noise-like dynamics, is not possible.

In spite of the presumed importance of the dynamic aspects of physiological system functioning, it is not always clear how oscillatory properties are important for the integrity of the organism. Sometimes, it is clear. For example, the utility of the oscillatory processes underlying locomotion and the transport of body fluids, gases, and food is obvious. The same is true for the adaptational advantage of circadian and circannual clocks which may serve to optimize the response of organisms to periodic changes in the environment (21). However, in other situations it is not obvious that particular dynamical characteristics do serve an adaptive function or confer any selective advantage to the system. For example, the "noise" seen in the electrical activity of the nervous system, it is argued by some, may have special positive effects on the ability of the nervous system to perform certain kinds of tasks. If variability is an intrinsic dynamic ingredient in the operation of normal physiological system, then its significance is far from clear. It is not difficult to see that an irregular oscillation encodes more information in its varying amplitudes and inter-event intervals than does a precisely periodic oscillation. However, it remains to be seen what the purpose of this information is and whether transmitting it by a noisy signal is more faithful in the face of ever-present biological noise. At this time an elucidation of the adaptive role of noise awaits a fuller understanding of the meaning of dynamic complexity and its alterations.

The work presented in this symposium highlights the importance of careful experimental documentation of the time-dependent behaviour of physiological systems, particularly in response to changes in the environment. Such observations not only provide valuable insight into the nature of the underlying control systems, but also place constraints on the features that proposed models must contain. Unfortunately, it is uncommon to find published time series for physiological phenomena, particularly in the recent clinical literature. It is quite possible that both interesting and relevant dynamical changes are often observed but not published because their significance is not fully appreciated, or the dynamical changes are wrongly ascribed to environmental noise and/or experimental error.

In mathematical models, changes in dynamics correspond to bifurcations which occur as one or more control parameters are varied. Dynamical diseases may similarly arise because of pathological alterations in underlying physiological control parameters. Clearly the hope is that it may eventually be possible to develop diagnostic techniques to identify dynamical diseases as well as the altered control parameters. Therapeutic strategies could then be devised to re-adjust these altered control parameters by, for example, using mechanical, electrical or pharmacological stimuli to reposition the control system in a range of parameter space associated with "healthy" dynamical behaviour.

5. References

1. H. Haken (Ed): Dynamics of Synergetic Systems (Springer, Berlin, Heidelberg 1980)
2. L. Rensing, N.I. Jaeger (Ed): Temporal Order (Springer, Berlin, Heidelberg 1985)
3. H.A. Reimann: Periodic Diseases, F.A. Davis, Philadelphia (1963)
4. M.C. Mackey, L. Glass: Science 197, 287-289 (1977)
5. L. Glass, M.C. Mackey: Ann. N.Y. Acad. Sci. 316, 214-235 (1979)
6. M.C. Mackey, U. an der Heiden: Funk. Biol. Med. 1, 156-164 (1982)
7. M.C. Mackey, J.G. Milton: Proc. New York Acad. Sci., in press
8. L. Glass, M.C. Mackey: From Clocks to Chaos: The Rhythms of Life, in press
9. R.J. Konopka, S. Benzer: Proc. Natl. Acad. Sci. US 68, 2112 (1971)
10. J.P. Eckmann: Rev. Mod. Phys. 53, 643-654 (1981)
11. E. Ott: Rev. Mod. Phys. 53, 655-671 (1981)
12. A. Lasota, M.C. Mackey: J. Math. Biology 19, 43-62 (1984)
13. M.C. Mackey: In Temporal Order ed. by L. Rensing and N.I. Jaeger (Springer, Berlin, Heidelberg 1985) p.315

14. M.C. Mackey, M. Santavy, P. Selepova: In Nonlinear Oscillations in Biology and Chemistry, ed. by H. Othmer (Springer, Berlin, Heidelberg in press)
15. M. Kobayashi, T. Musha: IEEE Trans. Biomed. Eng. 29, 456-457 (1982)
16. A.L. Goldberger, L.J. Findley, M.R. Blackburn, A.J. Mandell: Amer. Heart J. 107, 612-615 (1984)
17. T.R. Chay, J. Rinzel: Biophys. J. 47, 357-366 (1985)
18. P. LeBrun, I. Atwater: Biophys. J. 48, 529-531 (1985)
19. J.-P. Eckmann, D. Ruelle: Rev. Mod. Phys. 57, 617-656 (1985)
20. A. Lasota, M.C. Mackey: Probabilistic Properties of Deterministic Systems. (Cambridge University Press, Cambridge 1985)
21. L. Rensing: Biol. Rdsch. 24, 5-15 (1986)

Part I

Theoretical Concepts

Coupled Oscillators in Health and Disease

L. Glass

Department of Physiology, McGill University, 3655 Drummond Street, Montreal, H3G 1Y6, Quebec, Canada

All major organ systems of the body display rhythmic activity. These rhythms interact with one another and with the external environment to provide complex dynamics which underly fundamental life processes. The point of this presentation is to provide a brief summary of the role of coupled oscillators in normal and pathophysiology (Section 1), to sketch out experimental approaches to the study of coupled oscillators and indicate some main results (Section 2) and finally to indicate mathematical approaches and problems involved in the analysis (Section 3).

I. Coupled Oscillators in Normal and Pathophysiology

The various bodily rhythms can all be influenced by environmental periodicities such as the day-night cycle, eating, exercise and therapeutic interventions. As well, the bodily rhythms can interact with one another through multiple feedback paths through the blood, nerves and anatomical structures of the body. Although we are often aware of the various bodily rhythms, we are less frequently aware of their interactions. In this section I list several of the interactions of physiological oscillations with the external environment and with each other.

A. Interactions of Physiological Rhythms with the External Environment

There is a normal circadian (about 24 hours) rhythm which interacts with the periodic light dark cycle [1,2]. The coupling is generally thought to arise through influence of light on neural structures (e.g. the suprachiasmatic nucleus). The actual physiological basis of the circadian rhythm is controversial. Some think that there are two internal oscillators, one controlling the sleep-wake cycle and the other the bodily temperature and that the synchronization or lack thereof of the two rhythms plays a fundamental role in a person's circadian functioning [1,2]. Lack of entrainment of the intrinsic rhythms to the normal 24 hour rhythm may play a role in insomnias and affective illness [3]. Principles of phase resetting of oscillations may be useful in minimizing jet lag [4] and treating insomnia [5] and affective illness [3].

Many drug therapies are administered periodically (take two red pills every six hours!). Drug doses are usually determined on the basis of therapeutic drug levels and drug half-lives. Since such parameters may be difficult to assess administration of many drugs is "titrated" in a particular individual. Thus, drugs are gradually increased until desired therapeutic effects are achieved or adverse side-effects preclude further drug increase. Detailed consideration of the periodic drug administration on the intrinsic bodily rhythms may often not be carefully assessed [6]. One expects, a priori, possibility of complex interactions of drugs with the intrinsic rhythms. For example, one area in which it is often difficult to stabilize rhythms is in brittle diabetics. In such patients the fluctuating blood glucose and insulin levels may not be easily stabilized using periodic insulin administration [7].

Dramatic therapeutic measures are undertaken in patients with cardiac and respiratory arrest or failure. In such patients it may be necessary to use artificial pacemakers or mechanical ventilators to maintain adequate oxygenation of tissues. In both instances periodic stimulation is delivered to physiological systems which themselves may be potentially oscillating. This may lead to potentially complex interactions as will be sketched out in Section 2. In the clinical situations there may be sensing mechanisms so that the bodily rhythms feed back to influence the functioning of the pacemaker or ventilator. This adds a further level of mathematical complexity.

An unusual example, not well understood, is the periodic rocking of infants to put them to sleep. Presumably, the periodic stimulation of the vestibular system acts centrally, perhaps to entrain respiration. As a final example, consider the coupling between intrinsic and external periodicities during intercourse. This is not usually analyzed from a standpoint of the physiology and mathematics of coupled oscillators.

B. Interactions of Intrinsic Physiological Rhythms

In some systems, the coupling of multiple oscillators of the same tissue plays a key role in stabilizing and controlling the intrinsic rhythm. This is true for example for the sinus node [8], the gut [9] and locomotory [10] rhythms. Interactions between oscillators in a single tissue can also be associated with pathology. Thus, the appearance of spontaneous pacemakers in abnormal locations in the heart leads to cardiac arrhythmias such as parasystole [11].

There are also well-documented interactions between different organ systems. An entrainment between the breathing rhythm and locomotory rhythm has been found in humans and other species [12]. The heart rate is usually slightly increased during the inspiratory phase of respiration (respiratory sinus arrhythmia) [13]. There is an interaction between breathing and swallowing rhythms which is apparent in nursing infants.

Despite the above examples in which there are clear-cut interactions between oscillators in different physiological systems, the interactions between multiple endogenous rhythms are often not carefully considered or analyzed. Thus, there is periodic sympathetic activity associated with the respiratory cycle [14] but the influence of any of this on the many rhythms of endocrine secretion does not appear to be well documented. There is periodic afferent activity from baroreceptors, chemoreceptors, stretch receptors in the lungs, and elsewhere in the musculoskeletal system. In each case, these periodic inputs play a role in modulating the intrinsic rhythmic activity of the system which activates them, but the effects on other organ systems are not as well known. Likewise, it is not easy to document the effects of endocrine periodicities on other rhythms of the body. Thus, it seems that elucidation of the coupling between multiple physiological oscillations is a rich area for future studies.

2. Experimental Studies of the Periodic Forcing of Physiological Rhythms

One experimental paradigm for studying physiological oscillators is to subject the oscillator to periodic stimuli while maintaining physiological conditions as constant as possible. As the frequency and amplitude of the periodic stimulus are varied, a variety of different coupling patterns are set up between the stimulus and the spontaneous oscillator. In some situations the spontaneous rhythm is entrained or phase locked to the forcing stimulus so that for each N cycles of the stimulus there are M cycles of the spontaneous rhythm, and the spontaneous oscillation occurs at fixed phase (or phases) of the periodic stimulus (N:M phase locking). In addition to phase-locked rhythms, it is also possible to observe irregular or aperiodic rhythms in which fixed phase relationships and regular repeating cyclic patterns are not observed. I discuss two illustrative systems that have been studied at McGill: the mechanical ventilation of animals, and the periodic stimulation of cardiac oscillations using an intracellular microelectrode. Generalizations can be drawn from the work which are broadly applicable in a wide variety of experimental systems.

It has been known since the time of Hering and Breuer that periodic lung inflation by a mechanical ventilator can lead to phase locking between the ventilator and the intrinsic respiratory rhythm in mammals. The entrainment is believed to be mediated by the Hering-Breuer reflexes in which expansion of the lungs inhibits inspiration and prolongs expiration [15].

Experiments were performed on paralyzed, pentobarbital-anesthetized adult cats, and central respiratory activity was monitored by recording from a branch of the phrenic nerve [16]. In a normal unparalyzed animal, the phrenic nerve innervates the diaphragm and phrenic nerve activity causes the diaphragm to contract (lower), thus leading to inspiration. In the paralyzed animal, neuromuscular transmission between the phrenic nerve and the diaphragm is blocked and lung inflation is solely due to the mechanical ventilator. However, afferent activity from stretch receptors in the lung is still carried by the vagus nerve. CO_2 was added to the inspired gas in order to maintain constant physiological levels of CO_2 even at high ventilator volumes and frequencies.

As the ventilator volume and frequency are varied, a number of different rhythms are established between the ventilator and phrenic activity. These different rhythms are organized in an orderly fashion in the ventilator volume-ventilator frequency plane shown in Fig. 1. Insets show representative traces of ventilator volumes and phrenic nerve activity corresponding to different

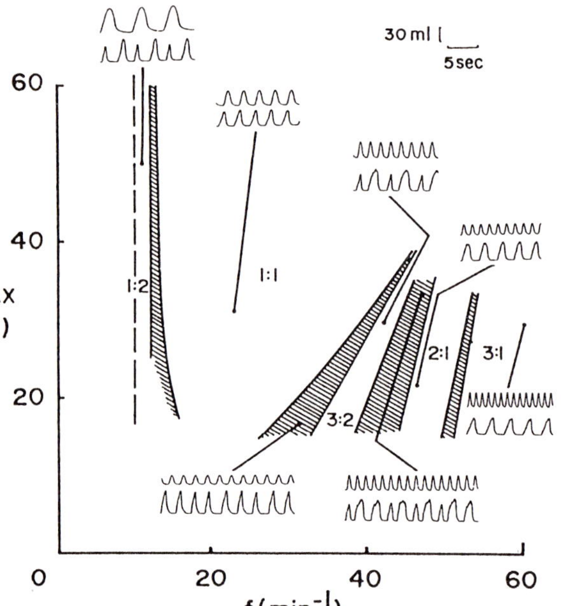

Fig. 1 Schematic diagram of phase locking zones obtained from paralyzed anesthetized mechanically ventilated cats with intrinsic respiratory frequency of about 20 min^{-1} and constant end-tidal CO_2. In each inset the upper trace is lung volume and lower trace is "integrated" phrenic activity. In regions between stable phase locked zones (shaded regions) irregular dynamics are found. V_{max}, maximal volume of ventilator, f, frequency of ventilator. Figure reproduced from [26].

stable phase-locked rhythms, as well as non-phase-locked rhythms (which occur in the shaded regions). In these experiments low ventilation frequencies and volumes could not be studied since adequate ventilation must be maintained. Likewise, very high volumes and frequencies could not be studied because of mechanical limitations of the ventilator, and the limited lung capacity of the cat.

Another series of experiments studied the effects of pulsatile electrical stimuli delivered to spontaneously beating cells derived from the ventricles of embryonic chick heart [17,18].

As the frequency and current intensity of the electrical stimuli are varied, a variety of different rhythms between the stimulator and the heart cells are established. The results of these experiments are summarized in the composite in Fig. 2. In this figure the insets represent the different observed phase-locking patterns, and the solid lines represent the results of theoretical computations based on phase-resetting experiments using single pulses. As well as the stable phase-locked rhythms, there are also a number of irregular rhythms. Theoretical techniques have been used to compute the phase-locking zones and associate the observed irregular rhythms with chaotic dynamics.

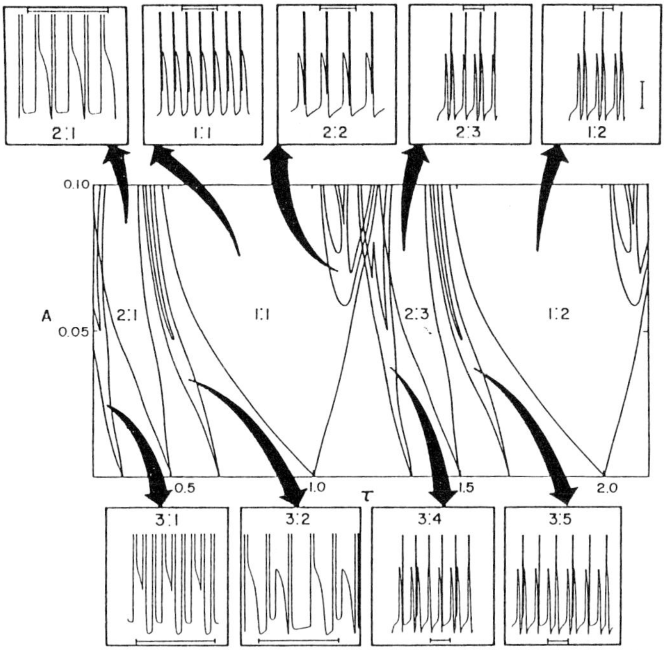

Fig. 2 Theoretically computed phase locking zones (solid lines) and experimental traces (insets) for periodically stimulated aggregates of embryonic heart cells. The ordinate is stimulus amplitude in arbitrary units and the abscissa is the stimulation period divided by the intrinsic cycle length. Computations from [8]. Horizontal scale is 500 msec and vertical scale is 50 mV. Figure reproduced from L. Glass, M.R. Guevara, A. Shrier, Ann N.Y. Acad. Sci. (In the Press).

Although the results in Figs. 1 and 2 have been obtained from two very different physiological systems using different types of periodic stimulation, there are certain striking gross features which are common to both. The following generalizations are applicable to a large number of experiments of periodic forcing of biological oscillators.

i) The stable zones of phase locking which are most commonly observed correspond to low order ratios between the number of cycles of the forcing stimulus and the intrinsic rhythm (i.e. 2:1, 3:2, 1:1, 2:3, 1:2). Although other N:M ratios with larger values of N and M can also be observed, these occupy smaller areas in the frequency-amplitude parameter space, and they are consequently easily overlooked or obscured by noise.

ii) The stable rhythms are organized in the frequency-amplitude plane in an orderly fashion. It is common to associate a rotation number $\rho = M/N$ with an N:M rhythm. Then as the stimulation frequency increases at fixed stimulus amplitude, ρ decreases.

iii) At very low stimulation amplitudes it is difficult to maintain stable phase locking.

iv) If the regions of frequency-amplitude parameter space between stable phase-locking zones are studied, then it is generally possible to find stimulation parameters which give rise to irregular dynamics.

These conclusions are supported by a number of studies in diverse systems [19,20,21].

Despite their similarities, there are differences between the cardiac and respiratory systems. For example, the 2:2 region observed in the periodically stimulated cardiac cells was not observed in the mechanically ventilated cats. The goal of theoretical studies of phase locking is to provide a theoretical basis for understanding the similarities and differences between the different preparations. Ideally, one would like to be able to make predictions about the phase-locking as stimulation parameters vary, based on the mechanisms of rhythmogenesis and the coupling of the stimulator to the intrinsic rhythm. In practice, the mathematical analysis of periodically forced nonlinear oscillators is an extremely difficult problem, and detailed quantitative understanding of dynamics has only been obtained in a few special situations.

3. Mathematical Analysis of Coupled Oscillators

An appreciation of the mathematical difficulties associated with the analysis of coupled oscillators, and a good source of reference for further reading, can be derived from a recent collection [22]. In this volume, several of the articles deal with a mathematical analysis of coupled nonlinear oscillations, under various approximations. The source of the difficulties is easy to appreciate. Ordinary differential equations which support nonlinear oscillations must be at least two-dimensional (i.e. two variables) and therefore models with coupled oscillators must be at least four-dimensional. Qualitative dynamics of ordinary differential equations in four dimensions is a difficult and still poorly understood problem.

One of the tricks for mathematical analysis is to assume that the oscillators represent strongly attracting limit cycle oscillations and that to a first approximation one need only consider the phase of the cycle. Now, for the case of two coupled oscillators one need only consider the phases of the two oscillators and the problem is reduced to a two-dimensional differential equation. A further simplification is sometimes made by assuming that the coupling strength depends only on the phase difference between the two oscillators [23] and the mathematics of the resulting problem are straightforward. Extension of this approach to multiple coupled oscillators has been fruitful [10]. However, this work is limited to "weak" coupling and experimental verification of this assumption is not straightforward.

An alternate approach is to reduce the study of coupled oscillators to a problem involving finite difference equations. In the situation in which a strongly attracting limit cycle oscillation is perturbed by brief stimuli, the dynamics can be described by the equation

$$\phi_{i+1} = g(\phi_i, b) + \tau \qquad (\text{mod } 1) \qquad (1)$$

where ϕ_i is the phase of the ith stimulus in the ith stimulus in the cycle of the forced oscillator, b is a parameter related to the strength of the stimulus and τ is the time interval between stimuli, relative to the period of the forced oscillator [17-20]. The function g is called the phase transition curve and it maps points on the unit circle to itself (it is a circle map).

Another class of models, called integrate and fire models represents periodically forced biological oscillators by activities which rise and fall to periodically modulated thresholds [24-28]. In such models the dynamics can also be represented by a one dimensional map

$$t_{i+1} = f(t_i, \lambda) \qquad (\text{mod } 1) \qquad (2)$$

where t_i represents the phase of the forcing oscillator at which the activity reaches threshold for the ith time, λ represents one of more parameters and f is a nonlinear circle map.

Detailed theoretical analysis of several different mathematical models of the form in (1) and (2) has provided at least partial insight into the experimental observations discussed in Section 2 and shown in Figs. 1 and 2. Indeed, all the main experimental observations summarized in Section 2 can be found in the different mathematical models, and in some instances quantitative agreement between experimental studies and theory has been found [17,18,26]. This might lead one to surmise that there is a "universal" topological structure for the organization of entrainment zones in frequency-amplitude parameter space. However, theoretical studies have shown that although this is true at comparatively low levels of stimulus-oscillator coupling, as the coupling increases the topological structure of the different mathematical models varies considerably [28]. Experimental resolution of the expected difference between the different models is difficult, however, because the differences between the different models are often confined to comparatively small regions in parameter space. Consequently, the fine structure is difficult to observe in the presence of physiological "noise", which tends to obscure the delicate topology which is theoretically predicted in the absence of noise.

Despite its successes, the mathematical analysis of coupled oscillators still poses great problems. In situations in which there is finite relaxation time back to the limit cycle, the approximations which have proved so useful to date in reducing the dimensionality of the problem will no longer be valid. For example, periodic forcing of limit cycles by brief, pulsatile stimuli in which there is finite relaxation time to the cycle must be described by maps in two or more dimensions. The connections between the dynamics in such systems and systems described by one-dimensional maps remain to be clarified. Finally, the problems associated with bidirectional coupling outside of the "weak coupling" limit are very rich and are still not well understood.

4. Summary and Conclusions

Coupled oscillators are ubiquitous in physiological systems, and hence an understanding of the dynamics of coupled oscillators seems essential to the analysis of dynamics in both normal and pathophysiology. Systematic experimental studies have described dynamics arising as a function of the frequency and amplitude of a forcing oscillator. Such studies have revealed extremely rich dynamics which can be at least partially understood from an analysis of mathematical models of the experimental systems. Further experimental studies in diverse systems are required. As well, the oversimplifications present in current models must be relaxed in order to obtain more realistic mathematical models. Since the underlying physiological problems are important, and the mathematics poses many interesting problems, this is a rich area for further research.

Acknowledgments

This report summarizes work done with many colleagues including M.C. Mackey, M.R. Guevara, A. Shrier, G.A. Petrillo, T. Trippenbach, J. Keener, J. Bélair. Thanks to NSERC and Canadian Heart Foundation for support of this research.

References

1. R.A. Wever: The Circadian System of Man (Springer-Verlag, Berlin 1979)
2. M.C. Moore-Ede, C. Czeisler (eds): Mathematical Models of the Circadian Sleep-Wake Cycle (Raven, New York 1984)
3. T.A. Wehr, F.K. Goodwin (eds): Circadian Rhythms in Psychiatry (Boxwood Press, Pacific Grove, CA 1983)
4. A.T. Winfree: Nature 321, 114 (1986)
5. C.A. Czeisler, G.S. Richardson, R.M. Coleman, J.C. Zimmerman, M.C. Moore-Ede, W.C. Dement, E.D. Weitzman: Sleep 4, 1 (1981)
6. F. Halberg: Chronobiologia 1 (Suppl. 1), 27 (1974)
7. G.D. Molnar, W.F. Taylor, A.L. Langworthy: Mayo Clin. Proc. 47, 709 (1972)
8. D.C. Michaels, E.P. Matyas, J. Jalife: Circ. Res. 58, 706 (1986)
9. B.J. Bardakjian, S.K. Sarna: IEEE Trans. Biomed. Eng. BME-27, 193 (1980)
10. N. Kopell: In Nonlinear Oscillations in Biology and Chemistry ed. by H.G. Othmer, Lecture Notes Biomath., Vol. 66 (Springer, Berlin 1986) p. 160
11. J. Jalife, D.C. Michaels: In Cardiac Electrophysiology and Arrhythmias ed. by D.P. Zipes and J. Jalife (Grune & Stratton, Orlando, Fla 1985) p. 109
12. D.M. Bramble, D.R. Carrier: Science 219, 251 (1983)
13. S. Bellet. Clinical Disorders of the Heartbeat (Lea & Febiger, Philadelphia, 1971)
14. G. Preiss, F. Kirchner, C. Polosa: Brain Res 87, 363 (1975)
15. J. Breuer: Sbev. Akad. Wiss. Wien 58, 909 (1868)
16. G.A. Petrillo, L. Glass, T. Trippenbach: Can. J. Physiol. Pharmacol. 61, 599 (1983)
17. M.R. Guevara, L. Glass, A. Shrier: Science 214, 1350 (1981)
18. L. Glass, M.R. Guevara, J. Belair, A. Shrier: Phys. Rev. A29, 1348 (1984)
19. D.H. Perkel, J.H. Schulman, T.H. Bullock, G.P. Moore, J.P. Segundo: Science 145, 61 (1964)
20. T. Pavlidis: Biological Oscillators: Their Mathematical Analysis (Academic, New York 1973)
21. R. Guttmann, L. Feldman, E. Jakobsson: J. Memb. Biol. 56, 9 (1980)
22. H.G. Othmer (ed.): Nonlinear Oscillations in Biology and Chemistry, Lecture Notes Biomath., Vol. 66 (Springer-Berlin, 1986)
23. A.H. Cohen, P.J. Holmes, R.H. Rand: J. Math. Biol. 13, 345 (1982)
24. L. Glass, M.C. Mackey: J. Math. Biol. 7, 339 (1979)
25. J.P. Keener, F.C. Hoppensteadt, J. Rinzel: SIAM J. Appl. Math. 41, 503 (1981)
26. G.A. Petrillo, L. Glass: Am. J. Physiol. 245, R311 (1984)
27. S. Daan, D. Beersma: In Mathematical Models of the Circadian Sleep-Wake Cycle, ed. by M.C. Moore-Ede, C.A. Czeisler (Raven, New York 1984)
28. L. Glass, J. Belair: In Nonlinear Oscillations in Biology and Chemistry ed. by H.G. Othmer, Lecture Notes Biomath., Vol. 66 (Springer, Berlin 1986) p. 232

Periodic Signaling and Receptor Desensitization: From cAMP Oscillations in *Dictyostelium* Cells to Pulsatile Patterns of Hormone Secretion

A. Goldbeter

Faculté des Sciences, Université Libre de Bruxelles, Campus Plaine, C.P. 231, Boulevard du Triomphe, B-1050 Bruxelles, Belgium

1. Introduction

Why are so many hormones released in a rhythmic, pulsatile manner? Since KNOBIL and co-workers (1,2) demonstrated that pulsatile stimulation by the hypothalamic hormone GnRH at regular, physiological intervals elicits the release of the gonadotropins LH and FSH by the pituitary – whereas continuous signaling by GnRH fails to yield such response –, an increasing number of hormones have been found to exert their physiological effects only when delivered in a periodic manner.

Insight into the function of periodic hormone signaling may be provided by one of the most primitive intercellular communication systems, namely, that which governs the aggregation of cellular slime molds after starvation. In *Dictyostelium discoideum* amoebae, cells behaving as aggregation centers secrete pulses of cyclic AMP (cAMP) with a periodicity of several minutes; other cells respond chemotactically to these pulsatile signals (3,4). Continuous cAMP signals as well as periodic signals delivered with a frequency higher than physiological fail to promote aggregation and differentiation, in contrast to cAMP pulses of 5 min periodicity (5,6). The analysis of a model for the cAMP signaling system (7,8) shows that the effectiveness of periodic signaling with the appropriate frequency can be comprehended in terms of receptor desensitization.

The purpose of this paper is to relate the dynamic behavior of the cAMP signaling system of *D. discoideum* to pulsatile patterns of hormone secretion. In these and other systems subjected to receptor desensitization, periodic signaling may have a similar function and appears to be the most efficient mode of intercellular communication. Disorders of such communication systems may give rise to "desensitization diseases" due to a mismatch between the frequency of signaling and the rate of recovery from receptor desensitization.

2. Periodic Generation of cAMP Pulses in *Dictyostelium* Cells

To understand the role of pulsatile secretion of cAMP in *D. discoideum*, it is necessary to consider in some detail the molecular mechanism of this periodic process. Here, indeed, mechanism and function are closely intertwined. For periodic hormone secretion whose origin is generally neuronal, the mechanism generating the periodicity may be dissociated from the effect of the hormone on target cells.

D. discoideum cells possess a cell surface receptor for cAMP; binding of extracellular cAMP to this receptor results in the activation of adenylate cyclase (see Fig.1). The intracellular cAMP thus synthesized is transported into the extracellular medium, where it is hydrolyzed by phosphodiesterase; the role of the latter enzyme is to

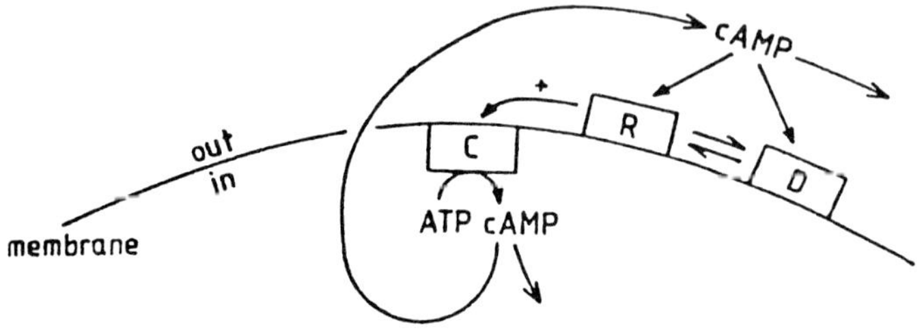

Fig.1. Model for the cAMP signaling system governing aggregation and differentiation in the slime mold *Dictyostelium discoideum* (7,8). Extracellular cAMP binds to a cell surface receptor (R) and thereby elicits the activation of adenylate cyclase (C). Upon binding cAMP, the R state of the receptor undergoes a transition into a desensitized state (D) unable (or less able) to activate cAMP synthesis. Arrows indicate transport of cAMP into the extracellular medium and hydrolysis by phosphodiesterase.

destroy the signal so as to make cells responsive to the next pulse (3,4).

Experiments show that the cAMP signaling system can either produce cAMP pulses in an autonomous manner, with a periodicity of several minutes – such behavior is that of aggregation centers – or it can amplify suprathreshold cAMP signals by synthesizing a pulse of cAMP (9). The latter behavior corresponds to the relay of chemotactic stimuli toward the periphery of the aggregation field. Relay allows one center to control the aggregation of as many as 10^5 amoebae over macroscopic distances (10). Other slime molds lacking the relay mechanism form much smaller aggregation territories; hence the name of *D. minutum* given to one of these species (11).

The mechanism of relay and oscillations rests on the positive feedback exerted by cAMP over its own production (see Fig.1), much as in the well-known example of glycolytic oscillations in yeast which originate from an autocatalytic enzyme reaction (12). The analysis of models for cAMP generation in *D. discoideum* shows that owing to the self-amplification properties of the signaling system, sustained cAMP oscillations occur in a range of values of enzyme activities and receptor concentration. Relay occurs for parameter values close to those producing oscillations.

In a previous model proposed for the cAMP signaling system (13), the rising phase of the oscillations, due to positive feedback, turned into a decreasing phase when substrate became limiting. Recent extension of this model indicates (7,8), in agreement with experimental observations, that the factor limiting the self-amplification may rather be located at the level of the receptor itself. Experiments indeed show that the decrease in cAMP synthesis upon prolonged stimulation by extracellular cAMP is associated with the reversible phosphorylation of the cAMP receptor (14,15). In the course of cAMP oscillations, the receptor alternates in a periodic manner between the phosphorylated and dephosphorylated states (16). Such periodic alternance between the active and desensitized states is also observed in the model based on receptor modification (7,8).

In many sensory systems, as in the case of *D. discoideum*, adaptation also occurs through receptor covalent modification. Thus, in bacteria, methylation of membrane receptors mediates adaptation of the chemotactic response to attractant stimuli (17,18). A general scheme for

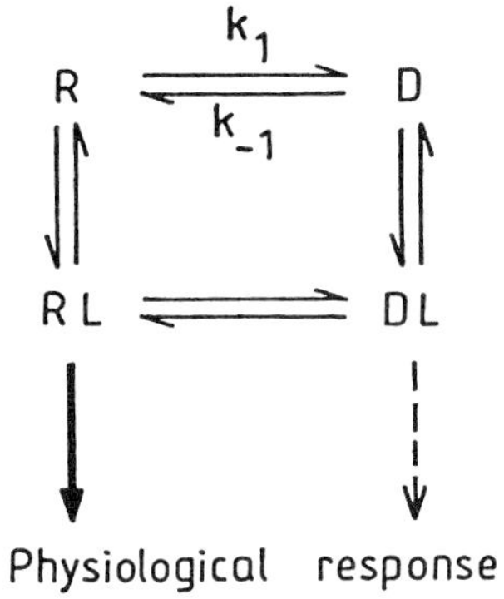

Fig.2. General scheme for receptor desensitization. Binding of ligand L to the active receptor state elicits the physiological response and induces the transition into the desensitized DL complex whose ability to evoke the response is weaker. The rate of recovery from the desensitized state upon removal of the stimulus is governed by constant k_{-1}. In molecular terms, desensitization may result from a simple conformational change, covalent modification, or down-regulation.

adaptation based on receptor desensitization is shown in Fig.2. Covalent modification is only one molecular basis for the transition between the two receptor states. In principle,as first envisaged by KATZ and THESLEFF (19), the two states R and D in Fig.2 could differ simply by their conformation, in which case the receptor would be an allosteric protein (20). Alternatively, the transition to the D state could correspond to a process of down-regulation.

3. Molecular Explanation for the Effectiveness of Periodic Signaling in *Dictyostelium*

The signaling system used by *D. discoideum* amoebae in the course of aggregation provides a convenient system for studying the role of periodic signals in intercellular communication. Moreover, the availability of a model based on receptor modification permits to investigate the molecular basis of such signaling process by means of numerical simulations.

Oscillations of cAMP in *D. discoideum* play a dual role. Besides controlling aggregation (5), they also promote cell differentiation by inducing the synthesis of specific proteins involved in signaling or in cell-to-cell adhesion (6).

The remarkable characteristic of intercellular communication in *D. discoideum* is that continuous cAMP signals fail to produce the responses evoked by signals delivered at the physiological frequency of one pulse every 5 min. Thus, mutants unable to aggregate do exhibit normal aggregation when subjected to pulses of cAMP delivered at 5 min intervals; no aggregation occurs, however, when cAMP is delivered continuously (5). Similarly, cAMP pulses delivered with a 5 min period accelerate differentiation in wild-type amoebae, in contrast to constant cAMP stimuli (6). Interestingly, periodic signals applied with a frequency of one pulse every 2 min also have no effect, much as constant stimuli (21).

A major question is therefore: what is special about the 5 min periodicity of the cAMP signal? What makes this frequency of periodic signaling efficient, in contrast to higher frequencies of stimulation? Numerical simulations of the model for cAMP synthesis show that the key to this puzzle appears to lie in the receptor modification process. These simulations suggest a molecular explanation for the effectiveness of periodic signaling.

When a pulse of cAMP is given to a suspension of slime mold cells, a biphasic response is observed: cAMP rises and thereafter subsides, owing to the increased phosphorylation of the cAMP receptor (14,15) (experimental evidence indeed suggests that as in the case of the β-adrenergic system (22), receptor phosphorylation is associated with a decrease in adenylate cyclase activity). Under physiological conditions, a pulse of cAMP is followed by a quiescent phase in signaling which lasts several minutes, before a second pulse is delivered. When this quiescent phase is sufficiently long, the receptor has enough time to fully return to the active, dephosphorylated state. Removal of the stimulus indeed instantly initiates a dephosphorylation process (15). Then, when the next pulse arrives, cells have recovered their full responsiveness and are thus capable of synthesizing cAMP to the same extent as for the previous stimulus. This situation is represented schematically in Fig.3a. Sketched in this figure are the periodic signal, the response (here, cAMP synthesis), and the time evolution of the fraction of active receptor (here, the amount of dephosphorylated receptor, divided by the total receptor concentration).

When the stimulus takes the form of a step increase in cAMP concentration (Fig.3c), the response occurs as a single peak, since the receptor reaches a new steady state corresponding to increased phosphorylation. In such conditions of constant stimulation, experiments (23) and numerical simulations (7,8) indicate that a new transient response can only be induced by a further step increase in stimulation.

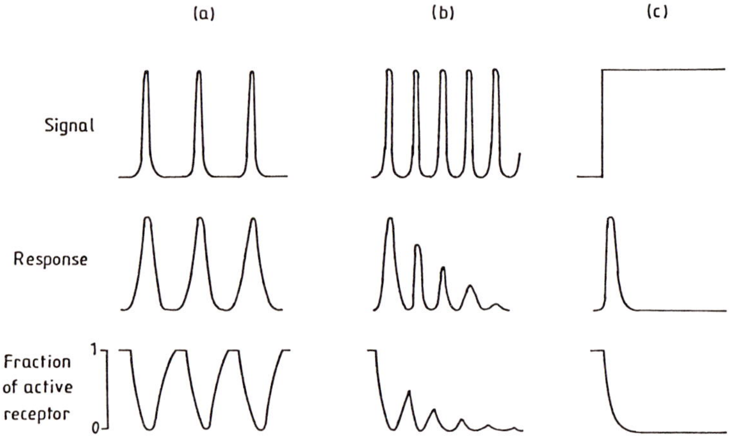

Fig.3. Patterns of receptor-mediated response to periodic stimuli. The three situations show, in a schematic manner, the response to (a) a periodic signal of physiological frequency, (b) a periodic signal whose frequency is higher than physiological, and (c) a constant signal in the form of a step increase in stimulus. Shown from top to bottom are the signal, the physiological response, and the fraction of receptor in active state. Decrease in this fraction is brought about by receptor desensitization (see Fig.2). The curves correspond to a stimulus of saturating amplitude which brings about a large decline in the fraction of active receptor. For stimuli of lower frequency or lower amplitude, the response in (b) may settle at a reduced but sizeable steady-state amplitude. It is suggested that the patterns of response apply to the cAMP signaling system of *D. discoideum*, as well as to the effect of GnRH pulses on the pituitary. In the former case, the signal is cAMP, and the response is cAMP synthesis and release; in the second situation, GnRH is the stimulus which elicits the release of the pituitary hormones LH and FSH.

An intermediate situation arises when cAMP pulses are delivered with a frequency higher than physiological, as represented schematically in Fig.3b. The response to the first pulse has a normal amplitude. However, when the second pulse arrives, the receptor has not yet fully recovered from its inactive state. The second response has therefore a smaller amplitude. This process repeats itself for the next pulses, so that the response either decreases more and more until it becomes vanishingly small, or settles at a reduced amplitude (J.L. Martiel and A. Goldbeter, manuscript submitted for publication).

The above results hold when the positive feedback loop (see Fig.1) is suppressed by controlling the extracellular cAMP level. Similar results are obtained when stimulation is applied in the presence of feedback; the recovery from refractoriness is then less gradual as an absolute refractory period exists in such conditions of excitability.

The above explanation accounts, in terms of receptor desensitization, for the effectiveness of cAMP pulses delivered every 5 min in *D. discoideum*, as well as for the ineffectiveness of pulses delivered every 2 min and of constant stimuli.

4. The GnRH-induced Secretion of Gonadotropins: a Prototype of Periodic Hormone Signaling

The secretion of the luteinizing hormone (LH) and follicle-stimulating hormone (FSH) by the pituitary is triggered by a decapeptide, the gonadotropin releasing hormone (GnRH) secreted by the hypothalamus (24). The hormones LH and FSH play a primary role in controlling follicular growth and ovulation in the female, as well as gonadal functions in the male. The pulsatory nature of the pituitary hormone secretion was first observed in ovariectomized rhesus monkeys where LH pulses occur approximately once every hour and were therefore termed "circhoral" (25). The frequency in humans is lower, i.e. one LH pulse every one to two hours (26). Besides these infradian episodes of hormone secretion, circadian variations in reproductive hormones also occur (26,27). Here we shall focus on the pulsatile release of gonadotropins which follows from the periodic release of GnRH pulses into the pituitary portal circulation (28). The function of GnRH pulses will be addressed, rather than the neural mechanism that produces these rhythms, i.e. the hypothalamic "pulse generator" (29,30).

What is the function of the rhythmic, pulsatile release of LH and FSH in the reproductive system? This question has been addressed in a series of experiments carried out by KNOBIL and co-workers (1,2) in the rhesus monkey subjected to specific hypothalamic lesions that suppress the autonomous generation of the GnRH signal.

When an exogenous GnRH signal is delivered at the physiological frequency of one pulse every hour, a normal ovarian cycle is restored, leading to ovulation. In contrast, a continuous GnRH signal fails to establish the appropriate LH and FSH levels and, therefore, does not induce ovulation. More surprisingly, GnRH pulses delivered at a frequency higher than physiological – i.e. two, three or five pulses per hour – also failed to elicit the normal response (2,31). Commenting on these results, KNOBIL (32) concluded: "It is tempting to speculate that an intermittent presentation of hypophysiotropic hormone to the pituitary gonadotrophs permits the regeneration of receptors to GnRH whereas the continuous mode of stimulation does not".

Support for this view is provided by the preceding discussion of the cAMP signaling system. The experimental results on the effect of various modes of GnRH delivery can, indeed, be accounted for in terms of the general mechanism schematized in Fig.3. Central here is the assumption that the receptor undergoes a transition into a physiologically less active (or inactive) state upon prolonged incubation with the ligand. When the GnRH signal is applied at a natural frequency of one 6 min-pulse per hour, the situation should be that of Fig.3a: the process of receptor desensitization is initiated as soon as the pulse begins, but the interval between two successive pulses is long enough for the receptor to recover from desensitization. The response to successive stimuli therefore does not diminish.

In the case of continuous stimulation (Fig.3c), the receptor reaches a steady-state level of desensitization. The unique, initial response can be followed by a second response only if the stimulus is raised to a higher level. Further response will, however, only occur if the first stimulus is not saturating.

The effect of an increase in the frequency of GnRH stimulation up to two or more pulses per hour should correspond to the situation depicted in Fig.3b. Here, the interval between two successive pulses is too short for the receptor to fully recover from refractoriness. Hence when the frequency of stimulation is large enough, the amplitude of the response to successive pulses progressively decreases in time, until the response completely vanishes or reaches a steady state of reduced amplitude. Such situation becomes analogous to that of continuous stimulation. This is expected as the periodic stimulus of Fig. 3b transforms into a step increase in stimulation when the frequency becomes sufficiently large.

As previously discussed, the desensitization process postulated in Fig.3 may take different – not necessarily exclusive – forms at the molecular level. Desensitization has been observed for the GnRH receptor (33), but the molecular basis of the phenomenon has not yet been fully characterized.

At first view, the mechanism of Fig.3 would predict that normal responses should occur for frequencies of GnRH signaling below the physiological value. The situation, however, is more complex and calls then for the consideration of additional factors. Experiments indicate (34) that lowering the GnRH frequency to one pulse every 2 or 3 hours fails to induce follicular development in the rhesus monkey. Such failure appears to be due to the establishment of an abnormal ratio of LH to FSH, because of differences in clearance rates for the two hormones.

The elucidation of the role of pulsatile GnRH secretion has recently led to the recognition of a new type of physiological disorder, both in males and females for whom regularly spaced GnRH pulses – and subsequently LH and FSH pulses – are essential for normal gonadal function. Thus, in the female, many reproductive disorders, such as idiopathic hypogonadotropic hypogonadism, are characterized by the absence of gonadotropin pulses or by an alteration in their frequency (35). Normal function of the pituitary-gonadal axis has been restored by the periodic delivery of GnRH pulses at a physiological frequency in a number of such disorders. This replacement therapy has led to the successful restoration of ovulation and to the induction of pregnancies in previously infertile women (36,37).

In the male also cases of hypogonadotropic hypogonadism have been successfully treated by application of GnRH pulses at a physiological frequency of one pulse every two hours (35). As demonstrated by the various clinical accounts in (38), both gonadal maturation and fertility can be restored with such pulsatile treatment by GnRH.

5. "Desensitization Diseases": a New Class of Temporal Disorders

The cAMP signaling system that governs aggregation and differentiation in the cellular slime mold *Dictyostelium discoideum* is often viewed as a primitive hormone communication system in which cAMP acts at the same time as first and second messenger (39). The relation of this process to hormone signaling may in fact be closer than the simple use of a chemical signal to stimulate a cellular response. A further property that cAMP signaling shares with many hormonal systems is its periodic, pulsatile nature.

The hypothesis presented here is that both in the case of cAMP pulses in *Dictyostelium* and in that of GnRH pulses in the reproductive system the periodic nature of the signal serves a similar function, which is to permit maximum responsiveness by avoidance of receptor desensitization. A similar mechanism permits to unify the behavior of the two systems, as well as the response of each of them to stimuli delivered with a physiological frequency, with a frequency higher than normal, or continuously.

As shown in Figures 2 and 3, the key factor in this mechanism is the magnitude of the interval separating two successive pulsatory stimuli, relative to the duration of receptor recovery from refractoriness upon removal of the stimulus. The latter recovery time is governed by the rate constant k_{-1} in Fig.2. Depending on the molecular nature of the desensitization process, this apparent first-order rate constant may relate to a conformational transition, a dephosphorylation reaction catalyzed by a protein phosphatase – as in the case of *D. discoideum* (15) –, or to the reappearance of functional receptor in the membrane, e.g. through *de novo* receptor synthesis.

Given the above mechanism, it is conceivable that physiological malfunction may arise from either one of several causes. The most obvious is, of course, that the stimulus may be absent or too feeble. When a pulsatory stimulus of sufficient amplitude exists, however, the frequency of stimulation may be too high for a given value of the resensitization constant; decrease or disappearance of the response will ensue. Conversely, a similar outcome will obtain if the frequency of stimulation is normal but the recovery of the receptor from its refractory state is too slow, i.e. k_{-1} has an abnormally low value.

Particularly relevant in this context is the discussion by WAGNER (40) of testosterone deficiency in a hypergonadotropic male patient. Rather than ascribing such disorder to the testis, this author suggests that it represents a "desensitization disease". This view holds well with the above described mechanism and with the previously mentioned comment by KNOBIL on the efficiency of pulsatile GnRH treatment in rhesus monkeys with hypothalamic lesions.

Rhythm-related disorders based on receptor desensitization can be viewed as a subclass of the broader category of pathological conditions referred to as "dynamic diseases" (41). The cAMP oscillations in *Dictyostelium* and the GnRH pulsatory secretion are only two examples of periodic signaling. It is probable that many hormones are, for similar reasons, delivered in a periodic manner. If so, many types of "desensitization diseases" reflecting a mismatch between receptor recovery from refractoriness and the frequency of stimulation should be observed. The interest of a detailed comprehension of periodic hormone processes is to make desensitization disorders amenable to a completely physiological treatment (40) based on natural parameters such as the amplitude and frequency of stimulation, or the dynamic properties of the hormone receptor.

References

1. P.E. Belchetz, T.M. Plant, Y. Nakai, E.J. Keogh, E. Knobil: Science 202, 631-633 (1978)
2. E. Knobil: Rec. Progr. Horm. Res. 36, 53-88 (1980)
3. P.C. Newell: In Microbial Interactions(Receptors and Recognition, Ser. B) Vol. 3 (ed. by J.L. Reissig), 3-57 Chapman and Hall, London, 1977
4. P.N. Devreotes: In The Development of Dictyostelium discoideum (ed. by W.F. Loomis) 117-168 Academic Press, New York, 1982
5. M. Darmon, P. Brachet, L.H. Pereira da Silva: Proc. Nat. Acad. Sci. USA 72, 3163-3166 (1975)
6. Gerisch, G., H. Fromm, A. Huesgen, U. Wick: Nature 255, 547-549 (1975)
7. Martiel, J.L., A. Goldbeter: C.R. Acad. Sci. (Paris) Sér. III 298, 549-552 (1984)
8. A. Goldbeter, J.L. Martiel: In Sensing and Response in Microorganisms (ed. by M. Eisenbach, M. Balaban) 185-198 Elsevier, Amsterdam, 1985
9. G. Gerisch, D. Malchow, W. Roos, U. Wick: J. Exp. Biol. 81, 33-47 (1979)
10. B. Shaffer: Adv. Morphogen. 2, 109-182 (1962)
11. G. Gerisch: Curr. Top. Devel. Biol. 3, 157-197 (1968)
12. A. Goldbeter, S.R. Caplan: Ann. Rev. Biophys. Bioeng. 5, 449-476 (1976)
13. A. Goldbeter, L.A. Segel: Proc. Nat. Acad. Sci. USA 74, 1543-1547 (1977)
14. C. Klein, J. Lubs-Haukeness, S. Simons: J. Cell Biol. 100, 715-720 (1985)
15. P.N. Devreotes, J.A. Sherring: J. Biol. Chem. 260, 6378-6384 (1985)
16. P. Klein, A. Theibert, D. Fontana, P.N. Devreotes: J. Biol. Chem. 260, 1757-1764 (1985)
17. D.E. Koshland, Jr: Physiol. Rev. 59, 811-862 (1979)
18. M.S. Springer, M.F. Goy, J. Adler: Nature 280, 279-284 (1979)
19. B. Katz, S. Thesleff: J. Physiol. 138, 63-80 (1957)
20. J.P. Changeux, A. Devillers-Thiéry, P. Chemouilli: Science 225, 1335-1345 (1984)
21. B. Wurster: Biophys. Struct. Mech. 9, 137-143 (1982)
22. D.R. Sibley, J.R. Peters, P. Nambi, M.G. Caron, R.J. Lefkowitz: J. Biol. Chem. 259, 9742-9749 (1984)
23. P.N. Devreotes, T.L. Steck: J. Cell Biol. 80, 300-309 (1979)
24. A.V. Schally, A. Arimura, A.J. Kastin, H. Matsuo, Y. Baba, T.W. Redding, R.M. Nair, L. Debeljuk: Science 173, 1036-1038 (1971)
25. D.J. Dierschke, A.N. Bhattacharya, L.E. Atkinson, E. Knobil: Endocrinology 87, 850-853 (1970)
26. R.W. Rebar, S.S.C. Yen: In Endocrine Rhythms (ed. by D.T. Krieger) 259-298 Raven Press, New York, 1979
27. F.W. Turek, J. Swann, D.J. Earnest: Rec. Progr. Horm. Res. 40, 143-183 (1984)
28. P.W. Carmel, S. Araki, M. Ferin: Endocrinology 99, 243-248 (1976)
29. R.C. Wilson, J.S. Kesner, J.M. Kaufman, T. Uemura, T. Akema, E. Knobil: Neuroendocrinology 39, 256-260 (1984)
30. D.W. Lincoln, H.M. Fraser, G.A. Lincoln, G.B. Martin, A.S. McNeilly: Rec. Progr. Horm. Res. 41, 369-419 (1985)
31. L. Wildt, A. Haüsler, G. Marshall, J.S. Hutchison, T.M. Plant, P.E. Belchetz, E. Knobil: Endocrinology 109, 376-385 (1981)
32. E. Knobil: Biol. Reprod. 24, 44-49 (1981)
33. P.M. Conn, A.J.W. Hsueh, W.F. Crowley, Jr: Fed. Proc. 43, 2351-2361 (1984)

34. C.R. Pohl, D.W. Richardson, J.S. Hutchison, J.A. Germak, E. Knobil: Endocrinology 112, 2076-2080 (1983)
35. W.F. Crowley, Jr, M. Filicori, D.J. Spratt, N.F. Santoro: Rec. Progr. Horm. Res. 41, 473-531 (1985)
36. G. Leyendecker, L. Wildt, M. Hansmann: J. Clin. Endocrinol. Metab. 51, 1214-1216 (1980)
37. R.L. Reid, G.R. Leopold, S.S.C. Yen: Fertil. Steril. 36, 553-559 (1981)
38. T.O.F. Wagner (ed.): Pulsatile LHRH Therapy of the Male (T.M. Verlag, Hameln, 1985)
39. T.M. Konijn: Adv. Cycl. Nucleot. Res. 1, 17-31 (1972)
40. M.C. Mackey, L. Glass: Science 197, 287-289 (1977)
41. T.O.F. Wagner: In ref. 38, pp 7 and 64

Oscillations and the Regulation of Spatial Order in Developing Systems

M.G. Vicker and L. Rensing

Fachbereich Biologie, Universität Bremen, PF 330440,
D-2800 Bremen, Fed. Rep. of Germany

Many authors seem convinced that the global order of patterning and cell positioning during development or some pathological situation is a consequence of supracellular processes, and have devoted considerable attention to the aesthetic virtues of morphogen concentration gradients. This notion rests on several principles including a) the evident graded form of organisms [1, 2], b) the concentration-dependent responses to inductive signals and c) the supposed ability of tactic cells to read spatial gradients of attractant molecules, an idea has been influential, if not appropriated wholesale. This view of taxis attained the status of a self-evident fact after investigations of neutrophil leukocytes [3] and the social amoeba *Dictyostelium discoideum* [4]. Subsequently, the signal form and cellular mechanisms of perception and response have been conflated into the wisdom "chemotactic gradient".

By analogy, morphogen signals are usually envisaged as gradients transversing embryonic fields. Cells respond not by moving but rather by differentiating to a new state depending on their "reading" of the ambient concentration [1, 2, 5]. Thus, gradient form is impressed upon the field, imparting "positional information" to the cells [5], a premise elaborated in models based, e.g., on Turing systems: the generation of morphogenic gradients from the autocatalytic synthesis of a short-range activator and a long-range inhibitor of a developmental process [6]. Morphogens have been found as peptides in *Hydra* [7] and as cyclic AMP (cAMP) in *D. discoideum* [8]; however, few have been identified elsewhere, and, consequently, the features of both signal form and effect remain generally puzzling. The question we shall address here is whether the analogy between attractant and morphogen gradient signals is justified,and what significance this may have for the role of oscillators in development.

Current models of morphogen gradients, e.g. [6], limit themselves to examining the generation of a spatial gradient and comparing predicted with empirical patterns, but assume that cells accurately read these signals. However, developing gradients also propagate temporal signals that confront cells as concentration impulses; a point hitherto ignored in previous discussions [9]. Newly identified responses of neutrophils and *D. discoideum,* the classical tactic eukaryotes, to controlled spatial or temporal attractant gradients indicate critical differences between their effects. The essential evidence that individual cells cannot read spatial gradient signals was obtained using cell populations that were initially randomly distributed across a limited territory to prevent spreading out [10, 11]. Equilibrium distributions are not perturbed by predeveloped spatial gradient of attractant. But a single, brief impulse, e.g. during gradient development, is a powerful tactic signal that increases cell motility and the proportion of motile cells, induces taxis and accumulation and immediately disrupts the equilibrium distribution (fig. 1). Thus, taxis, i.e. directed turning, requires a directed pulse or impulse signal. The time elapsed between

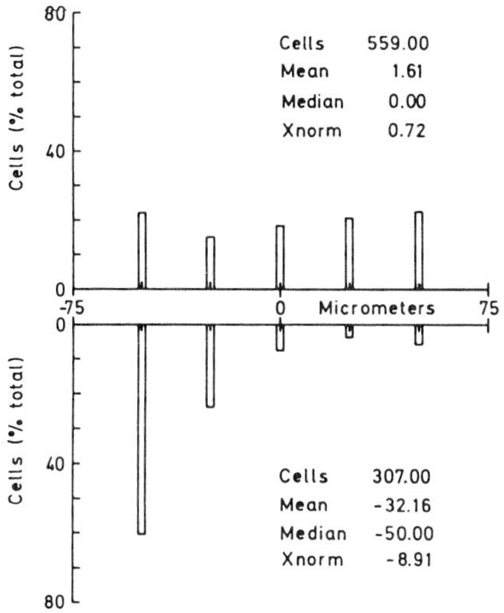

Figure 1. The behaviour of rabbit peritoneal neutrophil leukocytes in temporal and spatial gradient signals of formyl-Met-Leu-Phe. **Upper panel:** Cells were distributed evenly within a penetrable micropore filter (5 µm pore size). Ice-cold 2.5 pM fMLP was added on the left and ice-cold buffer on the right. After gradient development the cells were warmed to allow cell migration. Gradient predevelopment inhibited the effects of temporal signals. Cell positions were recorded after 38 min at 37°C. The relative gradient $\Delta C/C$ across a cell at X = 0 (mid-filter) is 20%. **Lower panel:** Motile cell responses to a temporal signal. fMLP was added warm, rather than cold, to confront sensitive cells as an impulse. The cell distributions are shown after 23 min. *Cells*, total counted; *Median* and *Mean*, of cell positions; *S.D.*, no meaning here; *Xnorm*, Wilcoxon statistic of the median shift: $>|2.56|$ indicates a shift from equilibrium at p = 1%. The behaviour of *D. discoideum* is identical to that of neutrophils [10, 11].

reception of a signal at a cell's proximal and distal ends is sufficient for the generation of reactions required for directed pseudopodial extension.

Therefore, attractant spatial gradients are not signals for taxis and temporal signals may play hitherto unappreciated roles as specific effectors of cell behaviour. Different intracellular reactions are generated by temporal and concentration signals. The accurate interpretion of concentrations in a spatial gradient requires the integration of cellular responses temporally or spatially, because the individual cell responses are highly variable to such signals [10]. Responses to temporal signals are qualitatively different from those to a concentration signal, being characterized by a series of adaptive reactions (see [10, 11]). Apparently, the rate of increase in cell-surface receptor occupancy in spatial gradients is too slow, even as a pseudopod projects up-gradient, to stimulate these reactions. The physiological responses excited by temporal signals are analogous to, or parts of, oscillatory systems and may perturb or entrain them. Thus, the motor reaction sensitivity in the "phototactic" *Halobacterium* varies with a period of 20 s [12], and a limit cycle has been used to model the cytoskeleton dynamics of higher cells [13]. Optimal exploitation of a temporal signalling system would require an oscillator to order signal and receptor perfomance.

The spatial and temporal sequences of morphogenesis are highly regulated, seemingly choreographed. Yet, they are known to be governed by oscillations only in the cellular slime moulds. Oscillations of 4-5 h in the cytoplasmic pH probably control the cell cycle during vegetative growth of *D. discoideum* [14]. Six hours after starvation a few cells begin periodically excreting pulses of cAMP (fig. 2), inducing chemotactic aggregation of cells that are simultaneously differentiating into prespore and prestalk cells [15, 16]. The aggregate moulds itself into a polarized, patterned, slime-coated slug, which wanders about before forming the fruiting-body. Rhythmic contractions and pulsitile cAMP signals arise at its anterior (presumptive-stalk cell) tip and are

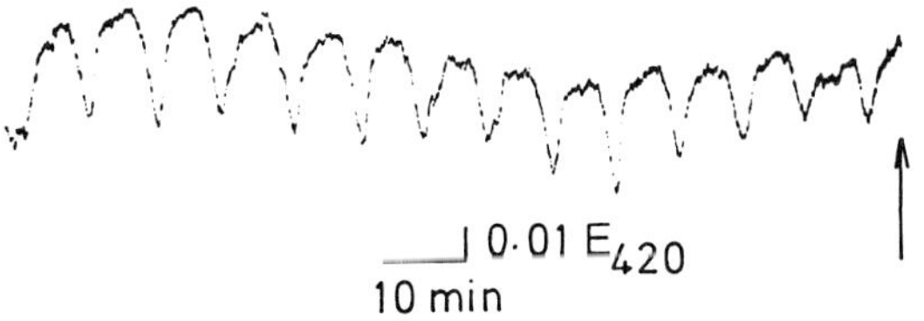

Figure 2. Spontaneous light-scattering oscillations, due to cell contraction and/or clumping, began in a suspension of *D. discoideum* after 316 min of starvation: arrow.

propagated along its A-P axis [8, 17]. cAMP in this organism is, perhaps fortuitously, both attractant and morphogen. Among the possible functions of pulsitile signaling are a) suppressing the maturation of other autonomous-signalling pacemaker cells [16], b) regulating the differentiation program [8] provided sufficient intercellular contact exists during aggregation [18], c) controlling cell orientation and motility, leading to the sorting-out of cells with different cAMP-responsiveness, i.e. the prestalk and prespore classes [19].

Stabilization of the prestalk state, adjacent to the pacemaker cell, requires cAMP [20], and upon inhibition of adenyl cyclase slug form breaks down [17]. Hydrolytic products of cAMP, notably adenosine, accumulate and inhibit the conversion of prestalk to prespore cells [8, 20]. Erratic rhythms induce differentiation; but morphogenesis fails at the aggregate stage in the mutants 91A and Fr17, which can not sustain a normal pulse frequency [21]. The oscillations of this amoeba have been described by a limit cycle [22], and the behaviour of Fr17 looks like autonomous chaos [23]. The cell cycle also appears to play a role in patterning in *D. discoideum,* where differentiation toward prespore or prestalk cells is determined by the cell's position in the cycle and its mitochondrial DNA content [20, 24]. Passage of slug cells through S-phase is regulated by cAMP. Adenosine regulates the proportions of prespore and prestalk cells [8, 20], perhaps by inhibiting DNA synthesis through pyrimidine starvation, and prevents conversion of prestalk to prespore cells. The head activator morphogen of *Hydra* is mitogenic for stem cells [7].

Many of the morphogenetic features of slime moulds find some analogy in other developing systems, suggesting that pulsitile morphogen signals or oscillators are also involved. For example, pulsitile signals regulate the tendency of prestalk cell grafts to shift within the host slug until they encounter a zone where their frequency dominates that of the host [16]. Similar shifts in graft position (rotations) occur in insects [25, 26]. Thus, temporal signals might control spatial patterning by regulating cell cohesion and directed locomotion in many systems. The intercellular relaying of temporal signals also occurs in organisms besides *Dictyostelium:* the glycolytic rhythm is entrained in yeast cultures by an unknown messenger [27], *Drosophila* tissue culture cells probably relay carnitine [28] and embryonic chick cells relay administered cAMP pulses [29], responding to it by increased cohesiveness [30] and attraction [31]. Temporal signals also induce differentiation in some systems. Feet are induced in the mid-gastric region of *Hydra* by local, brief electrical pulses each 2.5 min [32]. Injected pulses of cAMP and electrical current, e.g. each 5 min, synergistically induce lateral buds in *Hydractinia* [33]. Oscillations are evident in some developmental processes: protein synthesis [34] and Ca^{2+}-ATPase activity [35] in sea urchin embryos, in the intracellular Ca^{2+} level of mouse oocytes during activation by sperm or phorbol ester [36] and in the plasma membrane potential of mammary epithelial cells, with periods of up to 10 s several hours after treatment by epidermal growth factor (EGF) or insulin [37]. Human endocrine hormones are most efficient if delivered periodically, as they are *in vivo,* e.g. [33]. After fertilization in *Xenopus laevis,* 12 waves of cytokinesis 30 min apart cross the embryo from one region [39].

A simple example of patterning may suffice to suggest a role for oscillations in development. Spatial periodicities are salient features of fungal organization [40], and are often based upon endogenous temporal rhythms. These are particularly evident in *Neurospora crassa*, in which conidiation is restricted to the dark phase under a light-dark cycle [41]. The rhythm is expressed with an eigen-frequency of about 21 h in the *band* mutant upon agar. Spore differentiation depends on differential gene activation and repression [42]. The conidial pattern is extraordinarily analogous to the development of somite files in frogs (fig. 3). The linear pattern develops with a species-specific period, e.g. 140 min/somite in *Rana* [43, 44]. As cells emerge from and fall behind the zone of cell proliferation in the tail tip, a wave of somite determination and formation overtakes them, propagated from head to tail. The rhythm proceeds independently of the rate of tail growth. Thus, each cell seems preset to form part of a somite or furrow, like a clock, just as particular segments of *Neurospora* are ordained to develop conidia at circadian intervals once free of the growing end: each cell being in the same phase of the rhythm. Alternatively, as in the slime mould, the relay of a periodic signal from the tail tip might entrain those cells of a particular developmental stage (in the cell cycle?), which have just left the tip. These will then begin the coordinated sequences of cellular reorientation for somitogenesis. Two waves of ectodermal cell division proceed segmentation in the *Peracarida* (amphipods, *etc.*) [45]. Visible waves traverse the A-P axis of chick and fish embryos in periods decreasing, like in *D. discoideum*, from 11 to 2 min as development proceeds [46, 47]. Cells in developing vertebrate limbs become determined after leaving the cell proliferation zone at the apical ridge [48]. Growth declines in the cells left behind, and a tissue pattern unfolds behind a wave of determination sweeping along after the growing tip. These are familiar elements, common to fungi, slime moulds, frogs and insects.

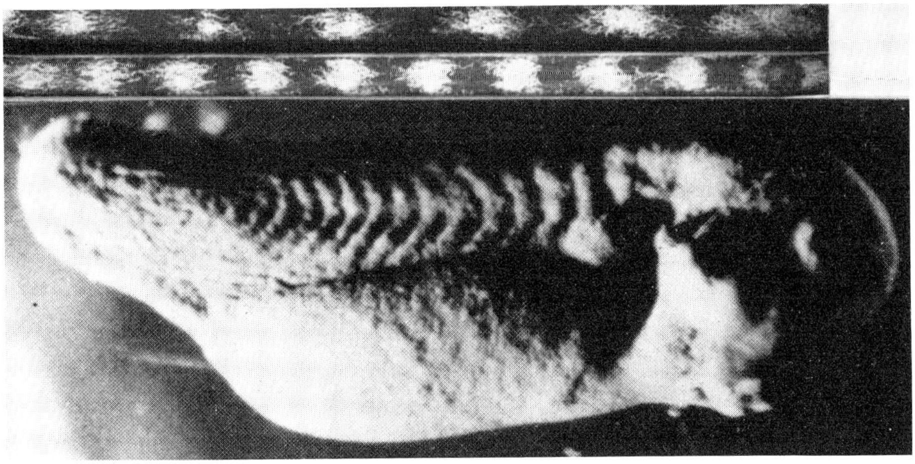

Figure 3 Above: *N. crassa* was seeded on nutrient agar at the right of each tube and incubated in the dark [49]. Conidia differentiate each 21 h under free-running conditions independently of the growth rate. The top tube is the long-period mutant *frq* 7 (29 h) and below it is *bd*. Below: A living 19 somite-stage embryo of *R. temporata*. Determination passes from head to tail as a wave 3 somites ahead of each visible somite. As somites form, cells turn as an ensemble and orient to the A-P axis. The rhythm is independent of the tail growth rate: from [44].

A further similarity between somitogenesis and rhythmic conidiation is the susceptibilty of both to heat shock. After a brief 37°C pulse, tip growth halts for 4.5 h, but somite formation continues for 3 periods before stopping. When tail development commences again the somite pattern is chaotic for several cycles before progressively returning to its usual form and rhythmicity. Tail development is completed normally. Heat shock shifts the rhythm in *Neurospora*, and the inducibility of its heat shock proteins (HSP) occurs as a circadian rhythm in liquid culture [50]. HSP synthesis accompanies ascospore development in the yeast *Saccharomyces* and oogenesis in *Drosophila melanogaster* and a specific pattern of HSP expression occurs in both cases [51]. Indeed, the induction of the mouse zygote begins with the synthesis of HSP [52]. These results indicate an inherent relationship between differentiation, HSP synthesis and various oscillations. Chemoattractants and heat shock both induce adaptive responses. Spatial periodicities appear prior to cellularization in *Drosophila* larva. Transcripts of the "paired-rule" loci appear in 7 belts 3-4 cells apart [53]. Later, the belts split in a process moving from head to tail. Homoeotic genes like these are interesting because of their wide distribution and selective involvement in critical developmental transitions, although their products have remained unknown [54]. But two such products, controlling the loci *Notch* in *Drosophila* and *lin-12* in the worm *Caenorhabditis elegans* may have indeed been identified. Their amino acid sequences are similar, but the finding of interest is that it may be homologous to EGF [55]. Perhaps these proteins are effective as switches in determination because they provide a growth-regulation signal at the cell surface.

Somitogenesis in frogs and the conidial pattern in *Neurospora* might both be determined by a synchronous rhythm in all cells. Feedback models provide an alternative explanation for frogs and flies, and have surprisingly general properties including the possibility that temporal signals are particularly effective. These models include a) the regulation of tissue proportions in the developing early chick embryo, where cells are diverted from differentiating toward particular states by signals from cells already there [56]; b) the cell-type ratio in *Dictyostelium* is regulated, because prestalk and prespore cells each produce an inhibitor (cAMP-adenosine) preventing conversion to its own type [20]; c) the accurate cell counting and periodicity of ovulation, which also has spatial relevance [57]; d) a general mutual activation model [6] suggesting that emissions from one group of cells invoke a complementary signal from a neighboring group. Each signal inducing the synthesis of the other at a distance but inhibiting it locally; thus, producing a pattern of two cell states like stripes. Pulse or impulse signals of morphogen may specifically maintain cell orientation (even in non-motile cells), establish a phase space in which the different endogenous frequencies of cells could guide them into a simple pattern by sorting-out, and entrain at its most efficient the dynamics of a) ligand receptor internalization, b) adaptive and oscillatory reactions and c) cell product synthesis, enhancing the feedback relation.

REFERENCES

1. C.M. Child: Patterns and Problems of Development (University Press, Chicago 1941)
2. K. Sander, K. Nübler-Jung: In International Cell Biology 1980-1981 ed. by H.G. Schweiger 1981) pp. 497-506
3. T. Leber 1888 Fortschr. Med. 6, 460-464
4. J.T. Bonner 1947 J. Exp. Zool. 106, 1-26
5. L. Wolpert 1971 Curr. Top. Dev. Biol. 6, 183-224
6. H. Meinhardt 1984 J. embryol. Exp. Morph. 83, 289-311 (Suppl.)
7. H.C. Schaller, H. Bodenmüller 1985 Hoppe Seyler's Biol. Chem. 366, 1003-1007

8. P. Schaap, M. Wang 1986 Cell 45, 137-144
9. M.G. Vicker 1981 Exp. Cell Res. 136, 91-100
10. M.G. Vicker, W. Schill, K. Drescher 1984 J. Cell Biol. 98, 2204-2214
11. M.G. Vicker, J.M. Lackie, W. Schill 1986 J. Cell Sci. 84, 263-280
12. A. Schimz, E. Hildebrand 1985 Nature (Lond.) 317, 641-643
13. W. Alt: In Temporal Order ed. by L. Rensing, N. Jaeger (Springer, Berlin 1984) pp. 163-174
14. R.J. Aerts, A.J. Durston, W.H. Moolenaar 1985 Cell 43, 653-657
15. G. Gerisch, D. Hülser, D. Malchow, U. Wick 1975 Phil. Trans. R. Soc. Lond. B 272, 181-192
16. H.K. MacWilliams: In Developmental Order: Its Origin and Regulation (Alan R. Liss, New York 1982) pp. 463-483
17. C.J. Weijer, C.N. Gottmann, C.N. David 1985 Eur. J. Cell Biol. 39, (suppl. 12), 35
18. R.E. Finney, C.J. Langtimm, D.R. Soll 1985 Dev. Biol. 110, 157-170
19. C.J. Weijer, S.A. McDonald, A.J. Durston 1984 Differ. 28, 9-123
20. C.J. Weijer, A.J. Durston 1985 J. embryol. Exp. Morph. 86, 19-37
21. A.J. Durston 1974 Devel. Biol. 37, 225-235
22. A. Goldbetter, L. Segel 1977 Proc. natn. Acad. Sci. USA 74, 1543-1547: and see the present volume
23. J.L. Martiel, A. Goldbetter 1985 Nature (Lond.) 313, 590-592
24. C.J. Weijer, G. Duschl, C.N. David 1984 J. Cell Sci. 70, 133-145
25. V. French 1976 Roux's Arch. Dev. Biol. 179, 57-76
26. K. Nübler-Jung 1974 Nature (Lond.) 248, 610-611
27. H. Jacobsen, H.G. Busse, B.N. Havsteen 1982 J. Biol. Chem. 257, 4001-4006
28. A.R. Gingle 1985 Comp. Biochem. Physiol. 82C, 235-241
29. A. Robertson, J.F. Grutsch, A.R. Gingel 1978 Science 199, 990-991
30. A.R. Gingle 1977 Dev. Biol. 58, 394-401
31. A. Robertson, A.R. Gingle 1977 Science 197, 1078-1079
32. B.C. Goodwin, M.H. Cohen 1969 J. Theoret. Biol. 25, 49-107
33. W.A. Müller 1984 J. embryol. Exp. Morph. 81, 253-271
34. Y. Mano 1970 Dev. Biol. 22, 433-460
35. C. Petzelt 1976 Cell Res. 102, 200-204
36. K.S.R. Cuthbertson, P.H. Cobbold 1985 Nature (Lond.) 316, 541-542
37. K.-I. Enomoto, M.F. Cossu, C. Edwards, T. Oka 1986 Proc. Natn. Acad. Sci. USA 83, 4754-4758
38. E. Loumaye, K.J. Catt 1982 Science 215, 983-985
39. E.C. Boterenbrood, J.M. Narraway, K. Hara 1983 Roux's Arch. Dev. Biol. 192, 216-221
40. S. Jerebzoff: In Temporal Order ed. by L. Rensing, N. Jaeger (Springer, Berlin 1985) pp. 246-247
41. J. Feldman, J. Dunlap 1983 Photochem. Photobiol. Rev. 7, 314-368
42. H.W. Sauer: Entwicklungsbiologie (Springer, Berlin, 1980)
43. J. Cooke, T. Elsdale 1980 J. embryol. Exp. Morph. 58, 107-118
44. T. Elsdale, D. Davidson 1983 J. embryol. Exp. Morph. 76, 157-176
45. G. Scholtz 1984 Zool. Jb. Anat. 112, 295-349
46. A. Robertson 1979 J exp Embryol Morph 50, 155-167
47. C.D. Stern, B.C. Goodwin 1977 J. embryol. Exp. Morph. 41, 15-22
48. D. Summerbell, J.H. Lewis 1975 J. embryol. Exp. Morph. 33, 321-643
49. L. Rensing, R. Schulz 1984 Biol. uns. Zeit 1, 13-19
50. G. Cornelius, L. Rensing 1986 Eur. J. Cell Biol. 40, 130-132
51. S. Kurtz, J. Ross, L. Petko, S. Lindquist 1986 Science, 231, 1154-1157
52. O. Bensaude, L. Babinet, M. Morange, F. Jacob 1983 Nature (Lond.) 305, 331-333
53. F. Kilchherr, S. Baumgartner, D. Bopp, E. Frei, M. Noll 1986 Nature (Lond.) 321, 493-499
54. A. Fjose, W.J. McGinnis, W.J. Gehring 1985 Nature (Lond.) 313, 284-289
55. W. Bender 1985 Cell 43, 559-560
56. J. Cooke 1983 J. embryol. Exp. Morph. 76, 95-114
57. M. Lacker: the present volume

Mixed Feedback: A Paradigm for Regular and Irregular Oscillations

U. an der Heiden[1] *and M.C. Mackey*[2]

[1]Faculty of Sciences, University of Witten/Herdecke, D-5810 Witten, Fed. Rep. of Germany

[2]Department of Physiology, McGill University, Montreal, H3G 1Y6, Quebec, Canada

1. Some Considerations on Biological Organization

One of the many striking features of living systems is their circular organization. Indeed, the essence of this property is captured in the old question: "Which came first, the chicken or the egg?".

Circular organization, or circularities, may be observed in biological systems from the microscopic molecular level to the macroscopic ecological level. At the molecular level, the most famous is the DNA - protein cycle. Thus, through several intermediate steps the DNA molecule produces protein enzymes which are, in turn, used in DNA synthesis. It is also important to note that during this process two DNA molecules may result out of one. Here, the circular organization is of an autocatalytic type which is just the condition that life can continue as a self-maintaining process. The necessity and importance of circularity and autocatalysis for living systems as parts of the self-generating and self-maintaining stream of life has been elaborated explicitly in the work of AN DER HEIDEN et al. /1 /, /2/.

At the cellular level, the circular organization of the cell cycle gives rise to two daughter cells out of a single mother cell.

Circular organization is not necessarily coupled to autocatalysis, e.g. generally there is a complicated circular interdependence between the organs of a multicellular organism. Thus the heart, liver, kidney and lungs are all highly dependent on one another for their individual integrity. Of course the number of organs in mature organisms is not increased.

The production of organisms is again autocatalytic. From one (or, in the case of sexual reproduction, from two) organism two or more additional organisms may result. At this level the autocatalytic principle has been pushed to its extreme. Thus, a single tree may have, in principle, millions of offspring.

Evidently, autocatalytic processes always produce populations (of molecules, cells, organisms etc.). Therefore, population dynamics generally includes autocatalytic feedback effects. Other nearly necessary effects are saturation (caused by environmental or internal, e.g. density, constraints) and destruction, which is unavoidable in any open system. Many types of destruction are known, e.g. mechanical, thermodynamic, chemical, and biological (death).

The interaction of autocatalysis, saturation and destruction is capable of generating dynamics ranging from the most simple to the most complicated. In this paper a simple model is presented which combines these three principles and demonstrates a variety of their effects.

2. A model for the interaction of autocatalysis, saturation, and destruction

Autocatalysis implies a circular dependence of a quantity x_1 (a single variable, a vector or a function of space) on itself. This dependence is not necessarily realized after a single step, but generally involves several intermediate steps which can be viewed diagrammatically as

$$x_1 \to x_2 \to x_3 \to \dots \to x_n \to x_1 \, .$$

The quantities x_i are assumed to be functions of time: $x_i = x_i(t)$. Each step requires a certain time for completion, so the time structure of the cycle is

$$x_1(t) \to x_2(t+d_1) \to x_3(t+d_1+d_2) \to \dots \to x_n(t+d_1+\dots+d_{n-1}) \to$$

$$\to x_1(t+d),$$

where $d = d_1+d_2+\dots+d_n$.

The detailed dynamics in each step may, in fact, be very complicated. A rather general Ansatz is given by

$$x_i(t) = \int_{-\infty}^{t} K_i(t,t',x_{i-1}(t'),x_i(t'))dt' - \int_{-\infty}^{t} G_i(t,t',x_i(t'))dt' \qquad (1)$$

$i = 1,2,\dots,n$

(in the case that $i=1$, set $i-1$ equal to n).

Here the delays d_i are implicit in the kernels K_i. The first integral describes production of the quantity x_i, while the second integral describes its destruction. A mathematical or numerical analysis of system (1) is not yet available.

The advantage of a general description like (1) is that many models in the literature may be recognized as special cases of this general system. In this way a definite relationship between these models may be established. Thus the well-known Goodwin model /3/ for the control of protein synthesis, closely related to early concepts of Jacob and Monod, is a special case of (1). Goodwin's system of equations, with delays introduced by LANDAHL /4/, is

$$\begin{aligned} dx_1(t)/dt &= f(x_n(t-d_n)) - a_1\, x_1(t) \, , \\ dx_i(t)/dt &= g_{i-1}\, x_{i-1}(t-d_{i-1}) - a_i\, x_i(t), \text{ for } i=1,2,\dots,n \, . \end{aligned} \qquad (2)$$

Here a_1, $a_2, \ldots,$ a_n and g_1, $g_2, \ldots,$ g_{n-1} are positive and constant rate factors. Only through the term $f(x_n(t-d_n))$ is nonlinearity introduced. Goodwin, and most other investigators of this system, have assumed the function f: $\mathbb{R}_+ \to \mathbb{R}_+$ to be either monotone increasing or monotone decreasing. In the first case system (2) represents a positive feedback loop, in the second case a negative feedback loop. Generally it is presumed that the function f is bounded (i.e. $f(x) \leq$ const. for all $x \in \mathbb{R}_+$), reflecting the principle of saturation. A review of mathematical results concerning the behavior of solutions to the system (2) in the situation where all delays $d_i = 0$, $i=1,2,\ldots,n$, can be found in TYSON & OTHMER /5/.

In case of negative feedback the essential result is that the system has a unique steady state which may be either (locally asymptotically) stable or unstable. In the first case the steady state is also globally asymptotically stable, meaning that all solutions approach the steady state as $t \to \infty$. If, on the other hand, the steady state is unstable then non-constant periodic solutions do exist (as proved for n=3 by TYSON /6/ and for arbitrary n by HASTINGS, TYSON & WEBSTER /7/).

For $n < 3$ and no delays, according to these results periodic solutions do not exist. Computer simulations suggest that periodic solutions, in cases where they exist, define a unique limit cycle which is attractive with respect to all solutions with the exception of the unstable steady state. However, no proof of this conjecture is available.

In the case of positive feedback there is either a unique globally asymptotically stable steady state or there are several steady states which are either locally asymptotically stable or unstable. Computer simulations suggest that no undamped oscillations do occur, normal hysteresis appears to be common. However, this question is not yet completely settled.

In considering situations with delays, let us return to the situation of negative feedback, i. e. f monotonic decreasing. The restriction $n > 2$ for the existence of periodic oscillations is not necessary when there are delays $d_i > 0$. This was proved by HADELER & TOMIUK /8/ for n=1 (in which case the system (2) reduces to a single differential-difference equation), by AN DER HEIDEN /9/ for n=2, and finally by MAHAFFY /10/ for arbitrary n.

These proofs only demonstrate that the system (2) has periodic solutions without addressing the stability of these solutions. However, in the case of positive delays extensive computer simulations always show stable limit cycles. These cycles are simple in the sense that within one period each of the variables x_i has a single maximum and a single minimum.

For n=1 the system (2) reduces to the single equation

$$dx(t)/dt = f(x(t-d)) - a\,x(t). \qquad (3)$$

Interestingly enough, this equation has been used in a variety of quite different areas. WAZEWSKA & LASOTA /11/, before 1974, used it for modelling the production of red blood cells. MACKEY and his co-workers /12-17/ have used it to explain the origin of a variety of haematological diseases including aplastic anemia and periodic haematopoiesis, COLEMAN & RENNINGER /18/ applied it to periodic excitations of neurons, MAY /19/ to the population dynamics of whales; MACKEY and GLASS /20/ to the respiratory cycle; KING et al. /21/ to psychiatric disorders like schizophrenia and panic attacks, AN DER HEIDEN et al. /22/ for inhibitory neural networks; MACKEY & AN DER HEIDEN /23/ to epileptic disorders; NISBET & GURNEY /24/ to blowflies; ANDERSON & MACKEY /25/ for commodity cycle oscillations. Solutions of equation (3) have also been used to explain the potential applicability of the concept of dynamical diseases /26/, /27/, /16/.

In some of these cases it cannot be claimed that (3) is a very realistic description of the underlying biology. What is important, however, is that a single equation of this type is sufficient to produce nearly all the phenomena observed in these different areas. For many of these phenomena, in particular for complex periodic oscillations (exhibiting more than one maximum per period) and irregular, chaotic-like oscillations, it is essential that the feedback function f is not monotone, i. e. f represents neither strictly positive nor negative feedback. Instead, the graph of f must have at least one "hump" as illustrated in Fig. 1a.

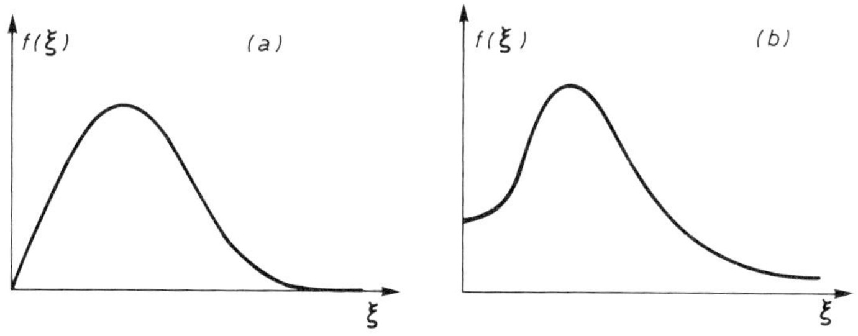

Fig. 1 Feedback nonlinearities of mixed type. It is essential that the functions are neither strictly decreasing (negative feedback) nor strictly increasing (positive feedback), but have at least one "hump"

Such a shape is quite reasonable for systems with autocatalysis and saturation. Since $f(x(t-d))$ describes the production of the quantity x, autocatalysis requires $f(0) = 0$: in the absence of x no new x can be produced (think e.g. that x is the concentration of red blood cells or the number of whales in a whale population). On the other hand, saturation implies that for large values of x no additional x is produced, i. e. $f(x) \to 0$ as $x \to \infty$. More generally it can be said that a function like that in Fig. 1 a or b represents positive feedback in its increasing part and negative feedback in its decreasing part. The functions of Figures 1 illustrate mixed feedback.

The fact that transition from single sign feedback to mixed feedback tremendously increases the complexity of the behavior of the system was first discovered by MACKEY & GLASS /20/ and independently by WAZEWSKA & LASOTA /11/. They used computer simulations to study behavior of solutions to (3) and found phenomena like period doubling bifurcations and chaotic oscillations (see e. g. GLASS & MACKEY /26/ for illustrations). AN DER HEIDEN /28/, /29/ showed numerically that system (2) without any delays (i. e. $d_i=0$ for $i=1,2,...,n$) also produces chaotic oscillations if f is assumed to be a humped function.

However, it is extremely difficult to give any mathematical treatment of the phenomena revealed by the computer "solutions". Thus, insight into why these complicated types of behavior occur is restricted. Recently, however, some progress has been made by choosing particularly simple feedback functions (AN DER HEIDEN & WALTHER /30/, AN DER HEIDEN & MACKEY /31/, AN DER HEIDEN /32/). In the following we give a simple approach to illustrate how complicated temporal behavior may arise from simple interactions, incorporating destruction, mixed feedback and delay.

3. A Paradigm for Complexity

In this section we show, step by step, how a complicated time series may arise from a simple limiting case of equation (3). To facilitate the analysis, the feedback function f has the simple humped form illustrated in Fig. 2., i. e.

$$f(x) = \begin{cases} 0 & \text{if } x < b \text{ or } x > 1 \\ c & \text{if } b \leq x \leq 1 \end{cases} \tag{4}$$

where the (constant) parameters b and c satisfy $0 < b < 1$ and $c > 0$.

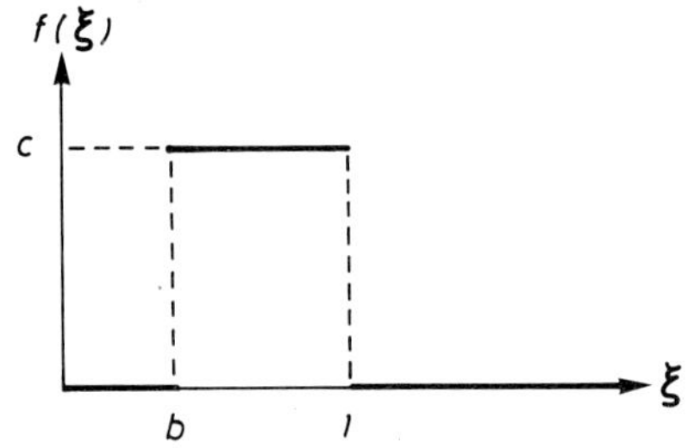

Fig. 2 Extreme case of a mixed feedback nonlinearity with a single hump

Combining equations (3) and (4) gives

$$dx(t)/dt = \begin{cases} -a\,x(t) & \text{if } x(t-1) < b \text{ or } x(t-1) > 1 & \text{(5a)} \\ c - a\,x(t) & \text{if } b \leq x(t-1) \leq 1 & \text{(5b)} \end{cases}$$

where we have set the delay, d, equal to 1 by choosing the unit of time t to be d.

The choice of such a step nonlinearity is purely for illustrative purposes. (The form of the nonlinearity suggests a process with two thresholds in production: a lower threshold (at x=b) for the onset of production; and an upper one (at x=1) for the cessation of production.) However, the type of behavior demonstrated here is not an artefact of the discontinuity in the function f, and in /30/ a mathematical argument is given why all results for the step function also hold for a class of smooth nonlinearities. The general case of a smooth nonlinearity requires substantially more effort in mathematical analysis, and also obscures understanding with a mountain of technical considerations. By considering the simpler situation we illustrate the principal aspects which may be important for understanding complexity in the applied sciences.

Since f is either 0 or c, Eq.(5) says that any solution x(t) obeys, alternately in successive time intervals, either

$$x(t) = x(\bar{t})\, e^{-a(t-\bar{t})} \qquad \text{if } x(s)>1 \text{ or } x(s)<b \text{ for all } s\in(\bar{t}-1,t-1) \qquad (6a)$$

or

$$x(t) = \gamma - (\gamma - x(\bar{t}))\, e^{-a(t-\bar{t})} \quad \text{if } b \leq x(s) \leq 1 \text{ for all } s \in (\bar{t}-1,t-1) \qquad (6b)$$

where $\gamma = c/a$.

Eq.(6a) (exponential decrease to 0) holds if, in the time between $\bar{t}-1$ and t-1, the values of x are larger than 1 or smaller than b. Correspondingly x obeys Eq.(6b) (exponential increase to γ) whenever, in the time interval from $\bar{t}-1$ to t-1, the values of x are between b and 1. Thus any solution of Eq.(5) is a piecewise and continuous composition of the functions of Eq.(6a) and Eq.(6b). A change between Eq.(6a) and Eq.(6b) takes place at any time t^* if, at time t^*-1, the variable x(t) crosses the level b or 1. Figures 3 through 6 show solutions of Eq.(5), and illustrate this pattern.

For simplicity, we restrict our attention to the case b = 1/2 and a fixed ratio $\gamma = 2$. Some remarks for arbitrary parameters are given in the end of this section. In the following, we show that increasing a from low to high values (thereby also increasing c because $\gamma = 2$) leads to a sequence of increasingly more complex oscillations.

The characterization of the temporal evolution of the process commences at time $t_o=0$. Because of the delay an arbitrary initial condition x(t), $-1 \leq t \leq 0$, must be given which uniquely determines x(t) for all t > 0. For simplicity start with the initial condition x(t)=1 for $-1 \leq t \leq 0$ (later it is shown that the following considerations hold equally well for a broad class of initial conditions). Then in the interval from t=0 to t=1 Eq.(6b) applies (take $\bar{t}=0$), resulting in

$$x(t) = 2 - \exp(-at) \qquad \text{for } 0 \leq t \leq 1 \qquad (7)$$

and thus, in particular, x(1) = 2-exp(-a). In Figs. 3 through 6 the time course of x(t) is plotted for various values of a. All of these plots show this initial rise of x(t) described by Eq.(7). In all of these figures the horizontal lines x=b=1/2 and x=1 are plotted as they prove to be important in understanding the solution: namely whenever they are crossed, then one time unit later an alteration between the equations (6a) and (6a) applies, i. e. an alteration between exponential increase and exponential decrease takes place.

Since $x(t)$ is larger than 1 between $t=0$ and $t=1$, Eq.(6a) applies for t between 1 and 2 (note that now $\bar{t}=1$) and thus

$$x(t) = x(1)\, e^{-a(t-1)} \qquad \text{for } 1 \leqq t \leqq 2 . \tag{8}$$

In particular $x(2) = x(1)\exp(-a)$.

The first maximum of $x(t)$ occurs at $t = 1$. Subsequently, $x(t)$ decreases exponentially, as described by (6a), until the level $x(t)=1$ is again reached. Denote the time at which this occurs t_1, so $x(t_1) = 1$ (see Fig. 3). Then because of Eq.(6a) (now with $\bar{t}=t_1$) $x(t)$ will still decrease exponentially until the time $t=t_1+1$, when it has the value $x(t_1+1) = \exp(-a)$. However, according to Eq.(6b) with $t=t_1+1$, once this point is reached $x(t)$ rises again, and therefore at t_1+1 a minimum is attained. As long as the parameters satisfy

$$\exp(-a) > b = 1/2 \tag{9}$$

this minimum is above the level b.

Assume inequality (9) to hold (as, e.g., in Fig. 3a for $a = 0.6$). After $t=t_1+1$, the variable $x(t)$ increases according to Eq.(6b) until a time $t=t^*+1$, where t^* is the first time when $x(t)$ crosses the level 1 from below. Clearly the time course of $x(t)$ in the time interval from $t=0$ to $t=1$ and in the interval from $t=t^*$ to $t=t^*+1$ coincide and so we have determined one period of a periodic solution of Eq.(5). Figure 3a shows a periodic solution (with period $\simeq 3.3$) of this type. It is simple in that there is just one minimum within one period.

The situation evolves in a different fashion if the inequality in (9) is reversed, i.e., if $\exp(-a) < b$. Then since $x(t)$ is below the level b for a certain time interval there is a decrease of $x(t)$ in the corresponding interval one time unit later. This decrease can be seen in Fig. 3b (for $a=0.8$) to occur between $t=3$ and $t=4$, and it is due to the undershoot by $x(t)$ of the level $b=1/2$ between $t=2$ and $t=3$. If a is not too large this undershoot lasts for a rather short time and consequently the short decrease of $x(t)$ in the time between $t=3$ and $t=4$ will not lead to a crossing of the level 1 from above. Afterwards $x(t)$ again increases until time $t=t^*+1$, where t^* again denotes the first time where $x(t)$ crosses level 1 from below. This increase is followed by an exponential decrease lasting until $t=t_2+1$, where $t_2= t^*+1$ is the time where $x(t)$ crosses 1 from above again. Obviously $x(t_2+1) = \exp(-a)$. Hence during the interval $t=t_2$ until $t=t_2+1$ the solution x behaves just as in the time interval from $t=t_1$ to t_1+1. Again we obtain one period of a periodic solution, where the period equals t_2-t_1 ($\simeq 3$ for $a=0.8$, see Fig. 3b). However, this solution is slightly more complex than found for low values of a, since now there are 2 minima within one period.

If a is further increased beyond 0.8 then the time when $x(t) < b=1/2$ becomes progressively more prolonged (compare Figs. 3b,c et. seq.). As a consequence, for values of a near $a=0.86$ the decrease of $x(t)$ one

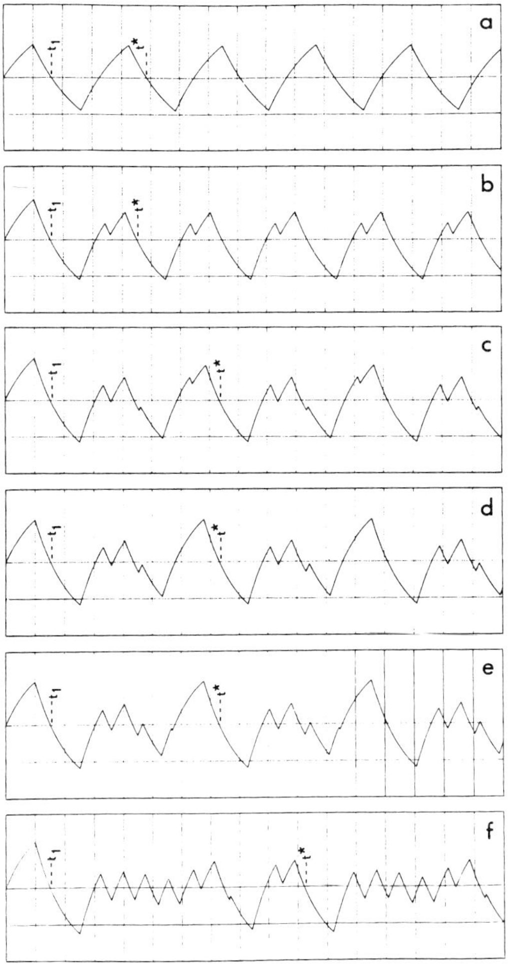

Fig. 3 The analytic solutions to Equation (3) in conjunction with Equation (4), and various values of the decay rate a. b=1/2, γ =c/a=2, x(t)=1 for $-1 \leq t \leq 0$, t=0 to 17 and x=0 to 2 throughout. The vertical lines here and in Figs. 4, 5 and 6 are spaced one time unit apart, and the horizontal lines are x=0, 1/2, 1 and 2. (a) a=0.6 (b) a=0.8 (c) a=0.86 (d) a=0.88 (e) a=0.9 (f) a=0.98 (AN DER HEIDEN & MACKEY /31/)

time unit later lasts so long that x(t) crosses the level 1 from above (for a=0.86 this occurs between t=3 and t=4, see Fig. 3c), ultimately giving rise to an additional minimum of x(t) in the interval between t=4 and t=5 (see Fig. 3c). This in turn implies that the duration of the second undershoot of the level 1/2 by x(t) becomes shorter, so short in fact that the decrease between t=6 and t=7 does not go beyond the level 1. Since between t=6 and t=7 the solution x(t) is larger than 1, x(t) afterwards decays exponentially to the value of exp(-a), completing one cycle which started at $t=t_1$ (see Fig. 3c). The important fact to note is that the crossing of 1 between t=3 and t=4 leads to a sudden increase of the period from about 3 at a=0.8 to about 6 at 0.86. A period doubling bifurcation is present at just that value of the parameter a for which the minimal value of x(t) between the times 3 and 4 equals 1. One period now contains 5 minima.

It may happen that a minimum will again disappear if a is increased still further. An example is shown in Fig. 3d, where a=0.88. There, the increase of x(t) between t=4 and t=5 has become so large that the undershoot of the level 1/2 present for a=0.86 between t=5 and t=6 is now missing. This, in turn, obliterates the minimum between t=6 and t=7. However, this change has no drastic influence on the period.

For a=0.9 (see Fig. 3e) the increase of x(t) in the time interval between t=4 and t=5 is so large that an additional minimum is again created between t=5 and t=6, though the periodicity remains unchanged and the period is still near 6 (remember that the time unit is just the delay time).

The next large change of period occurs between a=0.97 and a=0.98. For a=0.98 (see Fig. 3f) the maximum between t=5 and t=6 has become so large that the duration of the overshoot above 1 is sufficient to create a minimum between t=6 and t=7 which is below 1. The second exponential decay from 1 to exp(-a) occurs between t=10 and t=12 because x(t) is above 1 in the interval between t=9 and t=10. The periodic solution obtained has a period of about 8.8 time units and includes 9 minima. In this case the period of the new bifurcating solution is not twice as long as that of the original periodic solution.

As a is increased, progressively more complex solutions arise. The details of these behaviors may be reconstructed as in the above examples, using Eq.(6a) and Eq.(6b). Instead of discussing the details we briefly outline a criterion to demonstrate the existence of a stable periodic solution, which has already been applied several times.

3.1 A Sufficient Criterion for Periodicity

Whenever the solution x(t) exceeds the value 1 during a time interval longer than the delay (remember d=1 here), then afterwards the solution must decay exponentially to the value exp(-a). We have chosen the initial condition such that this decay occurs after one time unit. Therefore, if this occurs later on a second time we have ascertained that the solution between thes two events comprises just one period of a periodic solution, no matter what details the solution shows in between.

It is easily shown that the periodic solutions so far observed all obey this criterion. Its usefulness is seen directly from an example, as in Fig. 4a where a=1.0015. Here x(t) is larger than 1 in the interval from t=0 to t=1 and, for the second time, in the interval from t=12.3 to t=13.6. Therefore, there is a periodic solution between t_1 and t_2 (see Fig. 4a) with period $t_2 - t_1 \simeq 12.2$ (and 13 minima).

It is not a general rule that the length of the period, or the number of minima within one period, will increase when the parameter a is increased. For a=1.0125 (see Fig. 4b) the period is only about 7, a reduction by nearly a factor 2 from the period at a=1.0015 (Fig. 4a). The reduction is due to the fact that the seventh minimum shown in Fig. 4a, which is below 1, has a value above 1 for a=1.0125. Thus our criterion for periodic solutions applies in the interval between t=7 and t=8.

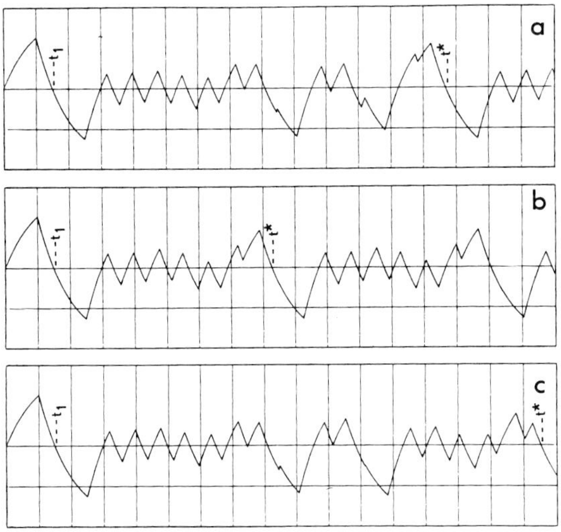

Fig. 4 As in Fig.3 with (a) a=1.0015 (b) a=1.0125 (c) a=1.001

Similar considerations hold for the pair a=1.001 (see Fig. 4c) and a=1.0015, where there is a reduction from a period of length 15 to a period of 12.2 (the example in Fig. 4c shows 16 minima within one period).

It should be noted that though this criterion is sufficient for the existence of a periodic solution, it is not necessary. Fig. 5a shows a periodic solution for a=2.75 which does not satisfy the criterion. However, a situation as in Fig. 5a is quite exceptional since it requires a very special composition and fitting of pieces of increasing and decreasing exponentials. Indeed Figs.5b (a=2.7) and 5c (a=2.775) again exhibit periodic solutions of the more general type (now with periods 72.4 and 20.2 respectively, count the number of minima!).

Figs.6a and 6b show two records of solutions where the period, if there is any at all, is longer than the time for which the solution has been computed. It is noteworthy that within time unit (i.e. the time delay) there occur many oscillations if a is large, and thus the time scale of the fine structure of the solutions for large a is much smaller than the time delay.

All of the periodic solutions satisfying the discussed criterion of periodicity are stable in the following sense: If $y(t)$, $-1 \leq t \leq 0$, is any other initial condition satisfying $b < y(t) < c/a$ (assuming $c/a > 1$) and not crossing the value 1 from above, then the corresponding solution $y(t)$, $t > 0$, converges to some time shift $x(t-t_0)$ of the periodic solution $x(t)$, $t > 0$ (as may be seen by following the solutions for two time units).

3.2 Existence of Stable Limit Cycles of Spiral Type

The previous sections give some intuition into how complexity may successively arise if some parameter is varied systematically. The

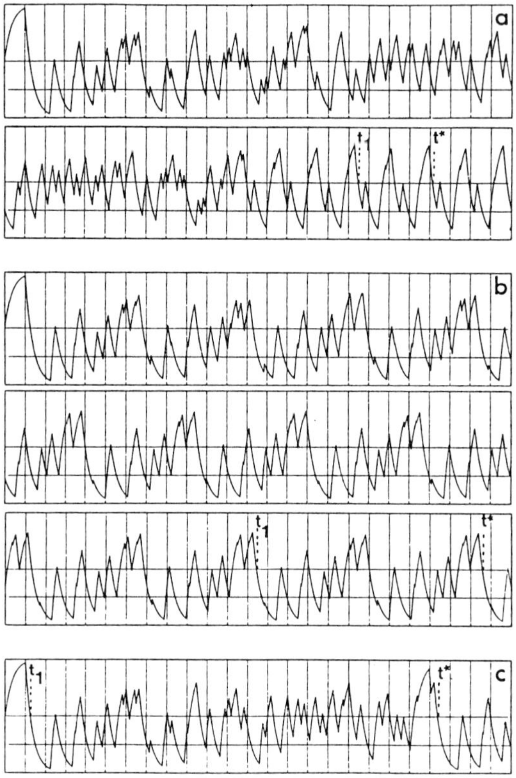

Fig. 5 As in Fig. 3 with 25 time units per panel. (a) a=2.75, t=0 to 50, (b) a=2.7, t=0 to 75, (c) a=2.775, t=0 to 25

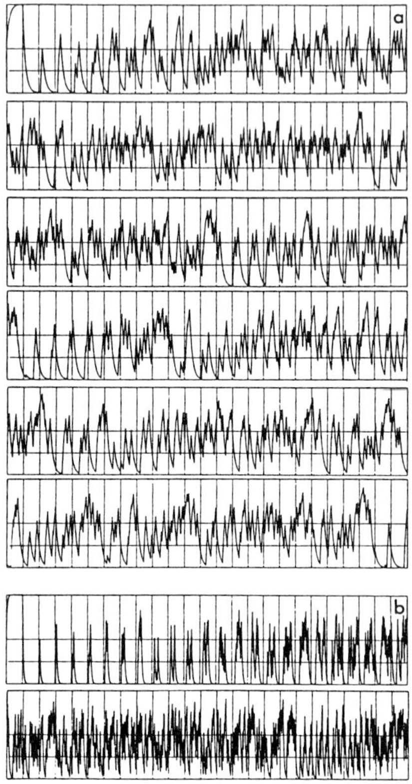

Fig. 6 As in Fig. 3 with 25 time units per panel. (a) a=6, t=0 to 150, (b) a=20, t=0 to 50

indicated techniques can be much more sharpened and extended such that it is possible to prove some far-reaching results. In the following sections we shall describe some of these results. For the proofs the reader is referred to the literature, essentially to the papers /30/, /31/, /32/.

A periodic solution is called of spiral type if one of its periods contains several maxima with increasing amplitude. In other words, during such a period the values of the solution at successive times of local maxima increase, and after this period the cycle repeats starting with a maximum with lowest value. It has been proved (see /31/) that there are values of the parameters a and c for which the following proposition holds:

There is a sequence of values (b_n), $n=1,2,\ldots$, $b_n < b_{n+1}$, such that for any b satisfying $b_n < b < b_{n+1}$ there exists an asymptotically orbitally stable periodic solution (limit cycle) of spiral type to Equations (3) & (4) having n maxima within one smallest period. As $n \to \infty$ the length of the period of the corresponding periodic solutions tends to ∞.

3.3 Existence of Chaotic Solutions

There are many different definitions of chaos in the literature. For nonlinearities f of the form

$$f(x) = \begin{cases} 0 & \text{if } x < b \\ c & \text{if } b \leq x \leq 1 \\ d & \text{if } 1 < x \end{cases} \tag{10}$$

the following type of chaos can be proved to exist for at least some of the parameter values a, b, c, and d (for specification see /31/).

Let (n_i), $i=1,2,\ldots$, be an arbitrary sequence of natural numbers satisfying $n_{i+1} > n_i$. Then there exists a solution x(t) of Equations (3) & (10) with the following properties:

x(t) has infinitely many maxima occurring at times t_j, $j=1,2,3,\ldots$, $t_{j+1} > t_j$. At other times no maxima occur. The relations

$$x(t_j) > 1 \text{ if } j = n_i \text{ for some } i$$

and

$$x(t_j) < 1 \text{ if } j \neq n_i \text{ for all } i$$

are satisfied.

More loosely speaking, there are solutions with arbitrary mixtures of small oscillations (where values at the maxima do not exceed the value one) and large oscillations (where values at the maxima do exceed 1).

3.4 Statistical Behavior

There is at least one difficulty with this and similar types of chaos. Just as a limit cycle or a steady state may be stable or unstable, the chaotic domain in the state space may be stable or unstable (or equivalently attractive or repelling). If it is unstable and if, moreover, its measure in the state space is zero, then generally the chaotic orbits will not be observed in any physical realization of the system. Indeed, it can be shown that for certain regions of the parameters (a, b, c, d) the chaotic set exhibited in the previous section has the structure of a Cantor set, hence has measure zero, and is unstable. Therefore it is important to find other domains in the parameter space where the chaotic behavior is not exceptional. This problem is considered in the paper /32/. In fact, it could be proved that for certain parameter values (a,b,c,d) there exists an attractive set of solutions to (3) & (10) such that the values of these solutions at their (infinitely many) maxima are distributed according to a continuous probability distribution.

More precisely it could be proved /32/ that there is an interval I and a map $G: I \to I$ such that the following conditions are satisfied:

For each $s \in I$ there is a solution x_s of (3) & (10) with the following properties:

(i) There are infinitely many times (t_i), $i=1,2,\dots$, $0 < t_i < t_{i+1}$, such that x_s has a maximum at t_i

(ii) $x_s(t_1) = s$ and $x_s(t_{i+1}) = G(x_s(t_i))$ for $i=1,2,\dots$

(iii) There is a density $h: I \to \mathbb{R}_+$ such that G is invariant, ergodic, mixing, and exact with respect to h.

The notions of ergodicity, mixing, and exactness describe increasing degrees of random and chaotic types of behavior. For an extensive discussion of these notions the reader is referred to the book by LASOTA & MACKEY /33/. The notion of mixing is really adapted to and from the ordinary idea of turbulence: Take any (arbitrarily small) subinterval J of I. Applying iteratively G on the points of J these in the long run become distributed in a random fashion across the whole interval I (just like in a turbulent pool of water the molecules of any small volume become distributed randomly across the whole pool in the course of time). In particular the phenomenon of "critical dependence of time courses on initial conditions" is realized.

3.5 The Influence of Discontinuities on the Solutions

When viewing the solutions presented in the previous sections as a is varied, one naturally wonders if the results are in some sense artifactual and due to the discontinuities in the slope and value of the function f as given in Eqs.(4) and (10). That this is definitely not the case can be shown analytically by techniques which have been successfully applied for a class of nonlinearities and the same delay-differential equation in /30/. All of the described qualitative phenomena are also obtained with smooth feedback functions f, at least if these are in a certain sense close to the described discontinuous nonlinearities.

Of course there are even large quantitative differences between solutions to equation (3) with different functions f. In order to give an impression about the variability in the appearance of solutions in Fig.7 numerical solutions are shown with other types of functions f, some aspects of which are, however, related to the previously discussed f. All of these types are encompassed by

$$f(x) = \begin{cases} 0 & \text{if } 0 \leq x < \delta \\ c(x-\delta)/(\varepsilon-\delta) & \text{if } \delta \leq x < \varepsilon \\ c & \text{if } \varepsilon \leq x \leq \psi \\ c(x-1)/(\psi-1) & \text{if } \psi < x \leq 1 \\ 0 & \text{if } 1 < x \end{cases} \qquad (11)$$

In Eq.(11) the parameters satisfy $0 \leq \delta \leq \varepsilon \leq \psi \leq 1$ and $c > 0$. Eq.(11) reduces to Eq.(4) if $\delta = \varepsilon = b$ and $\psi = 1$. As in the previous sections time is scaled, so $d=1$. In all calculations we used $a=1.7$ and $c=3.4$ (thereby preserving the previous relationship $\gamma = c/a = 2$), and an in-

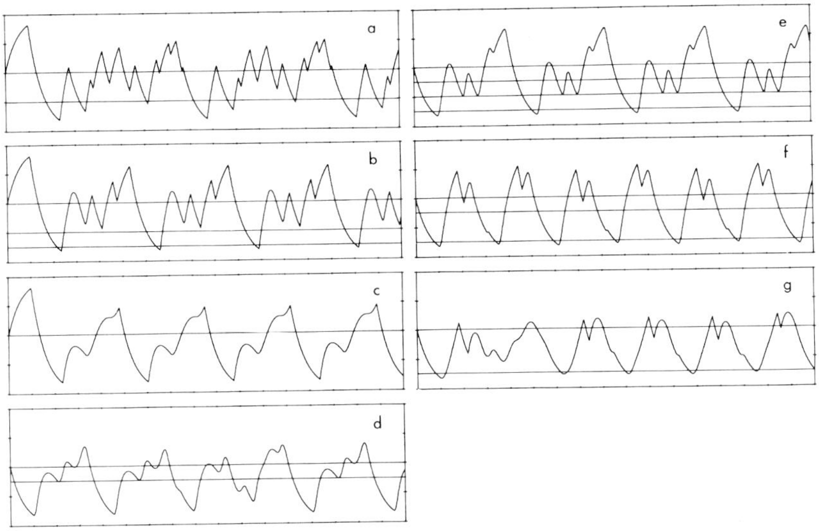

Fig. 7 Numerical solutions /x(t) vs. t/ to Eq.(3) in conjunction with Eq.(11) with various combinations of the parameters δ, ε, and ψ. In each panel t=0 to 17 and x=0 to 2. A predictor-corrector integration scheme with a step size of 5×10^{-3} was used, and a=1.7, c/a=2, d=1, and x(t)=1.0 for $-1 \leq t \leq 0$ throughout. In each case the values $x=\delta$, $x=\varepsilon$, $x=\psi$ are indicated by horizontal lines.
$(\delta, \varepsilon, \psi)$ =: (a) (1/2,1/2,1); (b) (1/4,1/2,1); (c) (0,1,1); (d) (0,3/4,3/4); (e) (1/4,1/2,3/4); (f) (1/4,1/4,3/4); (g) (1/4,1/4,1/4)

itial condition of x(t)=1 for $-1 \leq t \leq 0$. The other parameters (ε, δ, ψ) are different for each of the numerical solutions in Fig. 7a-g and are given in the legend. The interested reader may graphically realize which types of nonlinearities we captured by these choices of parameters. By help of the horizontal lines in Fig. 7, corresponding to the levels $x=\delta$, $x=\varepsilon$, $x=\psi$, the discussion of the first part of this section may be continued to obtain some understanding why the solutions behave as they do.

The essential points to note here are that: (1) the same techniques developed in the previous sections may be applied to understand the evolution of complex patterns; and (2) the removal of discontinuities in the values of f at x=1/2 and (or) at x=1 has smoothed the solutions. Further, the numerically generated solutions obey the general criteria for the determination of periodicity set forth previously (e.g. on this basis the period in Fig. 7b is approximately 4.3). Note, however, that some of the numerical solutions (Figs. 7d,g) are not periodic over the time displayed here.

4. Discussion

We have shown that simple mathematical tools (essentially knowing some qualitative properties of the exponential function) are sufficient to obtain insight into how complex, and at first sight somewhat unpredictable, temporal patterns may arise from simple deterministic mechanisms. As we pointed out, with somewhat more difficult mathematical techniques it has been proved that for a class of smooth nonlinearities f, Eq.(3) has infinitely many periodic solutions with differing periods (depending on initial conditions) and, moreover, infinitely many (so-called) aperiodic solutions. Aperiodicity may be defined in a way which incorporates properties essential for random processes /33/. Therefore deterministic and stochastic behavior are not mutually exclusive categories. For an observer not knowing the underlying deterministic structure (as given, e.g., by Eq.(3)) the process appears to be lacking in order despite the fact that all its details can be reproduced, and are determined by, a single equation.

It is important to note that in an experimental context the question of periodicity in a process is unanswerable if the period is longer than the period of observation. Moreover, as observed above, small changes in the parameters may lead to entirely different periodic patterns. Since in practice parameters are seldom absolutely constant, this is yet another potential source of complexity and irregularity.

Here, we have only discussed situations in which system dynamics are sensitive to the properties of the system some fixed time d in the past. However, there are two much more general situations which occur in a variety of applied sciences and which have received little attention.

1. State-dependent delays. In the first of these, the characteristic time delay d of the system is no longer constant but now depends on the state of the system at the current time, i. e., $d=d(x)$. Though this may seem to be a quite peculiar situation, a simple example will suffice to illustrate how it may occur.

In mammals, platelets are produced from cells in the bone marrow known as megakaryocytes. The production of immature megakaryocytes is controled by the number of circulating platelets, probably mediated by a poorly characterized hormone known as thrombopoietin. As megakaryocytes age, they undergo repeated rounds of DNA synthesis and nuclear division but without cytokinesis, so they may exist at ploidy values of 2 N, 4 N, 8 N, 16 N, or 32 N. Thus ploidy value is a convenient index of megakaryocytic age. In the normal situation, the vast majority of platelets are produced by megakaryocytes of 8 N ploidy, and the age of the megakaryocyte at this ploidy value is equivalent to a time delay in the platelet production system because of the platelet regulation of megakaryocyte production.

However, a variety of animal experiments as well as clinical observations in humans have shown that the ploidy value at which megakaryocytes produce platelets is proportional to circulating platelet numbers. Thus,the consequence of this is that the essential time delay in the platelet production system is a monotone increasing function of platelet number.

Numerical simulations of the platelet control system (BELAIR & MACKEY /34/) reveal that time delay differential equations with a state-dependent delay of this type may display an astonishing array of dynamical behavior. Many other biological and physical examples also exist in which state-dependent delays certainly exist and which may play a crucial role in determining dynamical behavior. Other than existence and uniqueness theorems of DRIVER /35/ there seems to be no analytic treatment of these problems in the literature. FELDSTEIN & NEVES /36/ have developed techniques for the numerical investigation of state-dependent delay differential equations.

2. Future effects. A second example of complicating behavior may arise in systems where the current dynamics depend, in some fashion, not only on the behavior in the present and in the past but also on future dynamics. Though we are totally unaccustomed to thinking about the possibility of the future affecting the present because of our perceptions of macroscopic causality, there are serious reasons for considering such possibilities. Two examples will suffice for illustration.

In the first instance, a wide variety of learned neural programs, e. g. catching a ball, walking on a treadmill, must integrate not only past and present system states but must also attempt to estimate future system states in order to operate smoothly. As a second example we might consider economic commodity markets in which the current market dynamics are a reflection of what has transpired in the past, what the current situation is, and what the anticipated future market position will be. All of these factors play a role in the operating of futures markets but have not, to our knowledge, ever been considered from a formal mathematical point of view.

Other examples from the physical sciences exist, and we mention only that arising in electromagnetic field theory in which, mathematically equally valid, advanced and retarded solutions to Maxwell's equations exist. Customarily, only the retarded solutions (with the time delay dependent on particle position, thus state dependent) are taken, though there is no a priori reason to reject the equally valid advanced solutions that are dependent on the future dynamics. Again, this is a poorly explored area in the mathematical literature.

Acknowledgement MCM would like to thank J. D. Murray, Centre for Mathematical Biology, University of Oxford, for his hospitality during the time this paper was written, and to the SERC (Great Britain) and to the NSERC (Canada) for their support.

References

1. U. an der Heiden, H. Schwegler, G. Roth: Acta Biotheoretica 34, 125 (1985)
2. U. an der Heiden, H. Schwegler, G. Roth: Funkt. Biol. Med. 5, 330 (1985)
3. B.C. Goodwin: In Advances in Enzyme Regulation, Vol. 3, ed. by G. Weber, (Pergamon Press, Oxford 1965)
4. H.D. Landahl: Bull. Math. Biophys. 31, 775 (1969)
5. J.J. Tyson, H.G. Othmer: Progr. Theor. Biol. 5, 1 (1978)
6. J.J. Tyson: J. Math. Biol. 1, 311 (1975)

7. S. Hastings, J.J. Tyson, D. Webster: J. Diff. Equs. 25, 39 (1977)
8. K.P. Hadeler, J. Tomiuk: Arch. Rat. Mech. An. 65, 87 (1977)
9. U. an der Heiden: J. Math. Analysis & Appl. 70, 599 (1979)
10. J.M. Mahaffy: J. Math. Anal. Appl. 74, 72 (1980)
11. M. Wazewska-Czyzewska, A. Lasota: Matematyka Stosowana 6, 23 (1976)
12. M.C. Mackey: Blood 51, 941 (1978)
13. M.C. Mackey: In Biophysical and Biochemical Information Transfer in Recognition, ed. by J.G. Vassileva-Popova, E.V. Jensen (Plenum Publ. Corp., New York 1979
14. M.C. Mackey: Bull. Math. Biol. 41, 829 (1979)
15. M.C. Mackey: In Biomathematics and Cell Kinetics, ed. by M. Rotenberg (Elsevier, North-Holland 1981)
16. M.C. Mackey, J. Milton: Ann. N. Y. Acad. Sci., in press (1986)
17. M.C. Mackey, J. Belaire: submitted to J. Math. Biol.
18. B.D. Coleman, G.H. Renninger: J. Math. Biol. 103 (1976)
19. R.M. May: In Lectures on Mathematics in the Life Sciences, Vol.13 (Amer. Math. Soc. 1980)
20. M.C. Mackey, L. Glass: Science 197, 287 (1977)
21. R. King, J.D. Barchas, B. Huberman: In Synergetics of the Brain, ed. by E. Basar, H. Flohr, H. Haken, A.J. Mandell, Springer Ser. Syn., Vol. 23 (Springer, Berlin, Heidelberg 1983)
22. U. an der Heiden, M.C. Mackey, H.-O. Walther: In Mathematical Aspects of Physiology, ed. by F.C. Hoppensteadt, Lect. Appl. Math. Vol.19 (Amer. Math. Soc., Providence, Rhode Island 1981)
23. M.C. Mackey, U. an der Heiden: J. Math. Biol. 19, 211 (1984)
24. R. Nisbet, W.S.C. Gurney: Nature 263, 319 (1976)
25. R.F.V. Anderson, M.C. Mackey: submitted to J. Math. Econ.
26. L. Glass, M.C. Mackey: Ann. N. Y. Acad. Sci. 316, 214 (1979)
27. M.C. Mackey, U. an der Heiden: Funkt. Biol. Med. 1, 156 (1982)
28. U. an der Heiden: In Zelluläre Kommunikations- und Kontrollmechanismen, ed. by L. Rensing & G. Roth (Universitätsverlag, Bremen 1978)
29. U. an der Heiden: J. Math. Biol. 8, 345 (1979)
30. U. an der Heiden, H.-O. Walther: J. Diff. Equs. 47, 273 (1983)
31. U. an der Heiden, M.C. Mackey: J. Math. Biol. 16, 75 (1982)
32. U. an der Heiden: In Delay Equations, Approximation and Application, ed. by G. Meinardus & G. Nürnberger, Internat. Ser. Num. Math., Vol.74 (Birkhäuser, Basel, Boston, Stuttgart 1985)
33. A. Lasota, M.C. Mackey: Probabilistic Properties of Deterministic Systems (Cambridge University Press, London, New York 1985)
34. J. Belair, M.C. Mackey: Ann. N. Y. Acad. Sci., in press (1986)
35. R.D. Driver: In Nonlinear Differential Equations and Nonlinear Mechanics (Academic Press 1963)
36. A. Feldstein, K.W. Neves: SIAM J. Numer. Anal. 21, 844 (1984)

Part II

Neural and Neuromotor Systems

Strange Attractors in the Human Cortex

A. Babloyantz and A. Destexhe

Faculté des Sciences, Université Libre de Bruxelles, Campus Plaine, C.P 231, Boulevard du Triomphe, B-1050 Bruxelles, Belgium

1. Introduction

The electrical activity of the brain can be recorded by electroencephalographic techniques (EEG) and is widely used in medical diagnosis. This electrical information may be analysed in various ways in order to obtain some clues regarding the structure and function of the brain. The recent developments of nonlinear dynamics (1-6) have provided new methods which are particularly interesting for the analysis of data obtained from complex systems such as the EEG. From the successive measurements at regular time intervals (time series) of a single time dependent property of the system, one tries to reconstruct the underlying dynamical processes (7-11).

In the framework of this nonlinear dynamic theory, one may find answers to the following questions : does the system under consideration obey a deterministic dynamics, with reproducible phase relationships, or does the great variability seen in a given complex system reflect random, therefore irreproducible, processes? For example, Fig.1c shows the EEG recorded during an instance of epileptic petit-mal seizure. Although at first sight the phenomenon appears periodic in time, a closer scrutiny shows pseudoperiodes with obvious variabilities. It is interesting to know if this variability is due to random noise or is determined by a deterministic dynamics.

Figure 1a represents a few seconds of alpha rhythm which is an instance of EEG recorded from a relaxed individual with eyes closed. Assuming for the moment that our analyses indicate the presence of deterministic dynamics for both 1a and 1c waves, is it possible to quantify the difference seen in the etiology of these two

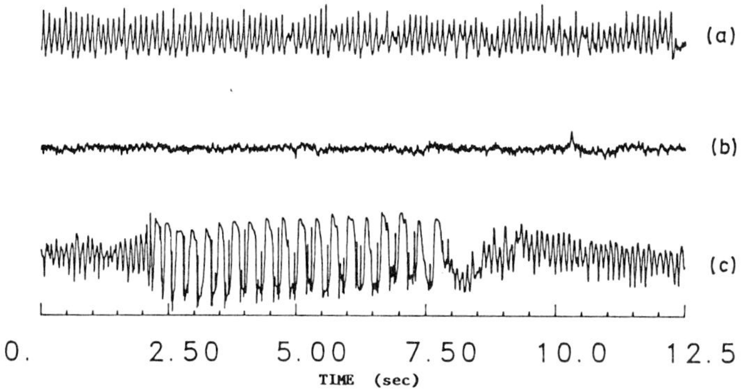

Figure 1. EEG of human brain activity recorded from three different stages: (a) alpha rhythm (eyes closed), (b) beta rhythm (eyes open) and (c) petit-mal (epilepsy). Both alpha and beta are taken from the same normal individual. These EEG signals represent the electrical potential differences between occipital and parietal regions of the scalp (P_4-O_2) and are identically scaled.

events ? Again, the framework of nonlinear dynamics provides an answer to this question.

One introduces the concept of dimension D of a dynamical system (12). The latter is a measure of the complexity of the system and may be evaluated from the original time series (13-19) (for example from the digitized EEG). The lower the value of D , the more coherent the dynamics. Moreover, the non-integer values of D greater than 2 indicate the presence of deterministic chaos (4-6). Such systems show a great sensitivity to initial conditions.

On the other hand, measured data in the form of a time series, particularly very long ones, may be expressed as phase trajectories which may be drawn in two or three dimensional euclidian space. Their shape is a visual indicator of systems dynamics. Change in form and extent of such phase portraits may be a useful clue indicating changes in the dynamics.

The dynamical approach described above is particularily valuable in problems where no obvious periodic or coherent pattern in time is seen in the measured quantities. For such cases, the usual power spectrum analysis does not shed much light on the system's dynamics. For example, systems characterized by broad band spectra are difficult to analyse. The evaluation of Lyapunov exponents is in principle appropriate for the analysis of complex dynamics (6,20), however in practice when dealing with time series the procedure is not easy to handle.

Phase space construction and dimensional analysis has been used in several fields such as hydrodynamics (21-24), chemistry (25), climatic variability (26,27), biochemistry (28,29), human brain activity (30-36) and other fields (37-40). Here we report our results relative to the analysis of EEG data. In particular, we concentrate on the study of an episode of epilepsy and alpha waves.

Although the procedure described above is based on sound grounds and gives very satisfactory results for mathematical models and a class of experimental systems, its actual application to several experimental systems poses a few problems which will be illustated in the present paper in the course of study of alpha waves for which discrepancies is seen in various studies.

2. Phase Space

Brain waves are recorded using classical electroencephalographic techniques and are digitized according to appropriate sampling frequencies. Let us represent the electrical potential measured from the scalp by the variable $V(t)$. Now, if we assume that the dynamics of the EEG may be described by a set of m variables, then one can show that these variables may be obtained from the time series by introducing a lag τ in the signal (6-9). These variables $V(t)$ $V(t+\tau)$ $V(t+2\tau)$ ... $V(t+(m-1)\tau)$ span a phase space where the instantaneous state of the system is represented by a point. In time the latter describes a curve which defines the phase space portrait of the systems dynamics. This phase space is topologically equivalent to the portrait of the original system.

This procedure was applied to the time series obtained from the EEG of an epileptic patient (petit-mal) and also from other brain waves (see Fig.1). Figure 2c represents the phase portrait of an episode of epileptic seizure from Fig.1 whereas Fig.2d is the phase portrait corresponding to a periodic dynamics (limit cycle). The comparison of the two phase portraits shows that, although the dynamics of the epileptic seizure is extremely coherent, it is far from being a periodic phenomenon. The trajectories evolve in two different planes corresponding to the "spike" and the "wave" activities. This invariant subset is called a strange attractor. In general,in the case of strange attractors, the phase space trajectories do not show an apparent regularity but neverthless trajectories are confined to a given region of phase space. The dynamics manifeste a great sensitivity to initial conditions (4-6).

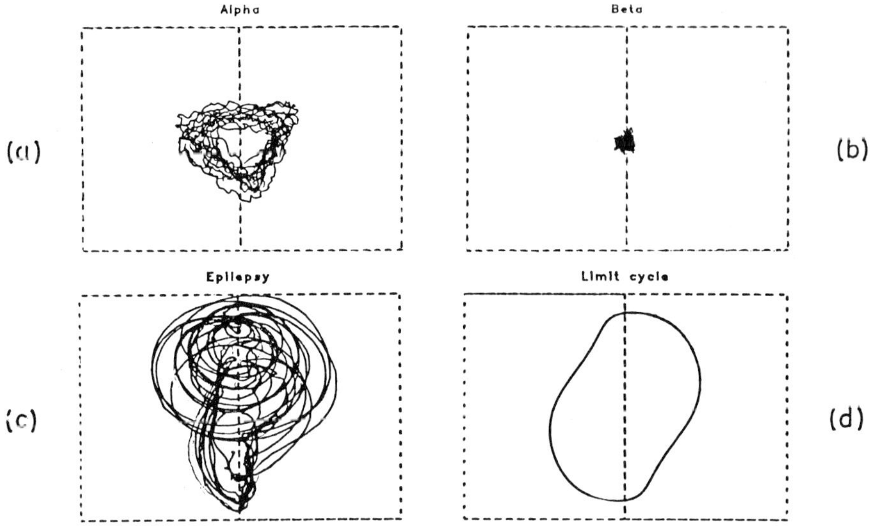

Figure 2. Phase portraits of brain waves constructed from the EEG of Fig.1: (a) alpha rhythm (3 sec, τ = 33 msec), (b) beta rhythm (3 sec, τ = 33 msec) and (c) petit-mal (6 sec, τ = 8 msec). These are the two dimensional projections of the three dimensional phase space. (d) A limit cycle.

The phase portraits of alpha and beta waves are shown in Fig.2a-2b. We see that the trajectories form a far more diffuse object than those of epilepsy. Therefore this low coherence may indicate deterministic dynamics of relatively large number of variables or a very "noisy" brain activity.

3. Correlation Dimension

In order to discriminate between a deterministic and a random activity, we must turn to another property of dynamical systems, namely the dimension **D** of their attractor (13-17). **D=1** shows the presence of periodic oscillations and the phase portrait is a limit cycle. **D=2** indicates quasi-periodic dynamics with two incommensurable frequencies and the corresponding phase portrait is a torus. If **D** has non-integer values greater than 2, it defines chaotic or strange attractors (4-6).

Instead of **D**, it is more convenient to evaluate the correlation dimension ν ($\nu \leqslant D$) from a time series of finite length **N** (13,14,18). Notice that if **m** represents the embedding dimension of the attractor, then necessarily $D \leqslant m$.

The correlation dimension of the attractor in **m** dimensional phase space may be evaluated by the construction of an **m** dimensional vector $\underline{V}$ (see above) by introducing a time lag τ ; $\underline{V}(t)$ designates a point in the phase space. We choose a reference point $\underline{V}_i$ from the data and its distances $|\underline{V}_i - \underline{V}_j|$ from the **N-1** remaining points are computed. In this way we count all data points which are within a prescribed distance **r** from the reference point $\underline{V}_i$ in the phase space. The operation is repeated for all points V_i and one constructs the correlation integral **C(r)** . The non-vanishing of **C(r)** measures the extent to which the presence of a given data point affects the position of its neighbors.

One shows (13,14) that for small **r**

$$C(r) \sim r^{\nu}$$

The correlation dimension ν of the attractor is therefore obtained from the slope of **Log C(r)** versus **Log r** .

In experimental situations where the embedding dimension of the phase space is not known, following the above cited procedure we compute the dimension ν by considering successive higher embedding dimensions m . If the ν versus m dependence is saturated beyond some relatively small m (m_0), it means that each supplementary degree of freedom added to the dynamics is not necessary for the characterisation of the system. Therefore one may say that the system is deterministic and may be described by m_0 variables. The saturation value ν_α is the dimension of the attractor and m_0 is the minimum number of variables necessary for modeling the dynamics represented by the time series.

Table 1 shows the embedding dimension and the correlation dimension of an episode of epileptic seizure, alpha waves and other stages of brain activity. We also report results from other research groups who have studied alpha waves (31,33-35) and the activity of simian motor cortex (30). One sees substantial differences in the dimensionality of these attractors. The beta rhythm (eyes open) shows a dimensionality of the order of 10. This value must be taken with extreme care as we are not sure that the algorithm is still valid for such high dimensions. For the same individual in an awake and relaxed state (alpha waves), we find an attractor of rather high dimension. However as sleep sets in, the brain activity shows dynamics of increasingly lower dimension (31). Finally in severe pathologies such as epilepsy, the dimension drops to a value close to two (32) which is comparable to those obtained (20) for three variable differential equations (41,42).

Table 1. Dimension of cerebral attractors. This table summarizes the various evaluations of attractor dimension from human EEG and simian neurons. (*) indicates that no saturation was found. (**) present paper.

Brain dynamics		Dimension ν	Dimension m_0
Sleep stage 2	(31)	5.0 -5.03	6
Sleep stage 4	(31)	4.05-4.4	5
REM sleep	(31)	(*)	(*)
Petit-mal	(32)	2.05	5
Slow neurons	(30)	2.2-3.5	10
Fast neurons	(30)	(*)	(*)
Alpha rhythm	(31)	(*)	(*)
Alpha rhythm	(34)	6.6 ± 5.	20
Alpha rhythm	(33)	2.6 ± 0.2	15
Alpha rhythm	(35)	7. ± 1.	15
Alpha rhythm	(**)	6.1 ± 0.5	10
Beta rhythm	(**)	9.7 ± 0.7	15

When the phenomenon in its totality is of short duration and if the dynamics is characterised by a rather low dimension, the above analysis may be performed without much difficulty. This is the case if we consider the EEG of a patient undergoing an epileptic seizure of the petit-mal type. However in other instances such as alpha waves, several problems may arise.

These difficulties are at the origin of discrepancies seen in the analysis of alpha waves performed by various groups. In a previous paper (31), we had found that such waves either could not be described by a low dimensional attractor or they are characterized by a high dimension ν . In parallel studies (35), it has been shown that a high dimensional attractor $\nu_\alpha = 7 \pm 1$ represents the dynamics of alpha waves. However in another study (33), a low dimension $\nu_\alpha = 2.6 \pm 0.2$ has been found for short streches of alpha waves. Here we want to show the origin of such discrepancies and also show how other factors may influence the value of ν_α in a given problem.

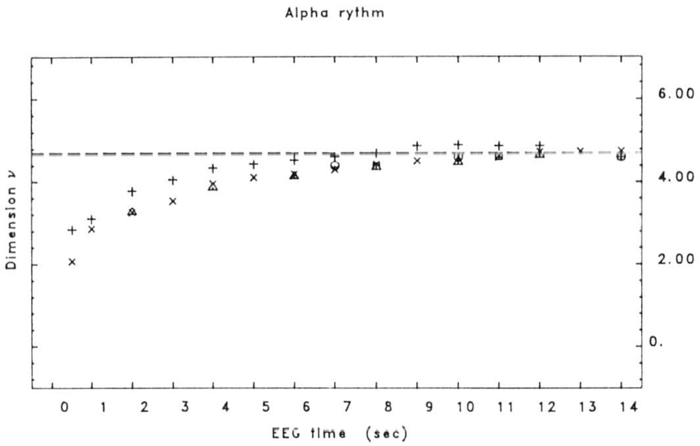

Figure 3. Dependance of the dimensionality of alpha rhythm upon the length of the time series. Several instances of alpha rhythm from the same individual are represented by different symbols (sampling frequency is 600 Hz).

Alpha waves like many other physiological phenomena occurring on relatively long time scales are almost never completely stationary. Therefore great care must be taken in choising the appropriate number of data points (13,14). Long time series necessitate costly computations and small data sets may not represent the dynamics completely. Figure 3 displays ν_α as a function of the EEG recording used to reconstruct the dynamics. The graph shows that computation with short episodes of EEG leads to an inevitable underestimation of the correlation dimension. We see that at least 6 sec EEG data are needed to extract consistent results. Therefore one may argue that the observed low dimension for alpha waves is the result of using short time series.

The choice of the sampling frequency is another source of concern. Since the computation time approximately scales as $N*(N-1)$, oversampling has to be avoided. In the case of spectral analysis, the usual rule adopted to avoid any loss of frequencies due to digitization is derived from the Shannon rule (43) which says that the lowest sampling frequency is $2*f_{max}$ where f_{max} is the higher peak in the power spectrum. Can similar rules hold for dimensional analysis ? We studied the same alpha waves sampled at three different frequencies (200 /s , 400 /s and 1200 /s). In these cases, the power spectrum does not show significant peaks higher than 100 Hz. Oversampling leads to substantial deformations of the spatial correlation integrals and to an underestimation of the dimension. Recent algorithms have been proposed which prevent the onset of such deformations (19).

From the content of Fig.4, it is seen that a sampling frequency of the order of 200 Hz seems to be the most appropriate time series for the evaluation of the dimension of alpha waves. For practical reasons, our data have been digitized using 240 Hz sampling frequency.

Although in principle all values of the time-delay τ are acceptable for an infinite number of data points (8), in practice only a narrow range of τ will give correlation integrals with sufficiently large streches of linear regions.

In spite of lack of rigorous theoretical evidence, a recent procedure seems to provide an acceptable value for the delay τ (44). It simply postulates that the best value is the one for which the variables are sufficiently uncorrelated (generalized independence) such that minimum common information is present in the dynamics.

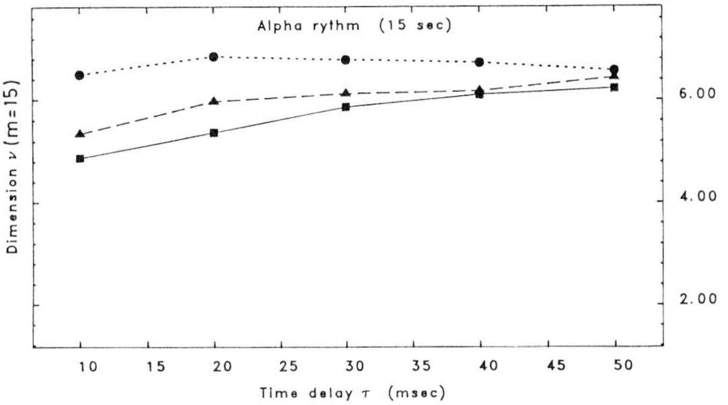

Figure 4. Dimensionality of alpha rhythm from three different sampling rates. The smoothest curve is the one obtained at 200 Hz (●), the 400 Hz (▲) and 1200 Hz (■) curves show a higher variability in function of τ (the same 15 sec EEG were used for the three attempts).

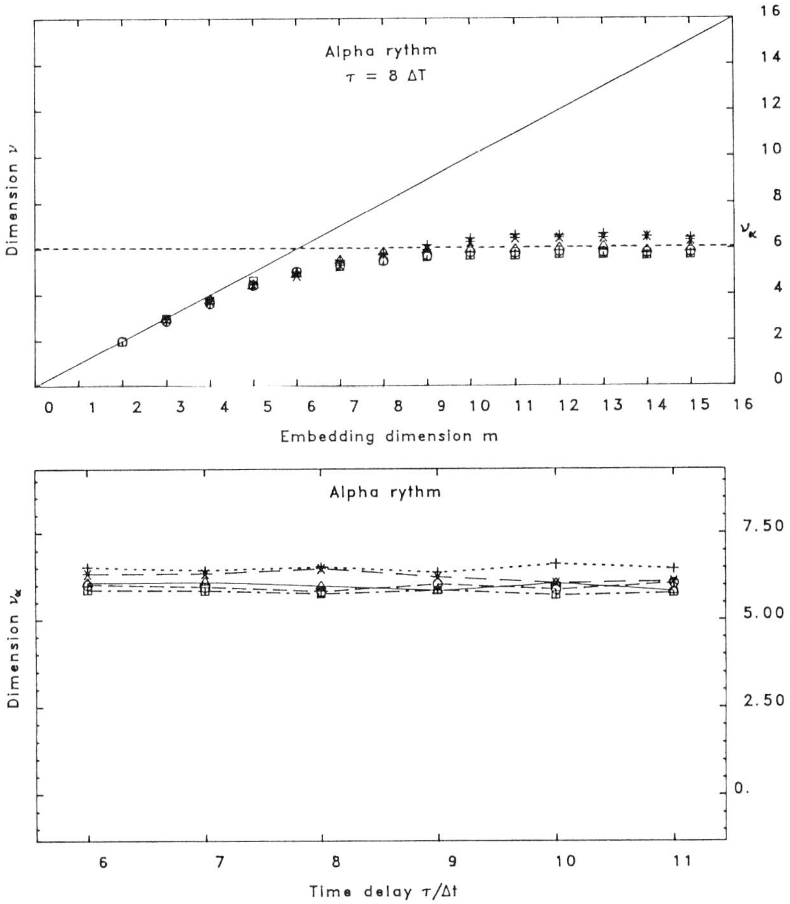

Figure 5. (a) Saturation curves obtained for five episodes of 15 sec (□ , Δ , O) 13 sec (✱) and 12 sec (✕) of alpha rhythm (240 Hz, τ = 8 Δt.). (b) Dependence of the dimensionality upon the delay τ for the same episodes.

As the best value of τ , some authors prefer to choose the first zero of the autocorrelation function (linear independence). In any case, a check for stationarity for this parameter is strongly recommended. The dependence of the dimension ν_α as a function of the parameter τ is shown in Fig. 5b for several episodes of alpha rhythm and it is seen that the dimension remains approximately constant in the range of 6 Δt to 11 Δt (25 to 46 msec). The minimum of mutual information (21 to 39 msec) and the zero of autocorrelation (29 msec) are both included in this range. So both methods seem to provide a good estimation of the delay τ for the alpha rhythm. It must be pointed out that the evaluation of the autocorrelation function is much more economical in computer time.

Finally, all these considerations were applied to the study of several instances of alpha rhythm from the same individual and we may see from Fig.5a that about 8-10 variables are needed for description of this rhythm together with an attractor dimension of $\nu_\alpha = 6.1 \pm 0.5$.

Figure 6 shows our attempt at the characterisation of beta waves. Although a very resonable saturation is obtained for $\nu_\beta = 9.7 \pm 0.7$, it remains to be seen whether the algorithm of Grassberger & Procaccia (13,14) still holds for such a high dimension.

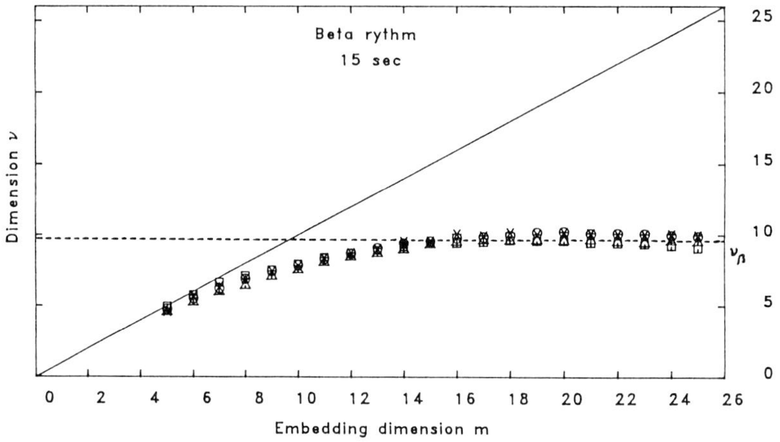

Figure 6. Saturation curves obtained from beta waves. 15 sec EEG are used with 240 Hz and with four different delays : 10 Δt (✱), 20 Δt(□), 30 Δt (△) and 40 Δt (O).

4. Conclusions

From the material of preceeding sections it is seen that phase space reconstruction and dimension analysis are new and extremely useful tools for the analysis of brain waves. The method provides radically new information about cerebral processes such as quantification of variability and assessment of brain determinism.

In particular, we have shown that brain activity with open eyes seems to obey either random processes or is described by an attractor of very high dimension. As eyes are closed and the subject drifts toward sleep, the brain activity jumps from one attractor to the next (31,32,45). For a normal brain, the lowest dimensionality is seen in the sleep stage 4. However in some pathologies such as epileptic seizures, extremely low dimensionalities are seen (32,36).

Although the method can be applied straightforwardly to model systems, in experimental situations some care must be taken in the handling of time series.

When dealing with physiological systems which are noise prone and usually non stationnary, the choice of data length, sampling rate and time-delays is very important. Great care must be taken in their choice, otherwise the algorithm fails to provide any valuable information. The knowledge of phase portraits, the attractor dimension and the minimum number of variables needed for the description of the brain dynami , in a given stage are valuable tools for model construction. On the other hand, the phase portraits with appropriate adjustments may be of help in medical diagnosis or compact storage of information.

Acknowledgments

We are grateful to Professor J.Korein for providing us with EEG data from normal individuals and for stimulating discussions. With the help of V.Lalieu from Digital Art Brussels and the use of their specialized graphical mini-computers, we were able to rotate the phase space portrait in a three dimensional euclidian space and follow its evolution in time. We thank him for his help. A.D. is a fellow from the Institut pour l'Encouragement de la Recherche Scientifique dans l'Industrie et l'Agriculture.

References

1. D.Ruelle & F.Takens: Comm. Math. Phys. 20, 167 (1971)
2. G.Nicolis & I.Prigogine: in Exploring complexity in press
3. N.B.Abraham, J.P.Gollub & H.L.Swinney: Physica 11D, 252 (1984)
4. P.Bergé, Y.Pomeau & C.Vidal: in L'Ordre dans le Chaos (Hermann Paris 1984)
5. H.Shuster: in Deterministic Chaos (Physik-verlag Weinheim 1984)
6. J.P.Eckmann & D.Ruelle: Rev. Mod. Phys. 57, 617 (1985)
7. N.H.Packard, J.P.Crutchfield, J.D.Farmer & R.S.Shaw: Phys. Rev. Lett. 45, 712 (1980)
8. F.Takens: in Dynamical Systems and Turbulence Eds. D.A.Rand & L.S.Young Lectures notes in mathematics 898, 366 (Springer Berlin 1981)
9. H.Froeling, J.P.Crutchfield, J.D.Farmer, N.H.Packard & R.S.Shaw: Physica 3D, 605 (1981)
10. H.G.E.Hentshel & I.Procaccia: Physica 8D, 435 (1983)
11. T.C.Halsey, M.H.Jensen, L.P.Kadanoff, I.Procaccia & B.I.Shairman: Phys. Rev. 33A, 1141 (1986)
12. B.Mandelbrot: in The Fractal Geometry of Nature (Freeman San Francisco 1982)
13. P.Grassberger & I.Procaccia: Phys. Rev. Lett. 50, 346 (1983)
14. P.Grassberger & I.Procaccia: Physica 9D, 189 (1983)
15. J.D.Farmer, E.Ott & J.A.Yorke: Physica 7D, 153 (1983)
16. Y.Termonia & Z.Alexandrowicz: Phys. Rev. Lett. 51, 1265 (1983)
17. R.Badii & A.Politi: Phys. Rev. Lett. 52, 1661 (1984)
18. A.Ben-Mizrachi, I.Procaccia & P.Grassberger Phys. Rev. 29A, 975 (1984)
19. J.Theiler: Phys. Rev. 34A, 2427 (1986)
20. A.Wolf, J.B.Swift, H.L.Swinney & J.A.Vastano: Physica 16D, 285 (1985)
21. A.Brandstater, J.Swift, H.L.Swinney, A.Wolf, J.D.Farmer, E.Jen & J.P.Crutchfield: Phys. Rev. Lett. 51, 1442 (1983)
22. B.Malraison, P.Atten, P.Berge & M.Dubois: J. de Phys. Lett. 44, 897 (1983)
23. P.Atten, J.G.Caputo, B.Malraison & Y.Gagne: in Dimensions and Entropies in Chaotic Systems Ed. G.Mayer-Kress (Springer Berlin 1986)
24. J.G.Caputo, B.Malraison & P.Atten: in Bifurcations et Comportements Chaotiques J. de mécanique numéro spécial (1985).
25. J.C.Roux, R.M.Simoyi & H.L.Swinney: Physica 8D, 257 (1983)
26. C.Nicolis & G.Nicolis: Nature 311, 529 (1984)
27. C.Nicolis & G.Nicolis: Proc. Natl. Acad. Sci. 83, 536 (1986)

28. M.Markus, D.Kuschmitz & B.Hess: FEBS Lett. 172, 235 (1984)
29. M.Markus, D.Kuschmitz & B.Hess: Biophys. Chem. 22, 95 (1985)
30. P.E.Rapp, I.D.Zimmerman, A.M.Albano, G.C.Deguzman & N.N.Greenbaun: Phys. Lett. 110A, 335 (1985)
31. A.Babloyantz, C.Nicolis & M.Salazar: Phys. Lett. 111A, 152 (1985)
32. A.Babloyantz & A.Destexhe: Proc. Natl. Acad. Sc. USA 83, 3513 (1986).
33. P.E.Rapp, I.D.Zimmerman, A.M.Albano, G.C.de Guzman, N.N.Greenbaun & T.R.Bashore: in Nonlinear Oscillations in Biology and Chemistry Ed. H.G.Othmer Lectures notes in Biomathematics 66, 175 (Springer Berlin 1986)
34. S.P.Layne, G.Mayer-Kress & J.Holzfuss: in Dimensions and Entropies in Chaotic Systems Ed. G.Mayer-Kress (Springer Berlin 1986)
35. I.Dvorak & J.Siska: Phys. lett. 118A, 63 (1986)
36. A.Destexhe & A.Babloyantz: to be published
37. J.Guckenheimer & G.Buzyna: Phys. Rev. Lett. 51, 1442 (1983)
38. C.D.Jeffries: Phys. Script. T9, 11 (1985)
39. M.H.Jensen & P.Bak: Phys. Script. T9, 64 (1985)
40. G.P.Puccioni, A.Poggi, W.Gadomski, J.R.Treddicce & T.Arecci: Phys. Rev. Lett. 55, 339 (1985)
41. D.E.Rössler: Ann. N.Y. Acad. Sci. 316, 376 (1979)
42. E.N.Lorenz: J. Atm. Sc. 20, 130 (1963)
43. J.Max: in Traitement du Signal (Masson Paris 1981)
44. A.M.Fraser & H.L.Swinney: Phys. Rev. 33A, 1134 (1986)
45. J.S.Nicolis: in Hierarchical systems (Springer Berlin 1985)

Analysis of the Human Electroencephalogram with Methods from Nonlinear Dynamics

G. Mayer-Kress[1,2] *and J. Holzfuss*[1,3]

[1]Center for Nonlinear Studies, Los Alamos National Laboratory, Los Alamos, NM 87545, USA

[2]Observatoire de Nice, F-63000 Nice, France

[3]Drittes Physikalisches Institut, Universität Göttingen, D-3400 Göttingen, Fed. Rep. of Germany

We apply several different methods from nonlinear dynamical systems to the analysis of the degree of temporal disorder in data from human EEGs. Among these are methods of geometrical reconstruction, dimensional complexity, mutual information content, and two different approaches for estimating Lyapunov characteristic exponents. We show how the naive interpretation of numerical results can lead to a considerable underestimation of the dimensional complexity. This is true even when the errors from least squares fits are small . We present more realistic error estimates and show that they seem to contain additional, important information. By applying independent methods of analysis to the same data sets for a given lead, we find that the degree of temporal disorder is minimal in a "resting awake" state and increases in sleep as well as in fluroxene induced general anesthesia. At the same time the statistical errors appear to decrease, which can be interpreted as a transition to a more uniform dynamical state.

1. Introduction:

For more than sixty years it has been known that the human brain exhibits electromagnetic activity which can be recorded externally as electro- or magnetoencephalograms (EEGs or MEGs).

The microscopic genesis of the EEG is not understood [1]. Macroscopically, electrical signals appear to originate from extensive dendritic arborizations on neurons. It is in this extensive overlap that excitations within one dendritic tree are conveyed to the arborizations of adjacent neurons [2]. These collective excitations, in turn, generate signals that are coordinated in space and time near the surface of the brain. Beyond this, there is some attenuation and, what is more important, a filtering of the brain's electrical activity by the intervening skull and scalp. A detailed discussion of the clinical problems related to EEG recording and possible error sources which are related to artifacts has been given elsewhere [3].

It has been known for a long time that the electrical signal of the EEG is in some way related to the mental activity of the brain. So, for instance it is possible for trained individuals to distinguish between sleep and awake states by visually inspecting the EEG. Thus there have been many attempts to find some quantitative observables which could measure these changes [4]. A limited success was achieved by fourier analyzing the EEG signal and specifying the different mental states according to the distribution of the power of the signal in different frequency bands. The most famous among them is the frequency band around 10Hz (alpha waves) which is in some way related to a relaxed state with eyes closed. The implicit assumption in this and similar ways of analysis is that the "active modes" in the brain which produce the electro-magnetic signal, are linear periodic oscillators. It is known, however that the number of these fourier modes can be much larger than the number of modes which actually are responsible for the physical, or in this case, biochemical processes [5].

Thus, while spectral methods which analyze frequency bands are optimized for regular periodic or quasi-periodic signals, the applicability of these methods becomes very limited in cases where the signal is intrinsically very irregular without very sharp and well defined frequency bands. This situation of deterministic chaos is known to be fairly common in nonlinear dynamical systems and is discussed as an origin of many biological and clinical cases of temporal disorders [6].

Therefore it appears to be of great importance to develop new methods for characterizing biological temporal signals. This should make it possible to classify them according to their degree of complexity or according to the number of nonlinear modes which are generating them.

2. Geometrical Reconstruction:

The main feature of this technique is to reinterpret time-signals as multidimensional geometrical objects [7]. This allows us to use notions from geometry to describe and characterize a time evolution. With methods based on these principles we obtain information which is in principle independent from the one we gain from the classical approaches using autocorrelation functions and power spectra. These are related via Fourier transformation, and therefore express the same kind of information about the presence of periodic oscillators in the signal.

The geometrical view of dynamical processes is based on the assumption that signals are generated by some deterministic and finite dimensional (generically nonlinear) dynamical system, which is not necessarily the superposition of periodic oscillators. The observed signal can then be interpreted as the projection of a multidimensional phase-space trajectory.

In the following analysis we reconstruct time-delayed vectors from EEG data with increasing values of the "embedding dimension" N , which specifies the number of components of the reconstructed vectors or the number of time delays. The general form of such a phase-space vector is given by:

$$\vec{x}_N(t) = (x(t), x(t+\tau), x(t+2\tau), \ldots, x(t+(N-1)\tau)).$$

These reconstructed phase-trajectories for EEG data can be plotted in different projections for different time delays and might be helpful in recognizing specific features in the data which are not so evident in the time series (see e.g. [3,8] for some examples). These objects in phase space (sometimes called "attractors") are the starting point for the following analysis.

In the next section, we give a quick review of the concept of "mutual information content" as a convenient tool for finding an optimal choice for the time delay τ.

3. Mutual Information Content:

In order to get a satisfactory reconstruction from time-series data, we require that the components $x(t + k\tau)$ of the vector $\vec{x}_N(t)$ be independent. The first idea that comes to mind concerning this optimum is to use a time delay for which the autocorrelation function of the time-series vanishes, i.e., the two coordinates are "uncorrelated". In the present context of nonlinear systems, however, this intuition might be misleading. There exist examples of low-dimensional deterministic systems which possess a power-spectrum which is identical with that of random noise [9].

Thus the autocorrelation function cannot distinguish between a purely deterministic process, where the dynamics is generated by just a few nonlinear modes and random noise, which represents a system where infinitely many (linear) modes are contributing to the dynamics.

SHAW [10] studied this problem from an information theoretical point of view, asking the question: *Assume we know the result x(t) of a measurement at time t. Under real experimental conditions with noise and finite resolution, what can be predicted about the outcome of the same measurement at time* τ *later?* FRASER and SWINNEY [11] developed this idea further and applied it to various experimental situations. By using the "mutual information content" as the criterion for choosing τ, rather than autocorrelation, we are able to obtain a better reconstruction in the sense that more details will become distinguishable at a given resolution.

Using codes developed by FRASER [11], which calculate mutual information content (MIC), we determine the "optimal" choice of time delay τ from a string of $\geq$ 4096 data-points and its copy shifted by τ. In general, we choose τ where the MIC has its first minimum. For some EEG data, however, there exists no distinct first minimum. In these instances, we choose a value of τ which is comparable to delays used in the other data sets. We find that the results are relatively stable within fairly large ranges of τ.

In the following section, we present the basic ideas behind dimensional analysis without going into the formalism that is reviewed in [12].

4. Dimensional Analysis:

In the strict sense, the dimension of a dynamical system is a measure of the number of independent variables needed to specify its state at a given instant and therefore, it is also a measure of complexity [13]. A method introduced by P.GRASSBERGER and I. PROCACCIA (we shall refer to it as "G-P"), which requires minimal computer time and memory, is now in wide use [14]. Here we want to present only the general ideas which facilitate the interpretation of our results. Details of the algorithms and a discussion of their reliability and error estimates are reviewed in [15]. A fast implementation of the code is also described in [16].

The original idea of G-P was to calculate how the number $n(r)$ of pairs of vectors $\vec{x}_i = \vec{x}_N(t_i)$, which are separated by distances less than r, changes as a function of r. They call this quantity "correlation integral" and in the general case it should scale like:

$$n(r) = r^d$$

where d is the "correlation" dimension of the set. The way it is usually obtained is by taking the logarithm which yields the linear function:

$$\log n(r) = d \log(r)$$

Thus if we plot the *dimension curve* $\log n(r)$ vs. $\log(r)$ we expect to observe a straight line, where the slope d corresponds to the dimension of the set. In practice, this method will never result in a perfectly straight line over the entire region $\log(r)$, because of the finite size of the vectors and other effects which are discussed in [18]. However, there is usually a smaller region over which a "straight line" may be fitted and therefore, a slope can be read off which is then called "dimension".

In our opinion, a major drawback of this algorithm is that by fitting a straight line to a portion of the dimension curve, it is always possible to get a result, namely a slope d, but it is not trivial to decide whether this value is really significant or purely due to artifacts.

After calculating time-delayed coordinates from normalized EEG data, we reconstruct phase space vectors $\vec{x}_N(t_i)$ for increasing embedding dimensions $N = 1, 2, \ldots, 20$. However, to use the original G-P algorithm, which calculates distances between all pairs $(\vec{x}_N(t_i), \vec{x}_N(t_j))$ of data points, would be too time consuming. Therefore, we choose a smaller set of n_{ref} equally spaced (in time) reference points $\vec{x}_N(t_k)$ and compute distances between reference points and the rest of the data points. Typically, we use 200 reference points and 3000 - 20000 data points.

To compute the correlation dimension we determine for each value of $\log(r)$ the average number $\log n(r)$ of pairs which are separated by $\hat{r} \leq r$. The error bars in Fig. 1 indicate the width of this distribution for each discrete value of $\log(r)$. In [15] we showed how this method can produce systematically small

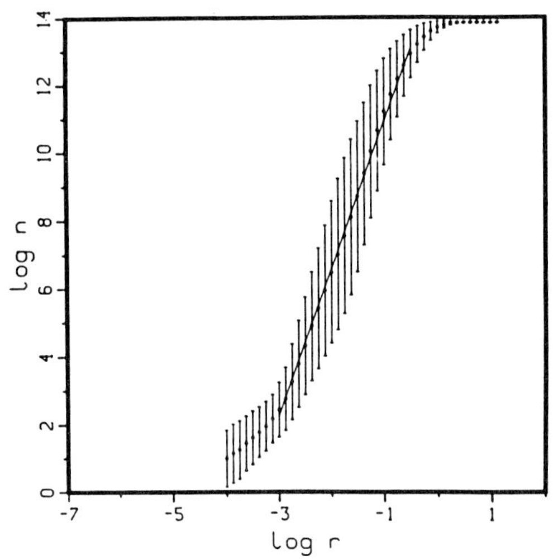

Fig. 1: "Dimension function" $\log n(r)$ vs. $\log(r)$ for lead P3-O1 while the subject was awake but quiet. We have 15000 points at a sampling rate of 500Hz. Time delay: τ = 20msec, embedding dimension N = 20, n_{ref} = 200 reference points

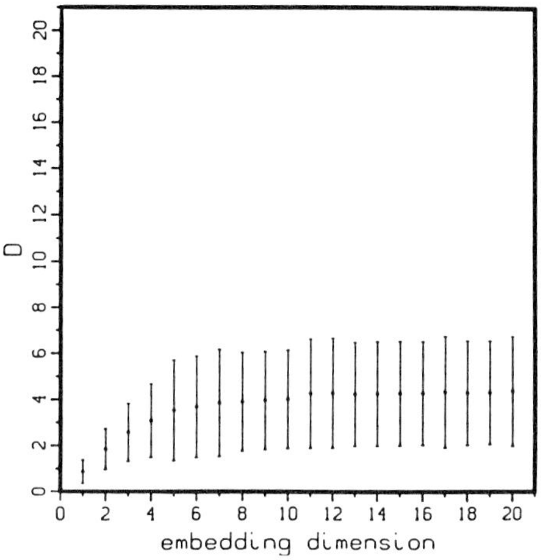

Fig. 2: G-P "Dimension" for increasing embedding dimensions. Same data as in Fig.1

values for the correlation dimension in the case of finite data sets from strongly non-uniform attractors. These error estimates indicate the maximal variations in slope for line segments in the "scaling region." For each data set, the overall error is proportional to the average size of the error-bars in the dimension curve and inversely proportional to the length of the "scaling region." Therefore, fitting over large "scaling regions" with large error bars yields similar results to fitting over small "scaling regions" with small error bars (see [15] for details). In the literature, errors based on a least squares fit are often quoted. We think this is far too optimistic, especially for small scaling regions.

If we look at the dimension-curves for each individual reference point, we see that many of them are displaced along the horizontal axis due to variations in scale as described in [15]. Their slopes correspond to the "point-wise dimension" of the different reference points and their average determines the

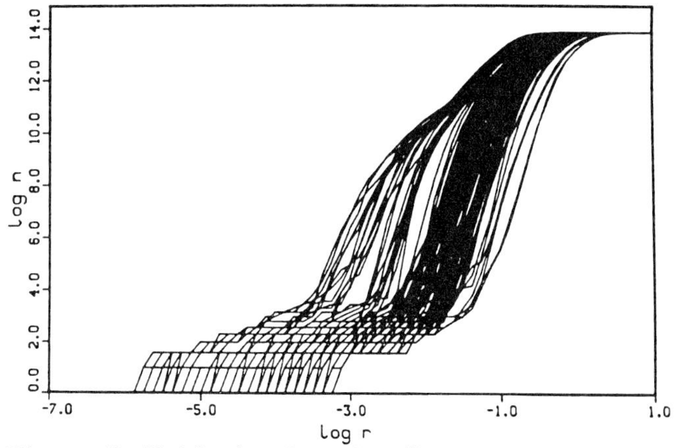

Fig. 3: Individual point-wise dimension curves for $n_{ref} = 200$ reference points. Same data as in Fig. 1

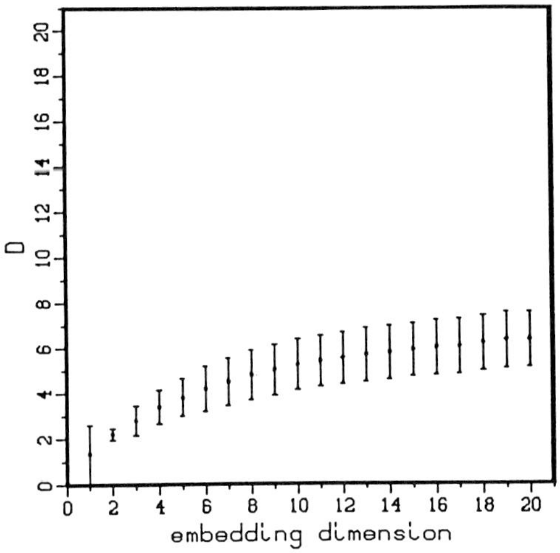

Fig. 4: Averaged point-wise dimension for increasing embedding dimension. Same data as in Fig. 1

"information dimension" $D^{(1)}$ [13] (see fig. 3). In the case of a very large number of data points the averaging according to the correlation dimension $D^{(2)}$ would yield a result which gets close to $D^{(1)}$. With our EEG data, however, we find in the case of "low-dimensional chaos" (awake, quiet, eyes closed, see Fig. 1) a value for the G-P dimension of $D^{(2)} = 4.3 \pm 2.2$. For the same data set we obtain $D^{(1)} = 6.4 \pm 1.2$ (see Fig. 4). In Fig. 5 we show the frequency distribution of the measured values of the point-wise dimension of the set of $n_{ref} = 200$ reference points. The errors indicated in these plots are statistical and more reliable. They also seem to be consistently smaller. When the patient is under fluroxene induced general anesthesia the G-P dimension increases to $D^{(2)} = 8.0 \pm 3.8$ [3]. This uncertainty of 50% at such a high value

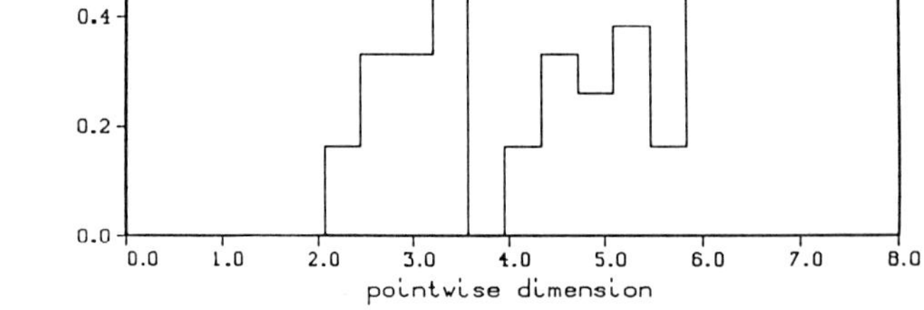

Fig. 5: Frequency of dimension values for $n_{ref} = 200$ reference points

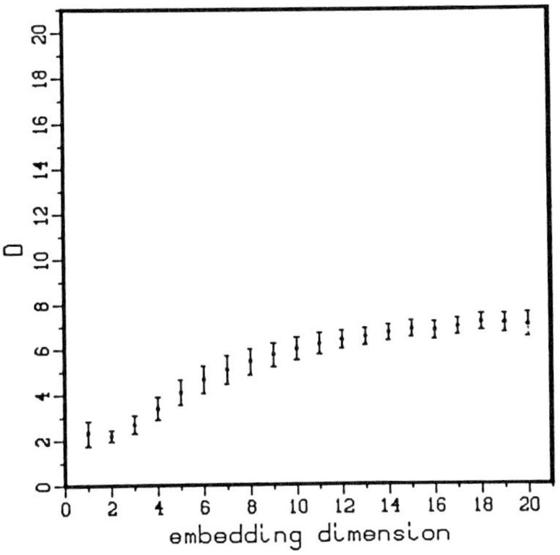

Fig. 6: Same as Fig. 4 for data from light, fluroxene-induced general anesthesia

for $D^{(2)}$ is very well compatible with the hypothesis of noise. For this data set we find for the information dimension $D^{(1)} = 7.1 \pm 0.5$ (Fig. 6). Thus we see a consistent increase in the dimensional complexity under the influence of fluroxene. Besides that it seems that the fluctuations in the dimension values have , decreased and the behavior has become more uniform (Fig. 7). We shall see below that this feature is also reflected in the observed Lyapunov exponents.

Similar behavior is observed in the sleep data, but the effect is not so pronounced there. We obtain dimensions, which are about the same for sleep onset ($D^{(2)} = 6.8 \pm 6.1$, $D^{(1)} = 6.8 \pm 0.3$) and rem sleep ($D^{(2)} = 6.4 \pm 5.1$, $D^{(1)} = 6.9 \pm 0.4$). For stage 4 sleep we get a decrease in complexity but an increase in the fluctuation level of the information dimension ($D^{(2)} = 5.9 \pm 4.4$, $D^{(1)} = 6.5 \pm 0.6$). Even though we think that these results do not correspond to the "actual dimension" of the EEG in the strict sense, we believe that they show a consistent dependence on the brain state.

In the following we'd like to discuss some of the common error sources found in dimension calculations.

Our EEG data were digitized at 500Hz, which is well above the maximal EEG frequency of $\leq$ 100Hz. Therefore, for very short distances r, neighboring vectors come from the same segment of trajectory and do not contribute to the dimensions which we want to extract. This is seen clearly in Fig. 1 where the slope d of the dimension curve is close to unity for $log(r) \leq -2.5$. This effect disappears when we reduce the sampling rate to 100Hz [3]. Thus there is a restriction on the accuracy of the dimension algorithm: it requires a large number of data points to fill a high dimensional phase-space volume. Roughly, the number of data points required to fill up an N-dimensional cube of given diameter goes exponentially with the embedding dimension N.

On the other hand it appears that the EEG is not stationary over the range of, say, minutes. This condition assigns an upper bound on the amount of EEG data that can be used for dimensional analysis. Generating a larger number of data points by increasing the sampling rate is not a solution, since these points are confined to low-dimensional subspaces and introduce the systematic errors described above. Therefore, we think that reports of "low-dimensional chaotic attractors" from EEGs [17,19] with dimensions less than three describe different phenomena which seem to be more related to the spectral than the dimensional properties of the system.

In order to calculate "dimension" automatically (for each embedding dimension N), we use an algorithm which fits a straight line to each point r_m of the dimension curve [15]. Then we calculate a goodness of fit for each line segment and located the point with the best fit. This point defines the center of the "scaling region." Subsequently, we increase the length of the "scaling region" until the goodness of fit reaches a chosen threshold value of 10%. We also require that our algorithm does not try to fit in regions of distances for which there are too few points (bad statistics) or too many (saturation). In Figs. 4-7 we have chosen $4 \leq log_2(n(r)) \leq log_2(\frac{1}{3} N_{dat})$.

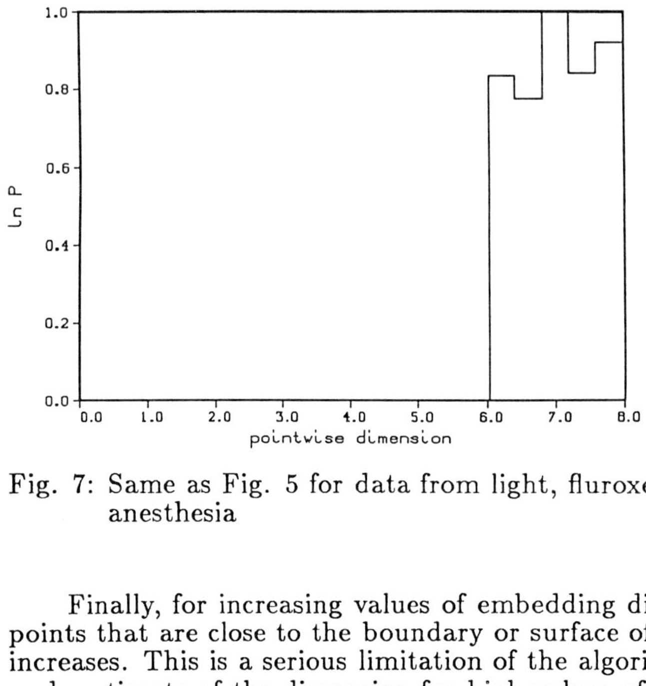

Fig. 7: Same as Fig. 5 for data from light, fluroxene-induced general anesthesia

Finally, for increasing values of embedding dimension N, the fraction of points that are close to the boundary or surface of the reconstructed data set increases. This is a serious limitation of the algorithm; it causes a systematic underestimate of the dimension for high values of embedding dimension [19]. We want to insure an asymptotic regime, by using large values of embedding dimension, but we also know that systematic errors due to boundary effects increase. Therefore, we consider any result of $d \geq 7$ to be indistinguishable from $d = \infty$.

5. Lyapunov Exponents

There are currently two basic methods available for estimating the sensitivity to an experimental system to initial conditions. For chaotic behavior it is characteristic that small perturbations get amplified exponentially fast. These growth rates of small perturbations can also be used for the quantification of the degree of temporal disorder.

In the algorithm of WOLF et al. [20] one computes the behavior of orbits which are close to a given reference orbit and measures their separation rates at each point of the attractor. With this method it is possible to extract the largest Lyapunov exponent.

In the second method we use a combination of algorithms of ECKMANN and RUELLE [21] and SANO and SAWADA [22], and try to reconstruct Jacobian matrices which yield information about the separation of nearby orbits. In this way it is possible in principle to compute all the Lyapunov exponents, i.e. the separation or convergence rates in all phase-space directions. We get a quite good convergence of the Lyapunov exponents with increasing matrix dimension (see [23] for a discussion and comparison of the methods).

The convergence or divergence rates of dynamical systems typically fluctuate to a large extent along the orbits. The Lyapunov exponents describe the average behavior of separation or convergence. The degree of fluctuations along the attractor orbits are quantified by the non-uniformity-factor [24] which corresponds to the standard deviation computed from the local divergence rates. In Figs. 8,9 we have the largest Lyapunov exponents together with the non-

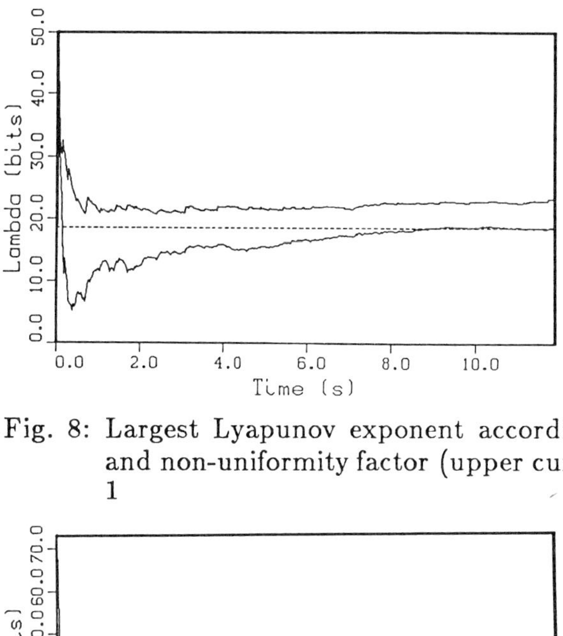

Fig. 8: Largest Lyapunov exponent according to [20] (lower curve), and non-uniformity factor (upper curve). Same data as in Fig. 1

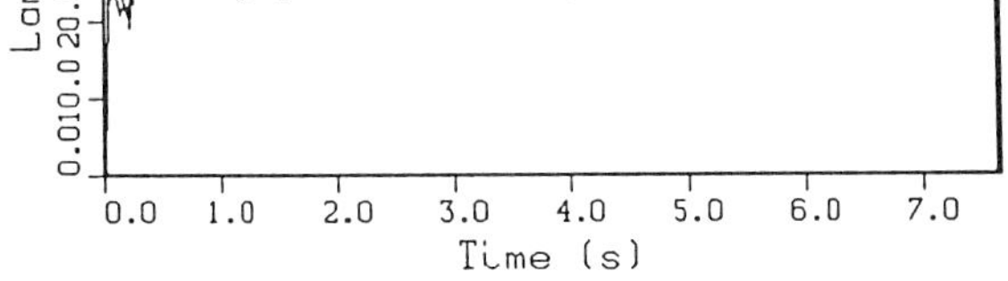

Fig. 9: Same as in Fig. 8 for data of Fig. 6

In Figs. 8,9 we have the largest Lyapunov exponents together with the non-uniformity-factor for the data sets of Figs. 4-7. The separation rates are given in bits per second. Notice that the non-uniformity-factor is always larger than the largest Lyapunov exponent.

We can see that again in the transition to anesthesia (Fig. 9) the Lyapunov exponent increases with respect to the resting awake state (Fig. 8) while the non-uniformity-factor is reduced. This, as mentioned above, supports the interpretation that the disorder increases but simultaneously the behavior becomes more uniform.

Again some error considerations: Since for bounded attractors the separation will only be exponential for small distances, the neighboring orbits have to be reset after a short evolution time. It appears that the values obtained for the Lyapunov exponents depend on the length of the time intervals between resettings.

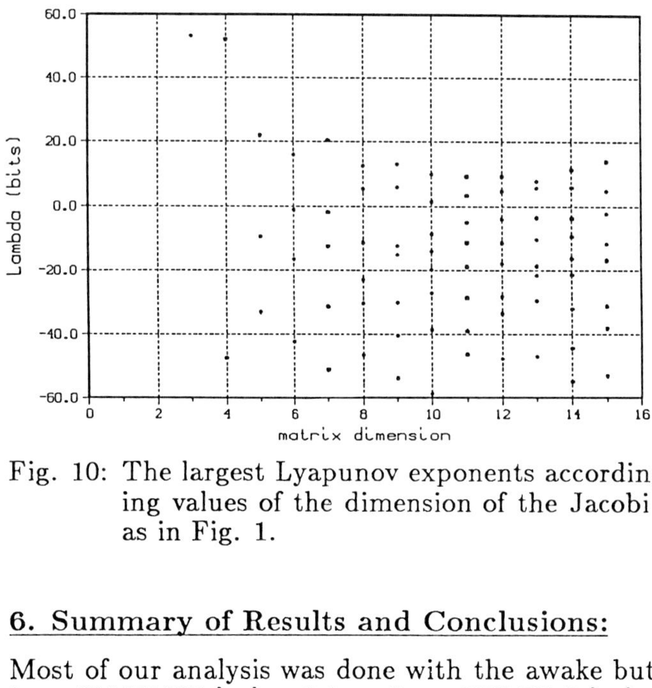

Fig. 10: The largest Lyapunov exponents according to [21] for increasing values of the dimension of the Jacobi matrix. Same data as in Fig. 1.

6. Summary of Results and Conclusions:

Most of our analysis was done with the awake but quiet, and anesthesia data from HANLEY [25] and data from EHLERS [26], which were recorded during several stages of sleep and wakefulness.

The power spectrum of our signals (see [3]) does not show a strong power law decay. This is an additional indication that we are observing "low dimensional chaos" and not "random noise with special statistics" as discussed by OSBORNE et al. [27].

We observe low "dimension" values, however, only in a resting state when the eyes are closed. When the subject opens the eyes, the dimension increases substantially. Also for the same subject, there seems to be a decrease in "dimension" for stage 4 sleep compared to the almost identical values for sleep onset and REM sleep. To our surprise we also find that the mutual information content varies significantly with different sleep stages (Fig. 27 in [3]). In stage 4 sleep the mutual information content decays very slowly which may reflect a slow rate at which new information is produced. For the cases of REM sleep and sleep onset, the mutual information curves lie close together, which possibly reflects the similarity between the two stages of sleep [28].

During light general anesthesia induced by fluroxene the "dimension" of leads P3-O1 and P4-O2 abruptly increase beyond our numerical limits. In the temporal leads this increase was not observed; the observed dimension is consistently very high. We don't see any changes during the transition from light to medium anesthesia. For this case, this indicates that "dimension" is not a sensitive measure of the depth of anesthesia. However, the relative increase in dimension is consistent with the excitatory action of the anesthetic fluroxene.

Finally, we want to mention that we also calculated the "dimension" of several MEG recordings [29]. These data reflect activity from a smaller volume of brain tissue than EEG. Nevertheless, it seems that the dimension of these MEG data is comparable to that of the EEG data we analyzed. This might support conjectures that the electromagnetic activities in the brain are coherently generated by large regions.

ACKNOWLEDGEMENTS: We are grateful to John Hanley, Cindy Ehlers, and Ed Flynn for providing us with clean experimental data. One of us (G.M-K.) would like to thank Arnold Mandell, Cindy Ehlers, and Jim Havstadt for stimulating discussions.

References

[1] R. Elul, "The genesis of the EEG.", Int. Rev. Neurobiol. 15: 227-272, 1972

[2] W.R. Adey, In Behavior and Brain Electrical Activity, ed. by N. Burch, H. Altshuler (Plenum, New York 1974) pp. 363-390

[3] S.P. Layne, G. Mayer-Kress, J. Holzfuss, In Dimensions and Entropies in Chaotic Systems ed. by G. Mayer-Kress, (Springer Ser. Syn., Vol. 32) (Springer, Berlin, Heidelberg 1986) pp. 246-256
G. Mayer-Kress, S.P. Layne, In Proc. NY Acad. Sci. Conf. on Biological Dynamics and Theoretical Medicine

[4] J. Hanley, "Electroencephalography in Psychiatric Disorders: Parts I,II". In Directions in Psychiatry. 4, 7: 1-8, 1984

[5] H. Haken, Synergetics- An Introduction, Springer Ser. Syn., Vol.1 3rd ed. (Springer, Berlin, Heidelberg 1983)

[6] U. an der Heiden, M.C. Mackey, this volume

[7] N.H. Packard, N.H., J.P.Crutchfield, J.D.Farmer, R.S.Shaw, "Geometry From a Time Series", Phys. Rev. Lett. 45: 712, 1982

[8] A. Babloyantz, this volume.

[9] S. Grossmann, S. Thomae, Z. Naturforsch. 32a: 1353, 1977

[10] R.S. Shaw, The Dripping Faucet as a Model Chaotic System, (Aerial Press, Santa Cruz, CA 1985)

[11] A.M. Fraser, H.L. Swinney, Phys. Rev. A 33: 1134-1140, 1986

[12] G. Mayer-Kress (ed.) Dimensions and Entropies in Chaotic Systems Springer Ser. Syn., Vol.32 (Springer, Berlin, Heidelberg 1986)

[13] J.D. Farmer, E. Ott, J. A. Yorke, Physica 7D:153-180, 1983

[14] P.Grassberger, I. Procaccia, Physica 9D: 189, 1983
[15] J. Holzfuss, G.Mayer-Kress, "An Approach to Error Estimation in the Application of Dimension Algorithms", In [12]
[16] W. Lauterborn, J. Holzfuss, "Evidence for a Low-Dimensional Strange Attractor in Acoustic Turbulence", Phys. Lett. 115A, 369, 1986
[17] A. Babloyantz, A. Destexhe, Proc. Natl. Acad. Sci. 83, 3513, 1986
[18] A.M. Albano, N.B. Abraham, G.C. de Guzman, M.F.H. Tarroja, D.K. Bandy, R.S. Gioggia, I.D. Zimmerman, N.N. Greenbaun, T.R. Bashore, "Lasers and Brains: Complex Systems with Low-Dimensional Attractors", In [12].
[19] J.G. Caputo, B. Malraison, P. Atten, "Determination of Attractor Dimension and Entropy for Various Flows: An Experimentalist's Viewpoint", In [12]
[20] A. Wolf, J. Swift, H.L. Swinney, J. Vastano, Physica 16D, 285 (1985)
[21] J.P. Eckman, D. Ruelle, Rev. Mod. Phys. 57, 617 (1985)
[22] M. Sano, Y. Sawada, Phys. Rev. Let. 55, 1082 (1985)
[23] J.A. Vastano, E.J. Kostelich, " Comparison of Algorithms for Determining Lyapunov Exponents from Experimental Data", In [12]
[24] J.S. Nicolis, G. Mayer-Kress, G. Haubs, Z. Naturforsch. 38a,1157 (1983)
[25] J. Hanley, Data taken at UCLA. The patient was a 45-year-old female. No medication prior to surgery. Anesthesia was induced by inhalation of fluroxene. The EEG record lasts for 15 minutes: 5 min. awake but quiet, 5 min. light anesthesia, and 5 min. medium anesthesia. Analog data from the EEG was digitized at 500 Hz.
[26] C. Ehlers, Data taken at UCSD. The EEG data were recorded from the same subject while performing various mental tasks and while sleeping.
[27] A.R. Osborne, A. Provenzale, L. Bergamasco. Preprint. Multivariate Scaling Portraits of the Lorenz Attractor.
[28] A. Mandell, private communication
[29] E. Flynn, Data taken at Los Alamos. The magneto-encephalogram data were recorded from the same subject while awake but quiet.

Studying Temporal Order in Human CNS by Means of "Running" Frequency and Coherence Analysis

M. Keidel[2], *W.-D. Keidel*[1], *W.S. Tirsch*[2], *and S.J. Pöppl*[2]

[1]University of Erlangen-Nürnberg, D-8520 Erlangen, Fed. Rep. of Germany
[2]Institute of Medical Informatics and Health Services Research, GSF, D-8042 Neuherberg/München, Fed. Rep. of Germany

1. INTRODUCTION

Within living systems, functions of the nervous system are not static but rather dynamic processes, exhibiting a well-ordered change of activity and of synergy in time. Such cyclic alterations of the CNS state form certain biological rhythms and oscillations with a great variety of period lengths ranging from milliseconds to months (e.g. cardio-vascular and respiratory 1-minute rhythm [1,2] or circa 90-minute 'Basic Rest-Activity Cycles' of the CNS;[3,4]). A survey of such ultra- and additional circa- and infra-dian human rhythmicities is given by HILDEBRANDT in this volume.

This report deals with faster 'ultra'-ultradian rhythms in man, which show predominant periods of circa 100 milliseconds. Such 10c/s oscillations generated by the neuraxis are generally known as the electrocortical fluctuations in the electroencephalogram (EEG), as mechanical oscillations of the body or body parts in tremor recordings (FREUND, in this volume) and as muscular vibrations in the vibromyogram (VMG; KEIDEL [5,6]). In this context tremor and VMG are considered to be the indirect and direct (damped) mechanical equivalents of the spinal (moto-) neuronal firing statistics, respectively.

The goals of the present study are (i) to discern an ultradian temporal order in the middle frequency range of each of the simultaneously recorded time series (EEG, VMG, tremor), as well as (ii) to demonstrate a temporal 'meta-order' of functional interplay between two of these biosignals. The following specific questions have been adressed: 1) Is there a rhythmic variation in amplitude (or frequency) of EEG, VMG or tremor, showing, for example, periods in the range of seconds or minutes and which can be quantified in form of a clear 'periodo- or cyclogram'? 2) (i) Does there exist a functional coupling in the sense of steady or transient synchronisation of the EEG with VMG or tremor? (ii) If this is the case, can a specific temporal pattern in (periodic) fluctuations of coupling strength be demonstrated ? 3) (i) Does the functional cooperation of different cortical brain areas increase during execution of a graded motor task and (ii) does this putative alteration differ with respect to specific EEG frequencies or scalp regions investigated.

2. MATERIALS AND METHODS

Eight healthy volunteers (mean age: 23.5 y. +/- 2.4 SD) were investigated. For data acquisition the subjects were in a reduced sound, electrically shielded room, free of disturbing vibrations with respect to the selected gain. In a waking state they were lying in a supine position with eyes closed. Scalp-EEG was recorded from Fz, C3, C4 and Oz (10/20-system;[7]). All 'active' electrodes were referred to linked earlobes (A1/A2; amplified by Nicolet Pathfinder II; bandwidth of 0.2 - 100 Hz). Artefact rejection was done by visual inspection. With a piezo-electric device (Bruel/Kjaer 4367) attached to the skin overlying the muscles of interest the acceleration curves of muscular vibrations were simultaneously measured, orthogonal to the surface (bandwidth: 0.2 - 100 Hz; for details see [5]). For recordings of physiological finger-tremor the subjects had to grip an accelerometer between the right thumb and forefinger with maximal force, which was monitored in addition to the tremor curve. All signals were recorded for 4 minutes and after appropriate amplification stored on a FM recorder (TEAC, XR-510). For off-line data analysis (FFT) a VAX-11/780 computer system combined with a Versatec plotter was used. The A/D-sampling rate was determined to be 2 kHz. On the basis of previously described analytical methods (KEIDEL [8]) special software was developed. This calculates, using a sliding analysis window, the 'running' auto- and cross-power densities, amplitudes as the root mean square of the power, as well as phase- and coherence-functions. The coherence was computed with respect to the questions formulated above since this algorithm (i.e. the ratio of the square of the cross-spectrum to the product of the auto-spectra, see [9]) verifies the strength of interrelation (e.g. of phase constancy or synchrony) between two biosignals, representing a standarized measure of frequency-specific covariance. Because a given analysis segment of e.g. 20 s was generally shifted over a long-lasting time course with a freely selectable Delta T of, e.g. 500 ms or 1 s, even short-lasting changes of frequency-related energies or coherence estimates could be discerned.

3. RESULTS

3.1. 'Running' Frequency Analysis

3.1.1. Brain Waves

A typical result of such 'running' spectral analysis of the ongoing EEG-activity (Oz - A1/A2) of an awake subject at rest is given in Fig.1. In this case a frequency range of analysis was selected from 1.6 - 32 Hz (x-axis). Fixed 20 s epochs sliding in 1 s steps over the total analysis epoch of 4 minutes were analysed. 220 single autospectra were yielded and were plotted pseudo-three-dimen-

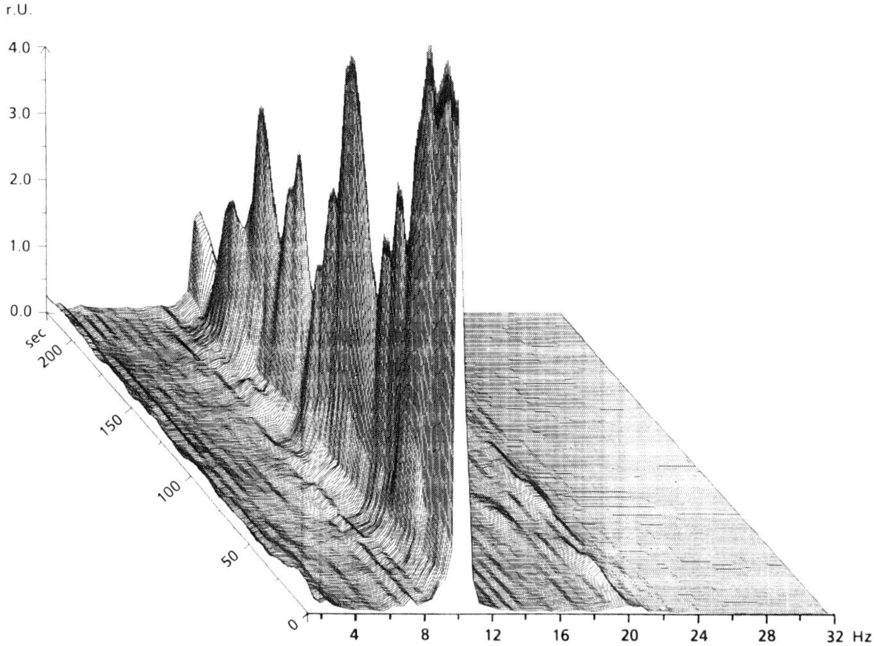

Fig. 1 Sliding spectra (see text) of ongoing EEG-activity (Oz - A1/A2). Prominent power (ordinate: relative units) lies in the alpha-range (abscissa: 8 - 12 Hz). A clear rhythmicity of the auto-power density with periods of 40 - 50 s and faster cycles of 20 s is evident.

sionally in the z-axis for each second. Main EEG-power lies in the alpha-range of 8 - 12 Hz. In this band the auto-power densities (resp. amplitudes) wax and wane with a periodicity of circa 40-50 s. The presence of additional faster cycles with approximately 20-s periods is clear.

3.1.2 Muscle Vibrations

The vibromyogram was Fourier transformed in the same way as described for the EEG. In the illustrated case of Fig.2 endogenous muscular vibrations of the right isometrically contracted biceps muscle (load of 30 N) were evaluated. The spectral pattern of such a gross mechanical muscle activity is composed of frequencies known from electrical brain activity. Dominant amplitudes as root mean square of power become evident in the alpha, beta1 and beta2 bands (8 - 12 Hz; 12.4 - 20 Hz; 20.4 - 32 Hz; z-axis of Fig.2). 4 - 5 periods of changes in amplitude (y-axis scaled in arbitrary units of acceleration) occur during the recording session of 4 minutes (x-axis). These amplitude cycles resemble a frequency of ca. 1.1 c/min.

3.1.3. Tremor

To obtain long-lasting recordings of oscillations of physiological finger tremor the subjects were lying in a supine position, the right arm was supported and an accelerometer was gripped between thumb and forefinger with maximal force (see methods). The autospectra show the widely described frequency dominance of tremor oscillations at about 10 Hz (circa 8 - 13 Hz in Fig.3). No 'higher' frequencies

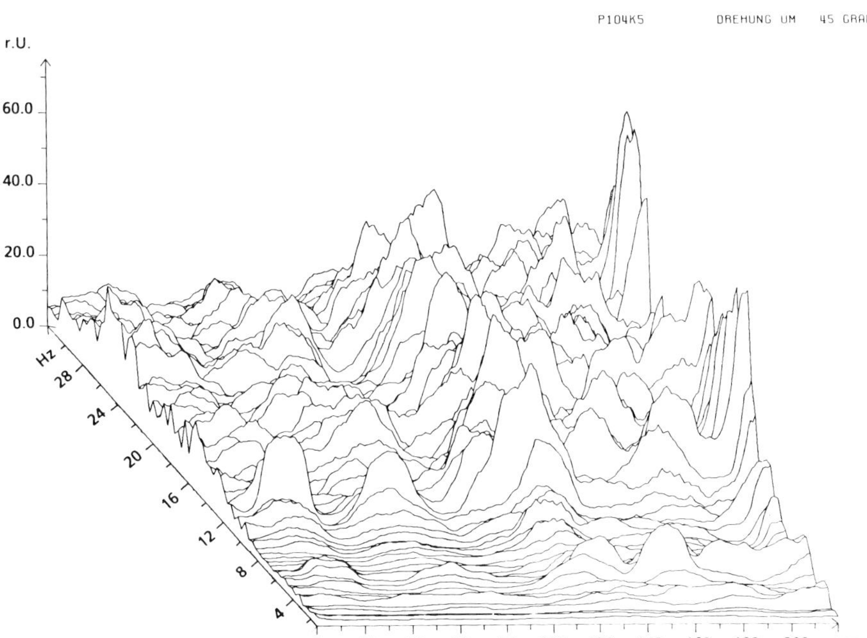

Fig. 2 Ca. 1-minute amplitude cycles of endogenous muscle vibrations of isometrically contracted right biceps muscle (load 30 N) revealed by 'running' spectral analysis. The vibration pattern shows frequencies within the EEG range (up to 32 Hz). During sustained (fatiguing) muscle contraction an increase of amplitude becomes evident. (From [10])

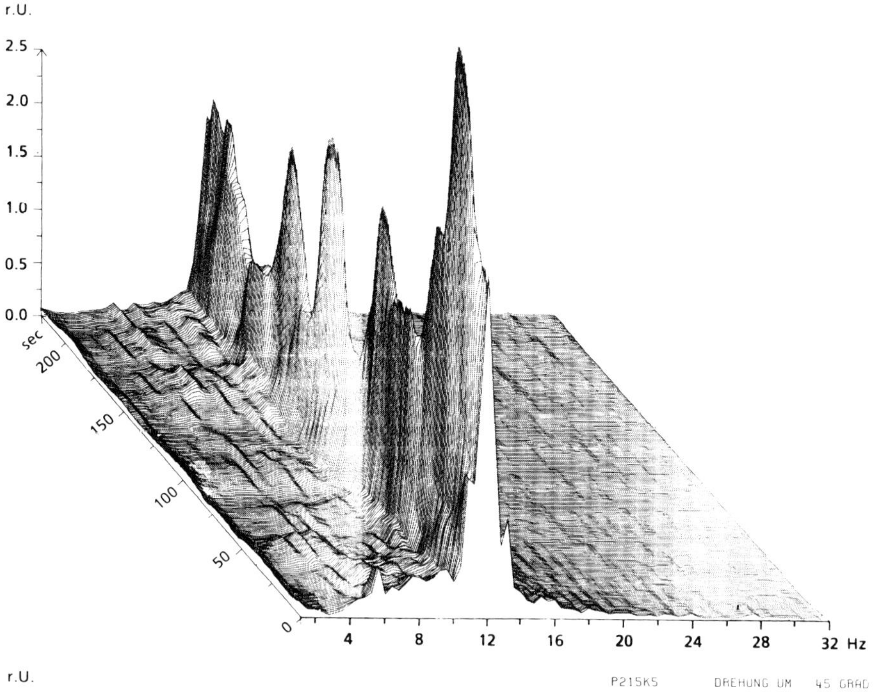

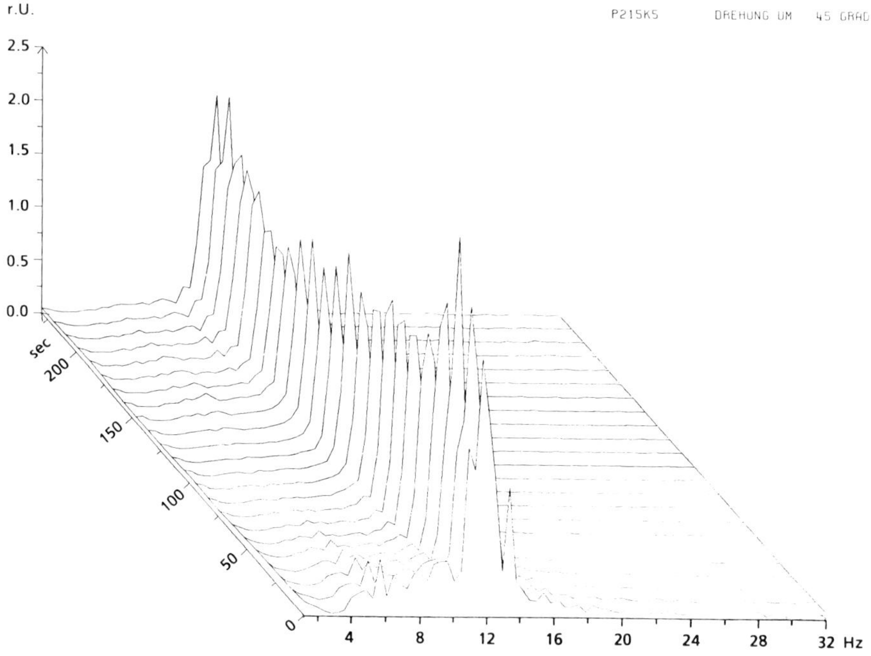

Fig. 3a Pseudo-3D plot of 'running' auto-power of spectrally analysed physiological finger tremor. Dominant power (y-axis: arbitrary units) lies in the range of 8 - 14 Hz (x-axis: 1.6 - 32 Hz). Note the rythmic variations in power densities with periods of circa 40 s during an analysis epoch of 4 minutes (z-axis: seconds). (From [10])
Fig. 3b Conventional FFT-analysis of the same data with successive analysis of 10-s segments does not disclose the clear rhythmicity shown in Fig 3a.

of 30 Hz up to a maximum of 100 Hz, which are a component of the muscular vibration pattern (see Fig.2), can be detected. As demonstrated for EEG and VMG, 'running' frequency analysis again reveals temporally well structured 'slow' oscillations and leads to this special type of 'tremor-periodogram' (TPG) as this rhythm imaging might be designated. Conventional successive frequency analysis of 10-s segments, resulting in 23 autospectra shown in Fig.3b does not disclose this rhythmicity.

3.2. 'Running' Coherence

3.2.1. EEG - VMG

As former correlation analyses of brief intervals of EEG and macro- or muscle-tremor did not show a stable interdependence [11], which might have been expected considering the comparable frequency ranges of these data, we hypothesized that there may exist a central neuronal network functioning as a common 'clock'. This should be responsible for transient short-lasting increases of synchronisation between brain waves (EEG), muscle vibrations (VMG) and corresponding coherence by driving cerebro-cortical and spino-segmental neuronal populations with a low but nevertheless temporally well-structured synchronisation rate. To confirm this hypothesis we computed continuous 'running' coherence values in 1-s steps according to the principle described for frequency analysis in Sect.1. We were able to monitor such a putative systematic change of the coupling strength between the EEG and VMG in all investigated subjects at rest and during sustained muscle contraction. A typical example from one subject is given in Fig.4. The 'running' coherence between the EEG of the left (dominant) motor cortex (C3) and the VMG of the isometrically contracted right biceps muscle (load of 30 N) was calculated. A cyclic variation of the band-related and integrated coherence is evident for all selected frequency bands (delta, theta, alpha, beta1, beta2). The cycle lengths vary from 20 - 70 s, rarely about 10 s, implying frequencies of 0.05 - 0.014 Hz or 0.1 Hz and indicating a temporal pattern in fluctuation of coupling strength. Normalized band coherence shows comparable values.

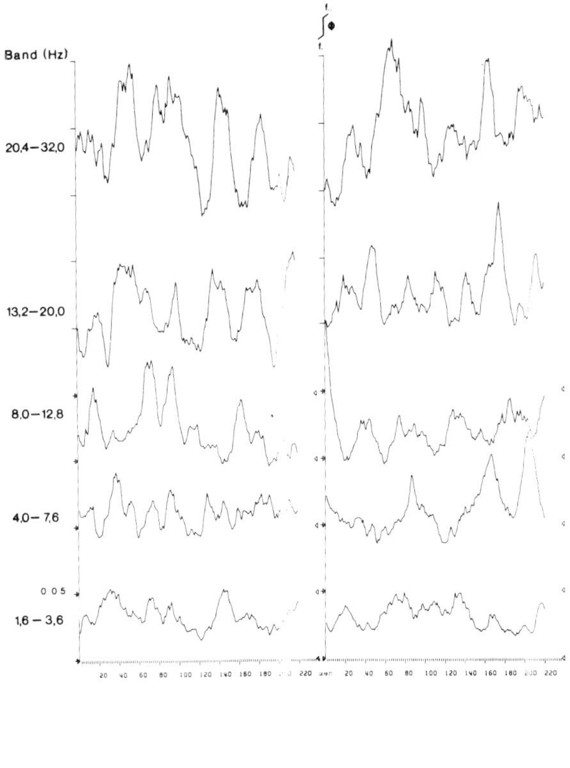

Fig. 4 Band-related and integrated 'running' coherence values from 2 typical subjects (EEG of C3; VMG of m. biceps, 30 N) according to 5 frequency bands plotted for each second of an epoch of 4 minutes. A cyclic variation of the coherence is evident (cycle length 20 - 70 s), suggesting transient changes in functional coupling strength of EEG and VMG activity as well as the existence of a central mechanism synchronising brain waves and muscle oscillations. (From [12])

3.2.2. EEG - EEG

Because we assumed that different brain areas show an increase of 'synergetic' cooperation during execution of a motor task compared to the 'resting' brain state, we computed the coherence function as a measure of the extent to which different EEG signals become synchronised, i.e. have common, time-locked frequency components. Homologous (motor) regions of the two hemispheres (C3-C4) and derivations within hemispheres (Fz-C3; Fz-C4; Oz-C3; Oz-C4) including an anterior-posterior montage (Fz-Oz) were investigated. Similar to the results described in Sect.3.2.1, the resting condition without any voluntary muscle contraction was compared with unilateral graded force development (of 10-40 N) by isometric contraction of the right forearm flexors. The initial data show that inter-hemispherical EEG-EEG coherence (left versus right motor cortex) changes in a manner parallel to the stepwise developed force level of, e.g., 20 up to 40 N as shown in Fig.5 (see above). In addition, the C3-C4 coherence increases the longer the (fatiguing) muscle contraction (of 240 s) is maintained. The higher the initial force level the steeper is the rise of coherence during the time course. Oscillations of this 'left-right' coherence with about 4 - 5 cycles per 220 s become evident as illustrated for the integrated coherence of the beta2 band (20.4 - 32 Hz; Fig.5).

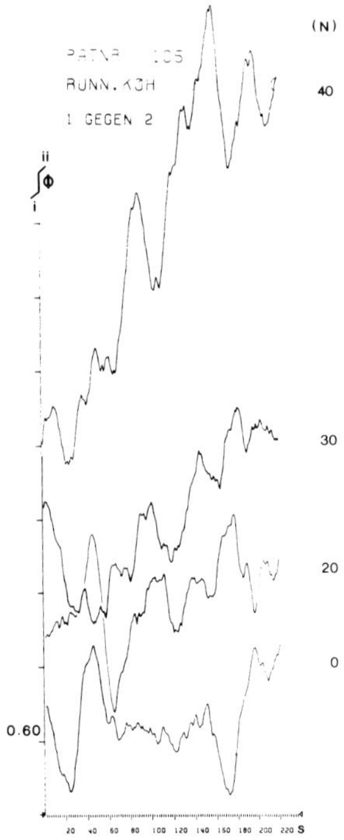

Fig. 5 The integral of the coherence values of the beta2 range (20.8 - 32 Hz) of the EEG recorded from left and right motor cortices (C3 - C4) are continuously displayed during isometric contraction of the right biceps muscle. Increasing development of force (20, 30, 40 N) showed an increase in interhemispherical coherence. During sustained muscle contraction at a given level of force a steep increase of the 'left-right' coherence of the motor areas can be observed. The steepness of rise depends on the initial load.

To verify time- and frequency-related alterations in EEG-coherence, the interhemispherical (C3-C4) coherence estimates of 77 adjacent individual frequencies spaced by 0.4 Hz steps were computed for a range of 1.6 - 32 Hz over an epoch of 220 s. Results obtained are shown in Fig.6a-c. The coherence at rest without voluntary muscle contraction (Fig.6a) is compared with the condition of activation of the motor system. In the case presented, the right biceps muscle had to maintain a given force level of 10 N (Fig. 6b+c). At rest the coherence shows an irregular behavior being stationary rather than oscillatory, even if some idea of a periodic change of coherence in time might be suspected preferentially for the beta2 band (20.4 - 32 Hz). Furthermore, in this range the coherence exhibits a greater magnitude than for the lower range of 1.6-20 Hz (Fig.6a). During motor

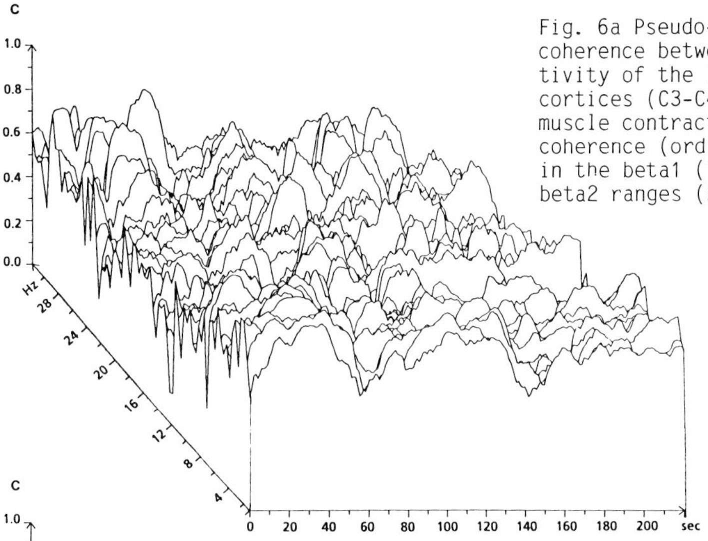

Fig. 6a Pseudo-3D plot of the running coherence between the ongoing EEG activity of the left and right motor cortices (C3-C4) without voluntary muscle contraction. Note the marked coherence (ordinate; C = coherence) in the beta1 (13.4 - 20.4 Hz) and beta2 ranges (20.8 - 32 Hz; z-axis).

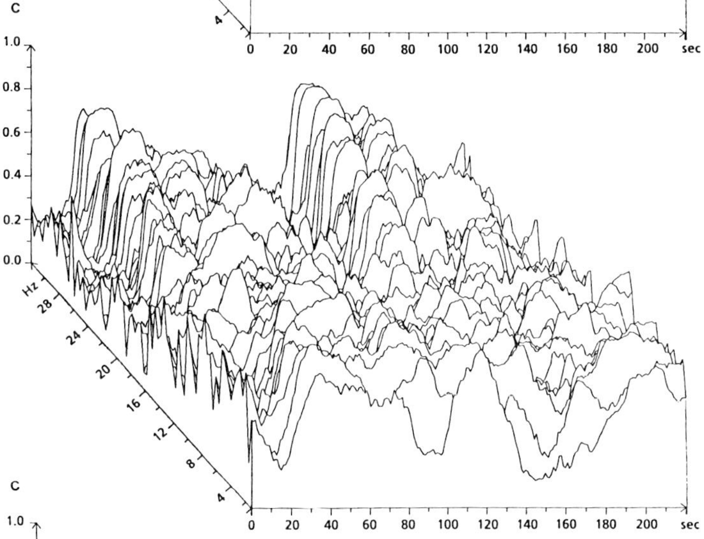

Fig. 6b During voluntary isometric contraction of the right biceps muscle (load: 10 N) an impressive oscillation (periods of circa 40 s) of the coherence (C) becomes evident, suggesting a higher temporal order of CNS-activity with a 'cyclic' change in synchronisation of left and right hemispheres.

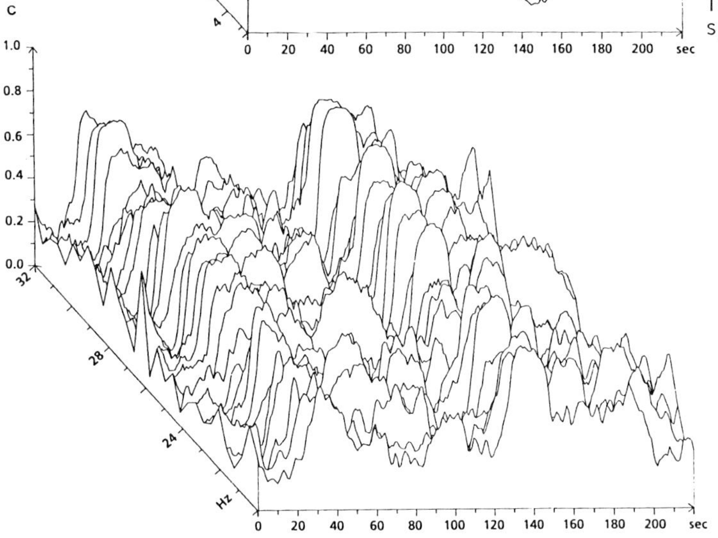

Fig. 6c Same results as shown in Fig. 6b, but z-axis is restricted to the beta2 range (20.4 - 32 Hz).

performance the coherence pattern develops an impressive temporal order and a clear transition from the 'chaotic' state (at rest) into a cyclic state occurs (Fig.6b + c). The coherence cycles show period lengths of about 40 s, are frequency- or frequency band-related and are accentuated in the beta2 range. These oscillations in EEG-coherence between homologous left and right motor cortices occurring just during performance of a motor task are finally emphasized in Fig.6c.

4. DISCUSSION

Coherence function is a measure of phase locking between two signals in the frequency domain and is considered as frequency-related covariance in mathematical terms (see methods). With respect to EEG analysis it quantifies synchrony of two EEG-curves or in the case of multi-electrode montage represents synchronisation of electrical activity recorded from different brain areas. A recent advance in scalp-topographic mapping of EEG coherence has been reported by RAPPELSBERGER et al. [13]. A high degree of synchronisation means a tight functional coupling of the recorded signals implying a large amount of cooperation or 'synergy' (in the context of Haken's concept [14]) between the various CNS parts generating the recordings as EEG, VMG or tremor. Thus we assume that high coherence values indicate a considerable negentropic order of the CNS state or, in terms of dynamic system theory [15,16], indicate a 'low-dimensional chaos'. In turn, loss of coherence seems to be the result of 'high-dimensional chaotic' neuronal behavior, resembling an increase in disorder in electrical (and mechanical) activity of the CNS and a transition to a state with higher entropy.

The approach of 'running' frequency and especially coherence computations in long term analysis describing the dynamical properties of CNS mechanisms enabled us to demonstrate that the human central nervous system does not hold the functional links of different systems and parts of its neural network at a constant level (Fig.4;6b+c). In contrast, it is apparently operating in an oscillating mode and there is a striking temporal order of cyclic change in the degree of coupling, e.g. between cortical and spinal neuronal populations (EEG-VMG coherence, Fig.4) or between different intra- or inter-hemispherical cortical areas (EEG-EEG, C3-C4 coherence, Fig.5,6b+c) with period lengths ranging from 20 s to 70 s, most frequently of 40 s (see results). As similar periods in amplitude (or power) cycles of EEG, VMG and tremor were discerned by running spectral analysis (Figs. 1-3), the stabilisation of such ordered transients of activity and synergy seems to be an important intrinsic property of the CNS which might be necessary for information processing by establishing a temporal meta-order. This structures the complex functional interplay of multiple parallel processing parts of the CNS. As one principal mechanism underlying the dynamics of the described circa 40-s biorhythms we propose the working hypothesis that a central oscillating mechanism such as the 'common brainstem system' (mainly formatio reticularis as arousal system; see [17]) and other subcortical structures (e.g. thalamus) may act as an ascending and descending synchronising clock, which is embedded in various loops and circuits. This may drive simultaneously and at a low frequency spinal and cortical neuronal assemblies, which function as coupled oscillators with their own rhythms [18], thus causing the demonstrated temporal pattern of EEG-EEG and EEG-VMG coherence. An intermittent fading out of phase would result in a transient decrease of coherence. Periodic oscillations in the brainstem arousal system(s) may be responsible for the amplitude cycles of VMG, tremor and EEG. A similar mechanism was discussed by KLEITMAN [4] for the 90-min cycles of vigilance and 'brain rest activity'. The circa 20-40 s EEG rhythm in amplitude (or power) was recently confirmed by LIPS et al. [19]. A further relation of the reported cycles to the autonomic nervous system seems to be feasible, since autonomic rhythms lie in the same frequency range (0.025 Hz;[1,2]). It is reasonable to suppose that the paced variation of coupling strength and synchronisation of neuronal assemblies is mediated via different fiber systems. This consideration is in line with the model described by THATCHER et al. in 1986 [9], explaining EEG coherence as a functional counterpart of the neuroanatomically clarified subcortical and cortical connectivity, making a distinction - based on

BRAITENBERG's experiments [20] - between long- and short-range fibered cells of types I and II. ELBERT and ROCKSTROH recently developed a comparable model with respect to scalp recorded DC-shifts of the human EEG [21]. Spontaneous low oscillations of the cortical DC-potential with 0.5 - 2c/min similar to those demonstrated for 'running' power and coherence in this study were reported in animal experiments by ALADJALOVA [22]. Nevertheless, whether or not the 'running' coherence changes in spatial coupling order of multiple EEG-recordings are related to temporal changes of electrical phenomena of single EEG-time series such as spontaneous ongoing and internal or external evoked potential- and/or frequency-changes (known as DC-shift, endogenous, event-related and evoked potentials) remains an open question. Our data so far suggest that EEG coherence is not solely increased by sensory input as observed by BASAR [18] but also during motor output (Fig.5;6b-c). Generally speaking, the receiving and delivering of information alters the coherence level and, with respect to the latter, the operation mode of the brain. This switches from a rather stationary state at rest (Fig.5;6a) to a periodic one (Fig.5;6b,c) during motor performance implying a capacity of the CNS to tighten and loosen the frequency-related coupling (of information processing) between distant neural generators, i.e. in this paradigm between the two brain hemispheres implicating ordered dynamics in functional dominance of one hemisphere. One is tempted to speculate that performance of a maintained motor action accompanied by increasing effort leads to an augmentation of cooperation between the dominant (C3) and non-dominant hemispheres (C4), (compare rise of coherence in Fig.5 during the time course of 220 s; subject was right-handed). It is remarkable that an increase of cycling coherence seems to correspond to a reported awareness of effort and will to fulfil the strain task (Fig.5,6). The use of 'running' coherence for investigating physiological correlates of such higher mental functions (see e.g. [23]) has to be proven by further controlled studies. Because our data so far show a task-dependent change in temporal pattern of cofunction of different brain areas, we consider the 'real time' analysis of the brain's 'synergy' by 'running' coherence computation to be a promising holistic approach to studying inherent (order) properties of the CNS with respect to psychophysiological issues [21,23], which cannot be solved completely by waveform analysis in a wider sense or by applying the theory of non-linear dynamics [15, 16] to EEG analysis. This latter is rather 'topistic' and commonly restricted to one single EEG channel, telling us something about order of function but not about 'meta-order' of cofunction. Thus a combined frequency, potential, 'dimensionality' and 'running' coherence analysis seems to be of special heuristic value. A study investigating a postulated relationship between coherence and attractor characteristics is in progress. We assume, that an increase in coherence may be combined with a decrease in dimension since BABLOYANTZ and DESTEXHE described a transition to 'low dimensional chaos' during epileptic EEG activity [24] and CONRAD for entrainment studies [25]. Both phenomena were coupled with increased synchronisation, which may be related to an expected rise of coherence estimates. With respect to the concept of 'dynamic diseases' [26,27] the introduction of the 'running' analysis methods discussed here, revealing the demonstrated periodograms, proves to be a promising approach to uncover temporal disorder of neurofunctional organisation and interaction. Further experiments may yield more detailed information about the functional significance in clinical application. The initial results of this longer term effort are encouraging.

5. SUMMARY

In man, three different time series such as Electroencephalogram, Vibromyogram and tremor were investigated by introduced 'running' frequency and coherence analysis. Coherence was calculated between EEG-EEG and EEG-VMG. Rhythmic variation in amplitude (or power) and coherence with circa 40-s cycles is demonstrated. The results suggest that the CNS periodically alters the level of activity and degree of 'synergy' between different (parallel processing) structures and systems rather than maintaining a steady state. A central oscillating mechanism (common brainstem system) is considered as being responsible for this well-structured temporal pattern. 'Running' frequency and coherence analysis provides a 'real time' imaging of the dynamics in temporal order and disorder of CNS function and spatio-temporal 'meta-order' of cofunction.

6. REFERENCES

1. H.P. Koepchen, S.M. Hilton, A. Trzebski: Central Interaction Between Respiratory and Cardiovascular Control Systems (Springer, Berlin Heidelberg 1980)
2. K.M. Einhäupl, C. Garner, U. Dirnagl, G. Schmieder, P. Schmiedek, G. Kufner, J. Rieder: In Intracranial Pressure VI, ed. by J.D. Miller (Springer, Berlin, Heidelberg) in press
3. C. Manseau, R.J. Broughton: J. Psychophysiol. 21, 265 (1984)
4. N. Kleitman: In Sleep: Physiology and Pathology, ed. by A. Kales (Lippincott, Philadelphia 1969) p.335.
5. M. Keidel, W.-D. Keidel: Functional Neurology, in press
6. M. Keidel, W.-D. Keidel: Electroenceph. Clin. Neurophysiol. 61, 126 (1985)
7. H.H. Jasper: Electroenceph. Clin. Neurophysiol. 10, 371 (1958)
8. W.-D. Keidel: In Handbook of Sensory Physiology, Vol. 5, The Auditory System-Part 3. Clinical and Special Topics, ed. by W.-D. Keidel and W. Neff (Springer, Berlin, Heidelberg 1976) p.105
9. R.W. Thatcher, P.J. Krause, M. Hrybyk: Electroenceph. Clin. Neurophysiol. 64, 123 (1986)
10. M. Keidel, W.-D. Keidel, W.S. Tirsch, S.J. Pöppl: In Proceedings Volume (Meeting of the German Neurological Society, Aachen 1986) ed by K. Poeck, H. Hacke (Springer, Berlin, Heidelberg) in press
11. O. Lippold: The Origin of the Alpha Rhythm (Churchill Livingstone, Edinburgh, London 1973)
12. M. Keidel, W.-D. Keidel, W.S. Tirsch, S.J. Pöppl: In Proceedings Volume (Meeting of the European Society for Chronobiology, Marburg 1986) ed by G. Hildebrandt, in preparation
13. P. Rappelsberger, H. Pockberger, H. Petsche: EDV in Medizin und Biologie 17, 45 (1986)
14. H. Haken: Synergetics, An Introduction. Springer Ser. Syn., Vol.1 (Springer, Berlin, Heidelberg 1977)
15. A. Holden: Chaos (Manchester University Press, Manchester 1986)
16. H. G. Schuster: Deterministic Chaos (Physik Verlag, Weinheim 1984)
17. P. Langhorst, B. Schulz, M. Lambertz, G. Schulz, H. Camerer: In [1], p.30
18. E. Basar: In Synergetics of the Brain, ed. by E. Basar, H. Flohr, H. Haken, A.J. Mandell, Springer Ser. Syn., Vol.23 (Springer, Berlin, Heidelberg 1983) p.183
19. U. Lips, A. Schultz, I. Pichlmayr: abstr. (German EEG-society 1986), Electroenceph. Clin. Neurophysiol., in press
20. V. Braitenberg: In Architectonics of the Cerebral Cortex, ed. by M.A.B. Brazier and H. Petsche (Raven Press, New York 1978) p.443
21. Th. Elbert, B. Rockstroh: J. Psychophysiol., in press
22. N.A. Aladjalova: Nature 179, 957 (1957)
23. M. Keidel: Naturwissenschaften 70, 180 (1983)
24. A. Babloyantz, A. Destexhe: in press (1986)
25. M. Conrad: In [15], p.3
26. M.C. Mackey, L. Glass: Science 197, 287 (1977)
27. R. King, J.D. Barchas, B.A. Huberman: Proc. Natl. Acad. Sci. 81, 1244 (1984)

Central Rhythmicities in Motor Control and Its Perturbances

H.-J. Freund

Neurologische Universitätsklinik, Moorenstraße 5,
D-4000 Düsseldorf, Fed. Rep. of Germany

1. INTRODUCTION

There is one prominent and striking oscillatory feature in motor control, tremor. Tremor is an inevitable side effect of any muscle activity, although the physiological tremor accompanying any movement or muscle contraction is usually not perceived.
This article will be structured into 3 parts.
1. The discussion of some relevant properties of physiological tremor as it appears in normal subjects.
2. The changes of these characteristics of physiological tremor under pathological conditions, and
3. The relation of these oscillatory phenomena to some major principles in the temporal organization of motor behaviour.

2. MECHANISMS UNDERLYING PHYSIOLOGICAL TREMOR

A number of different factors have been recognized as the major determinants of physiological tremor: Rhythmic changes due to pulsatial blood flow, breathing, mechanically and neurally determined oscillations.
Mechanical oscillations are due to the resonant frequencies of the different body parts, they are therefore subject to experimental manipulation. Changes in inertia or stiffness of the limb are associated with changes in the resonant frequency, as documented by the shift of the peak in the corresponding power spectra.
With respect to neural synchronization two types of physiological tremor must be distinguished. The first is non-activated physiological tremor which is not associated with neural synchronization. There is not more than chance synchronization between the motor units /1/, /2/, /3/. In this condition tremor is produced by the unfused parts of the twitches of the motor units firing at different rates /4/. The frequency range of the power spectrum of tremor force corresponds to the range of firing rates between recruitment and fusion of the muscle fibres (8-30 Hz). The decay of the peak of the power spectrum towards higher frequencies reflects the properties of a second order damped system due to the fusion characteristics of the muscle fibres.
The second type of physiological tremor is enhanced physiological tremor. In this condition motor units become synchronized. Their synchronized activity generates muscle unit contractions that are suprathreshold for the spindle receptors that in turn excite motor units so that a servo-loop oscillation comes into play. The almost unfused muscle twitches produced at the lowest maintained firing rates around 8 Hz (onset firing rates) represent the most powerful input for the muscle spindles. If a few motor units become synchronized at these frequencies the muscle spindles become excited so that the reflex loop comes into play. This

may be one mechanical reason why whenever synchronization occurs it takes place at the onset firing rates of the motor units for the given muscle. In the case of pathological tremor, which is characterized by abnormally low peak frequencies, the muscle fibre contractions are not even partly fused but remain unfused, representing the strongest possible muscle spindle input. Whether this increase in gain of the peripheral reflex loop represents one factor in the development of the abnormally low peak frequencies of pathological tremor is an open question. Typical power spectra of two patients with essential tremor of different amplitude are shown in fig. 1.

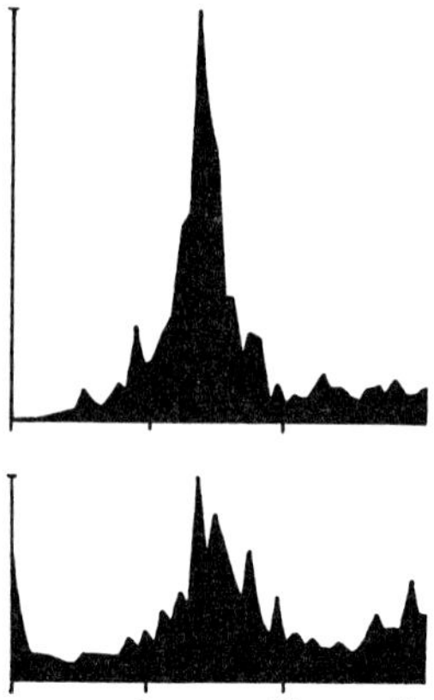

Fig. 1: Power spectra of two patients with essential tremor of different amplitude. Essential tremor is a familial variant of activated physiological tremor characterized by abnormally strong synchronization reflected by prominent peaks in the power spectra.

The interaction between the neural oscillation and the mechanically induced oscillations is complex. As long as the synchronization remains relatively weak, the repetition rate of this synchrony follows - within certain limits - the mechanically imposed alterations of inertia and stiffness: in enhanced physiological tremor the rate of synchronization is determined by the mechanical resonant frequency. Hence the mechanical resonance and neural synchronization are additive at the same frequency.

3. PATHOLOGICAL TREMOR

Pathological tremors are characterized by strong motor unit synchronization. This leads to a large amplitude tremor which becomes disturbing to the patient and interferes with movement. In addition to the increase in amplitude, pathological tremors are invariantly slower than physiological tremor (fig. 1B). The strong tremor oscillations are no longer subject to modification by comparable mechanical changes. Both the mechanical and the EMG peak remain unaltered. The lesions underlying pathological tremor are always in the central nervous system. They only appear if the pathological process damages one of the major extrapyramidal nuclei such as the basal ganglia or nuclei in the brainstem or in the cerebellum. Cooling, pharmacological influences and lesions of these structures can cause pathological tremors. Microelectrode recordings in

monkeys and in human patients during stereotactic operations have shown that these central structures show the same rhythmical burst activity of the neurones as those that can be recorded from the trembling muscles.
Although reflex loop oscillations are involved in the high gain of pathological tremor, the central oscillators do not depend on their integrity. This has been revealed by experiments where the trembling limbs were deafferented so that all the feedback signals from the muscle spindles were interrupted: tremor amplitude decreased significantly but still persisted at a larger than normal amplitude and lower than normal frequency, /5/; /6/; /7/.

4. The RELATIONSHIP between the OSCILLATORY PROPERTIES of TREMOR and INVARIANT PRINCIPLES of the TEMPORAL ORGANIZATION of MOTOR CONTROL

a) The frequency range of motor unit discharge rates

There are two remarkable features in the temporal organization of motor control. The first is the fact that movements are generally limited to a frequency range whose upper limit is demarcated by the peak frequency of tremor. This is different for the various body parts. For the hand, the frequency of physiological tremor lies in the 8-12 Hz range. Rapid alternating movements can only be executed up to these frequencies. The "movement range" is therefore confined to frequencies between 0 and 8-12 Hz.

A second consistent feature is that the firing range of the motor units is limited to the frequency range between 8 and 30 Hz for the hand and forearm muscles. Only during very fast contractions can the firing rates increase up to about 120 Hz but only for a few spikes. It is impossible to produce maintained firing rates below 6-8 Hz. Unlike the sensory systems, where firing rate modulation can be varied between 0 and the highest possible frequency, the motor neurones are limited to a remarkably narrow firing range. This firing range corresponds precisely to the range of partial fusion i.e. where the muscle fibre contractions start fusion at about 8 Hz and reach full tetanic fusion at about 30 Hz. The fusion properties represent a powerful force generating mechanism.

b) The frequency range of movement

If subjects are asked to move their fingers or hand with the largest possible amplitude but with slowly increasing alternation rates, the full amplitudes can only be maintained up to alternation rates around 2 Hz. At higher rates the amplitudes decrease continuously until the fastest movements are performed at approximately 8 Hz. The main reason for this decrease in amplitude is again mechanical in nature. The fastest possible single contractions require 50-80 msec for the time to peak of the muscle twitch. The time of the whole contraction is 350 msec. For a sequence of agonistic muscle contractions in one and antagonistic muscle contraction in the other direction the full amplitude can only be achieved when the antagonistic contraction does not start before the agonistic contraction terminates. Consequentially the amplitudes decrease by subtraction of counteractive forces as the antagonistic contractions become increasingly more overlapping. It appears that the mechanical requirements for force generation by the muscle are precisely inverse to those of the motor units.
Many rapid alternating movements employed in everyday motor skills

such as writing, shaving, hammering, typing or playing musical instruments lie at frequencies above 2 Hz which are already characterized by amplitude damping. This frequency range lies outside the frequency range of ocular pursuit so that these movements can not be sensory controlled, /8/9/. A remarkable property of their performance is that they follow an invariant time principle called isochrony, /10/. This isochrony implies that these movements require the same time irrespective of amplitude. These aspects can not be further discussed in the context of this treatise, but are more thoroughly discussed elsewhere /11/.
In summary, the simple involuntary oscillatory behaviour underlying tremor has a remarkable correspondence with frequency characteristics of invariant features of motor unit and muscle control. The major factors determining these frequency ranges are the mechanical properties of the muscle and muscle fibres. As illustrated in fig. 2, the movement and the firing range cover adjacent segments on the frequency domain. They overlap between 8-12 Hz, the range of peak frequencies of physiological tremor. The close matching between the temporal properties of the central nervous system and those of the contractile properties of the neuromuscular machinery represents a challenging issue for the understanding of such oscillatory systems. An intriguing aspect of the relationship between the time characteristics of tremor, motor unit and muscle activity is illustrated by the fact that if extrapyramidal lesions lead to the development of pathological tremor, the range of movements and the range of motor unit firing rates becomes abnormally low as well as that of rapid alternating movements.

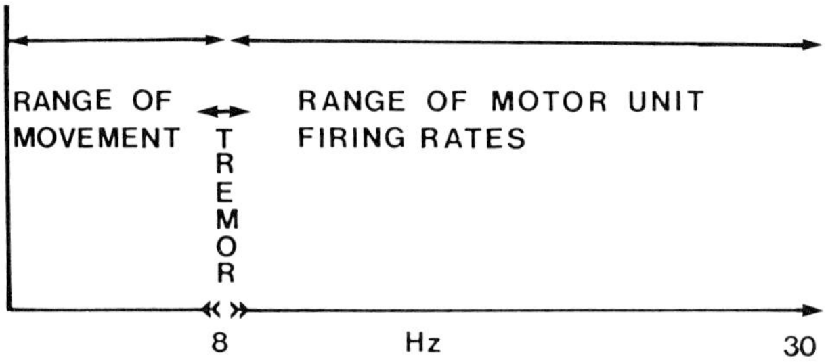

Fig. 2: Schematic illustration of the frequency ranges of motor unit firing rates and of movement. They cover adjacent segments on the frequency axis. The range of tremor peak frequencies lies precisely between these ranges.

1. H. Kranz, G. Baumgartner: Brain Res., 67, 324-329 (1974)
2. A. Taylor: J. Physiol. London, 162, 259-269 (1962)
3. V. Dietz, E. Bischofsberger, C. Wita, H.-J. Freund: Electroencephalogr. Clin. Neurophysiol. 40, 97-105 (1976)
4. J.H.J. Allum, V. Dietz, H.-J. Freund: J. Neurophysiol., 41, 557-571 (1978)
5. S. Gilman, D. Carr, J. Hollenberg: Brain, 99, 311-330 (1976)
6. C. Ohye, R. Bouchard, K. Larochelle, P. Bedard, R. Boucher, B. Raphy, L.J. Poirier: Exp. Brain Res., 10, 140-150 (1970)
7. C.N. Liu, W.W. Chambers: Acta Neurobiol. Exp., 31, 263-289 (1971)
8. H.-J. Freund: In The Oculomotor and Skeletalmotor Systems, ed. by H.-J. Freund, U. Büttner, B. Cohen, J. Noth, Progress in Brain Research, Vol. 64 (Elsevier Science Publishers B.V. (Biomedical Division)), pp. 287-294 (1986)
9. A. Leist, H,.-J. Freund, B. Cohen: Human Neurobiol., 5 (1986) in press
10. P. Viviani, C. Terzuolo: In Tutorials in Motor Behavior, ed. by G.C. Stelmach, J. Requin (Elsevier/North-Holland Amsterdam), pp. 525-533 (1980)
11. H.-J. Freund: Physiol. Rev., 63, 387-436 (1983)

Neurological Oscillations: Formulation of Mathematical Control Models and Applications to Clinical Syndromes

L. Stark

Neurology Unit, University of California, Berkeley, CA 94720, USA

1- INTRODUCTION

Oscillations are a closed mystery to the non-mathematical biologist. In this paper, we review the application of control theory to a number of different oscillatory mechanisms in neurology.

First, we deal with linear theory predicting occurrence of oscillatory behavior in the pupil reflex to light. This is then generalized to a root distribution criterion, gamma-B, for linear models of many different neurological systems. Sampled data behavior is present in complex movement control for limbs, head, and eyes; the resulting oscillations are square-waved. In addition, the cerebellum is suggested as the site of an adaptive mechanism continuously recalibrating gains of such systems.

The role of the muscle actuator and the load or plant is next shown to be important in shaping those peculiar eye oscillations known as as voluntary nystagmus. These, in turn, illuminate the sensory sensation of oscillopsia, an expression of the absence of space constancy. Nonlinear relaxation oscillator theory, of course, is neccessary for fuller explanation of the above quasi-linear oscillations.

However, the recent theory of strange attractors directs one's focus on the non-linear aspect of the oscillatory mechanism in the form of Poincare maps. These together with bifurcation diagrams and Lyapunov coefficients are shown to be adequate descriptions for feasible models for certain kinds of muscle tremor.

1-1 Clinical Applications

Throughout, we point out clinical applications after basic scientific analysis of these oscillations. The pupil oscillation has been used --- the relevant variable is the "cycle time" --- as a diagnostic quantity since Stark and Cornsweet (1958) analyzed Wybar's observations. Macrosaccadic oscillations are a sign of cerebellar failure, even though the brainstem, is generating Olympian saccades! Voluntary nystagmus continually bedevils the clinician, while oscillopsia as an important clinical sign must be distinguished from accommodative blur and migrainous shimmering.

2- PUPILLARY OSCILLATIONS

The classical anaylysis of the pupil as a control system indicates the difficulties in embedding a biological system in engineering terms. A feedback control system model is developed to encompass the light regulator features of the pupil. Linearization of this system enables a dimensionless open loop gain to be calculated (Stark and Sherman 1957). This formulation is important since, without a dimensionless gain, stability of the pupil system can be misinterpreted (Stegemann 1957). The transfer function equation, comprising a gain, a time delay, and a third order lag, approximates the Bode diagram data (Stark 1959; Sun et al. 1979; Varju 1964, Van der Tweel and Van der Gon 1959). It accounts for the neuromuscular plant dynamics that are frequently limiting, but omits subtler features such as low-frequency retinal adaption and various noise processes. Also, nonlinearities present in great variety in the pupil reflex to light are eliminated in this linearized approach.

The ability of the pupil transfer function to predict entirely different behaviors of the pupil--- high gain oscillations--- was of timely significance. Oscillations are almost always caused by abnormal function of a feedback control system, and an explanation in quantitative terms is essential. Thus, the quantitative prediction of the pupil high-gain oscillation represented an early contribution to mathematical biology (Stark 1959a, b). This theoretical and experimental success helped to convince biologists that the application of engineering principles of control and communication, named "cybernetics" by Norbert Wiener (1948) was possible in the biomedical world. A different display of amplitude-phase data, the Nyquist diagram, has gain, modulus length, as a function of phase angle; note that the polar plot has frequency only as an implicit function (figure 1, left). The Nyquist criterion for stability (figure 1, right) indicates how the high-gain operating condition transforms the pupil regulator for light into an unstable oscillating system (Stark 1959a, b; Stark and Cornsweet 1958; Stark and Baker 1959).

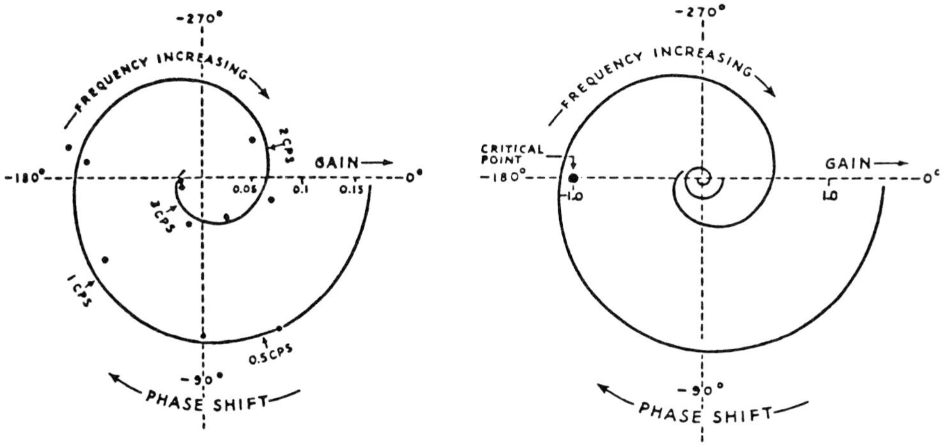

Figure 1 (left). Nyquist Diagram Of Pupil Response: vector plot of gain and phase shift; scale of modulus shown; and a few frequencies indicated; curve is derived from fitted lines from gain and phase frequency-response graphs, while points are experimental. (Stark and Sherman 1957)
Figure 1 (right). Nyquist Stability Criterion: Compare plot of unstable (large, outer curve) to stable (small inner curve) servosystem. Curve of stable system lies between Nyquist critical point and origin, indicating stability. Conversely, curve of unstable system encloses critical point, indicating instability. Critical point is that point in the graphical plot of open loop transfer function that represents gain of 1 at phase lag of 180 degrees. Since no frequency-dependent parameters have changed, 180 degree phase crossover frequency of high gain and low gain systems are identical. (Stark and Baker 1959)

The frequency of this oscillation is predicted by the 180 degree phase-crossover frequency of the normal pupil. An even more stringent test was carried out by using drugs to lower the bandwidth of the pupil transfer function. When the drugged pupil was made to oscillate using the high-gain operating condition, the lower frequency of oscillation was predicted by the lower 180 degree phase-crossover frequency of the drugged pupil (Stark and Baker 1959). The high-gain experimental operating condition was generalized by electronic means by Stark (1962) and was used for a number of other biological and neurological control systems (Stark 1968) (figure 2).

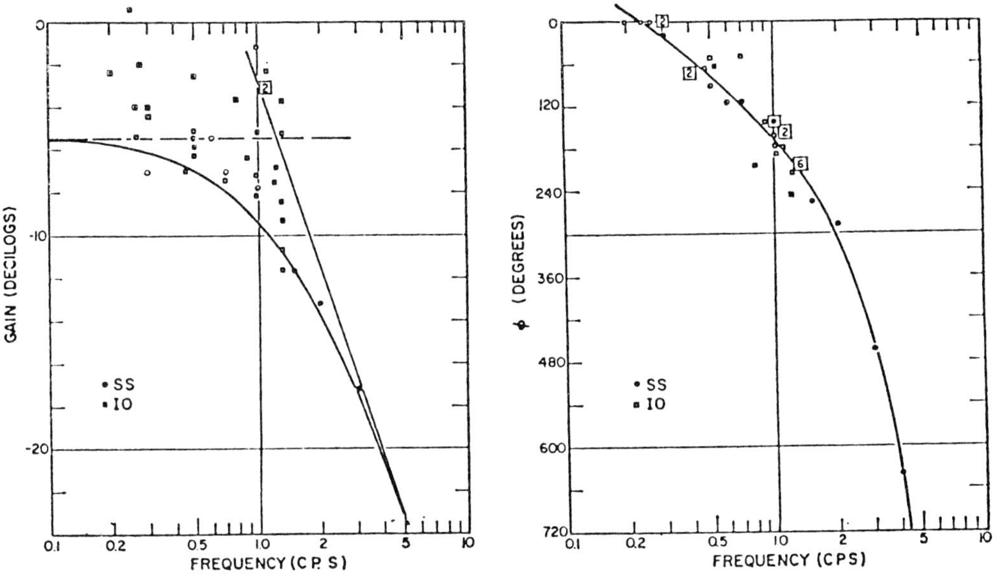

Figure 2 Frequency Characteristics as Bode plot of both high-gain instability-oscillation experiments (squares) and driven response experiments (filled circles). Heavy solid lines are empirical fits to steady experiments; dashed and thin continuous lines are asymptotes. Numerals indicate number of different experiments whose values fell too closely together to be plotted separately. (Stark 1962)

3- GAMMA-B: A ROOT DISTRIBUTION CRITERION

3-1 Introduction

Techniques of modeling and simulation are discussed as they relate to bioengineering systems. An Inners Criterion for checking the validity of a model is proposed to determine if its roots lie within a certain 'biologically realistic' region B, in the complex plane. This region was determined by a careful study of the roots of linearized models for a large variety of neuromuscular systems. Several algorithmic methods based on the "Jury Inners Test" are developed which calculate whether the model roots lie within the desired region, thereby circumventing tedious simulation on an unrealistic model with roots lying far outside this region.

Extensive simulations of unstable or biologically unrealistic models of neuromuscular systems may be avoided if a criterion can be developed to test the reasonableness of a proposed model. It is desirable therefore, to develop a generalized criterion, along with a computationally simple alogarithm to test it, that could be applied as a preliminary check on any such proposed model. The Inners criterion proposed here provides a simple preliminary check that indicates the validity or biological realism of the given neuromuscular model before extensive simulations of the model are carried out. For the class of neuromuscular systems studied, a region, gamma-B, in the complex plane has been proposed in which the roots of a linearized model shall lie: it is based on the physiological data as well as study of several previous models. The double convex lenticular shape of gamma-B is not sacrosanct: it is possible to define other equally valid boundaries to this approximate region. A main advantage of using this particular double convex shape lies in the simplicity of the algorithm used to check the criterion that all roots of a proposed model lie within gamma-B in this complex plane.

An attempt is made to compare the conditions for the general error-optimality of linear systems developed by Kalman with the conditions for feasibility of linear models of neuromuscular and physiological control systems.

Models of three actual physiological systems are tested for both the above criteria. Theoretical analysis presented here shows that there are no simple relationships between the two sets of conditions. Analysis carried out on the physiological systems models suggests the need for a general set of conditions for other optimality criteria, such as time and energy minimization, similar to Kalman's condition for error minimization.

3-2 Gamma-B

Modeling of human neuromuscular systems and some of the other biological systems has generally been approached from an input-output formulation , i.e. systems models are constructed on the basis of their outputs to some particular types of input functions. These models are developed using the standard transfer-function approach or the state-space approach; they are often then used to predict the behavior of the system under various input conditions. The idea of developing a criterion that could be used to check the general validity of a model was discussed earlier by Clark, Jury, Krishnan and Stark (1975b). A criterion that was applicable to linear or linearized systems models was developed and it amounted to testing whether the poles of the system transfer function were within a particular region of the s-plane. This region was termed the gamma-B region (figure 3) and is a bilenticular region in the left half of the complex plane with its major axis parallel to the imaginary axis; a simple test using the Inners method was developed for testing whether all the poles of the model transfer function fell within this gamma-B region.

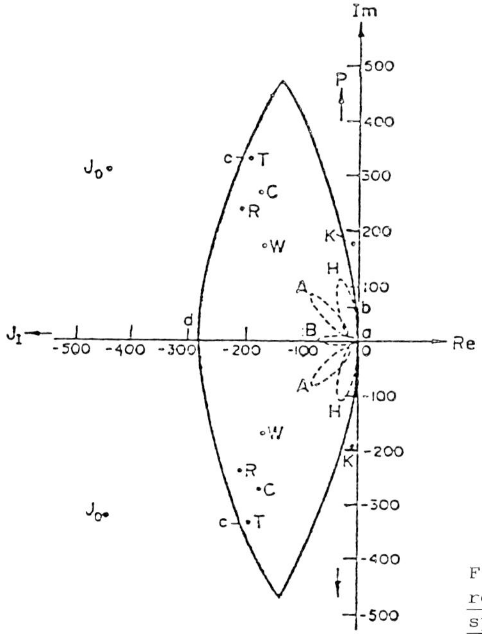

Figure 3 Gamma-B region within which lie roots of models for most neuromuscular systems (Clark, Krishnan and Stark 1975c)

3-3 Three bases for Gamma-B

A subsequent paper (Clark, Krishnan and Stark 1975c) discussed the bases for a region applicable to neuromuscular models. The criteria for determining the boundaries of the gamma-B region were the following: (i) experimental evidence: a number of linear models which successfully described the behavior of visual neuromuscular systems were analysed to determine the location of their poles. It was found that the roots were within a small region in the left hand plane, and this region was incorporated into Gamma-B; (ii) physiological basis: the outer boundaries of Gamma-B were determined on the basis of physiological data. These data were used to determine the fastest time constant (real axis limit) and the highest periodicity (approach to imaginary axis) that are physiological and gamma-B was so constructed that models which had poles outside the physiological limits were also outside of gamma-B. The origin of the s-plane was included in gamma-B since physiological control systems often contain integrators; (iii) mathematical simplicity: the bilenticular shape was chosen purely on the basis of ease of computation; it represented the intersection of two circular regions. It was specifically noted that the shape of gamma-B should really be based on some other considerations that are biologically more significant.

3-4 Comparison of Gamma-B and Kalman Optimality

Krishnan, Jury and Stark (1982) next reexamined the gamma-B region again to test whether or not it possesses any general optimality properties, i.e.if a system has poles that fall within the gamma-B region in the s-plane, does it possess any general and easily recognizable optimality properties? This particular approach is inspired by the work of Kalman (1964), who tackled a similar problem for linear systems. We attempt here to apply Kalman's formulation to a general second-order system which satisfies the gamma-B criterion. We also test it with examples of real physiological system models that are known to satisfy the requirements of the gamma-B region and obey the restrictions of the class of systems considered by Kalman.

In order to graphically illustrate how the gamma-B conditions and the Kalman conditions compare with each other, we have plotted the gamma-B region and the Kalman optimality region in K1 - K2 space (figure 4). The regions are not plotted to scale because of the very wide disparity in numerical values, but the approximate shapes of the gamma-B and the Kalman optimality regions in the K1 - K2 space should provide some information about the comparability of the two regions.

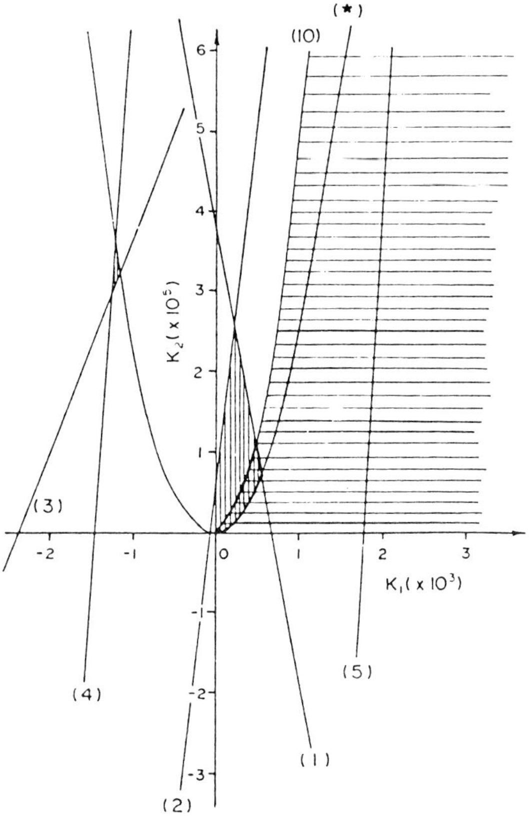

Figure 4 Comparison of the gamma-B and Kalman error-optimality conditions in the K1-K2 space.

K1 and K2 are the respective velocity and displacement feedback gains. For purposes of computation the two poles of the open-loop system have been assumed to be at -9.1 and -1.0, respectively. The gamma-B region in the K1-K2 space is shown as a vertically hatched region; the Kalman error-optimality region is shown as a horizontally hatched region. The boundary of the intersection of these two regions is shown as a thick continuous line. Because of the wide disparity of the numerical values, the figure is not to scale. (Krishnan, Jury & Stark 1982)

The 'overlap region' between the Kalman optimality region and the Gamma-B region, as indicated by thick boundary lines (figure 4), may at first glance seem small. Note, however, that Gamma-B is contrained to K1 less than or equal to 600 because of physiological frequencies set by realizable muscle accelerations. Thus the large expanse to the right of K1 = 600 satifies Kalman optimality, but is not at all available to biological systems. The small low-velocity region below the overlap region might well have been excluded from Gamma-B because of stability margin requirements. The admissible region for Gamma-B not in the Kalman region may indeed represent trade-off of time optimality for error and controller minimization. Thus we can see in this K1-K2 plane how biological optimality diverges from Kalman optimality.

4- SQUARE-WAVED OSCILLATIONS IN A SAMPLED-DATA CONTROL SYSTEM

Clinical recordings of patients with saccadic overshoot dysmetria (Selhorst, Stark, Ochs and Hoyt 1976) using photocell glasses (Stark, Vossius and Young, 1962) give an impression of a short series of sequentially diminishing square waves (Aschoff and Cohen 1971; Optican and Robinson 1980). In control system terms, square or flat-topped oscillations signify a discrete position-correcting mechanism, holding position during intersaccadic intervals; also, step discharge rate is precomputed along with saccade pulse duration, and that this rate does not change until the next corrective saccade occurs. More specifically, the system follows a discrete sampled data control rule (figure 5) and thus is in the 'open loop' mode between saccades (Young and Stark 1963a, b). These theoretical deductions are supported by EMG recordings in man and by microelectrode data in monkeys on the pulse-step envelope of discharges in ocular motor neuron during eye position changes.

Saccadic overshoot dysmetria in patients with cerebellar involvement may be related to the minor dysmetric errors recorded in normal subjects (figure 6, right panel). Occurrence of these minor undershoots and overshoots suggests that feed-forward gain normally fluctuates within narrow limits. The control system

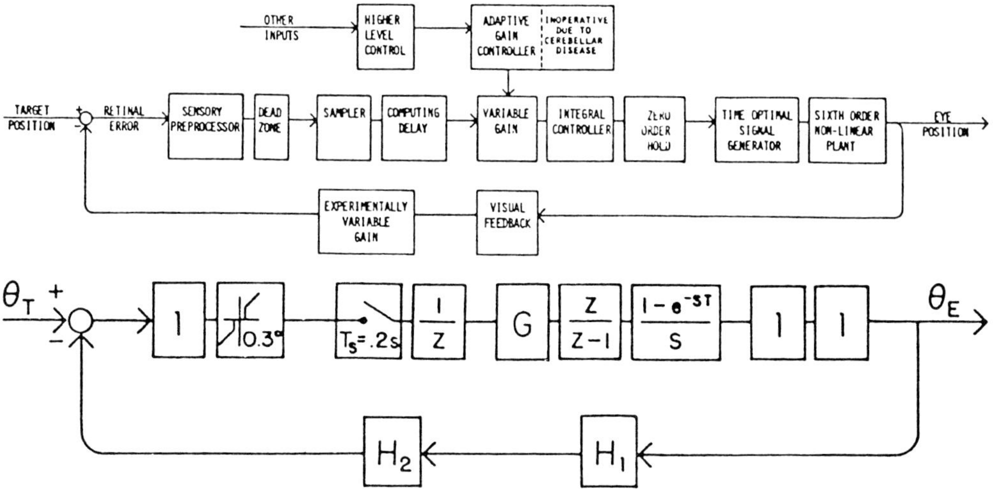

Figure 5 Sampled data control block diagram for human saccadic system (a) Descriptive model (b) Simplified quantitative model; Sensory preprocessor, time-optimal signal generator, and plant are all assumed to be unity. Adaptive gain controller is inoperative in patients with cerebellar disease. A nominal value of 0.2 sec is used for both sampling interval (Ts) and computing delay (1/z).

G represents fluctuating forward gain , uncontrolled in patients; H1 is normal external feedback gain, while H2 is experimentally variable external feedback gain. (Hsu, Krishnan and Stark 1976)

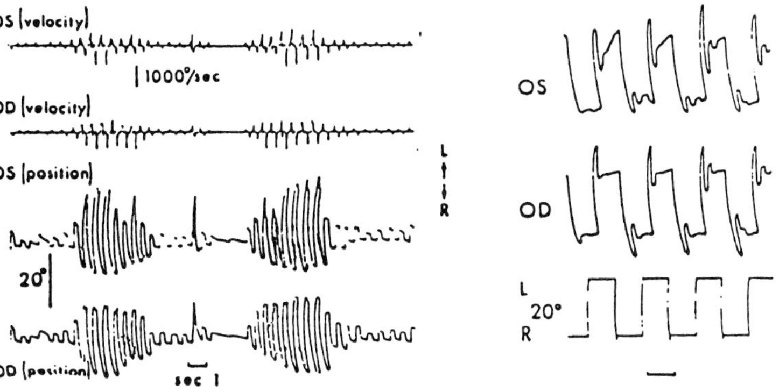

Figure 6 Clinical recordings of patient's eye movements of macrosaccadic oscillation (left panel) and saccadic overshoot dysmetria (right panel). An extreme dysmetria, macrosaccadic oscillation initially increased in amplitude (left panel) indicating that the gain in the feed-forward visual ocular motor path exceeded 2.0. After 3 to 6 cycles of oscillation, amplitude remained constant for several additional cycles. Amplitude then diminished, but the eye continued to overshoot the target, indicating a gain between 2.0 and 1.0 as in saccadic overshoot dysmetria. (Selhorst, Stark, Ochs, and Hoyt 1976a, b)

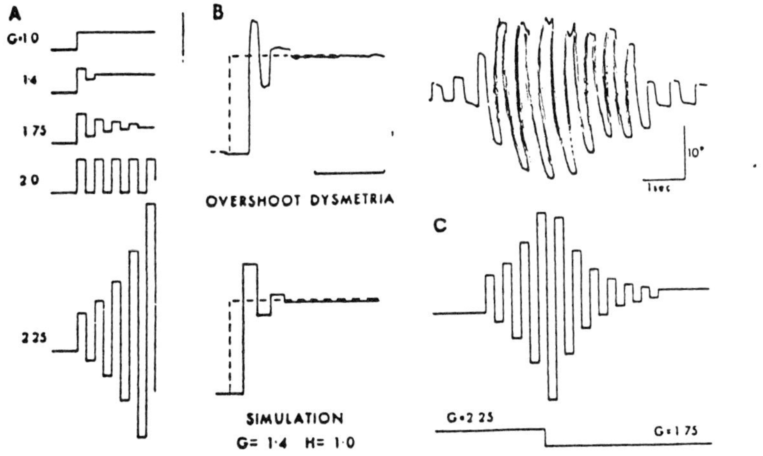

Figure 7. Computer simulations of sampled data model. (A) variable feed-forward gains; (B) simulation (lower) of overshoot dysmetria recording (upper); (C) simulation (lower) of monosaccadic oscillation (upper); note gain change switch below to account for spindle. (Selhorst, Stark, Ochs, Hoyt 1976a, b)

abnormality in saccadic overshoot dysmetria is an abnormally high gain in the brain's feed-forward path. We suggest that it is the cerebellum, the 'calibrator organ' that continuously modulates saccadic gain, although it may not lie directly in the visual ocular motor (feed-forward) path (Stark 1982). Thus rapid correction by saccades of off-foveal target position is possible, while longer-term adaptive modulation by the cerebellum provides parametric control over saccadic precision without interposing an additional delay in the saccadic system. Cerebellar gain control of VOR is perhaps similar.

Initial increase in gain occurred either suddenly after a large saccade or after a series of small oscillations of constant amplitude. Computer simulation approximated saccadic overshoot dysmetria (figure 7B) and macrosaccadic oscillation (figure 7C) using the variable gain forward loop model (fig. 5)

(Hsu, Krishnan, and Stark 1976). Macrosaccadic oscillation requires an intact visual feed-back loop; clinical evidence for this is its exacerbation by visually guided attempts at fixation or smooth pursuit. An elegant observation is that in the dark, the oscillation stops abruptly.

In the tradition of Hughlings Jackson, we emphasize that there are separable lower and higher levels of supranuclear ocular motor control acting in cerebellar macrosaccadic oscillation. At the lower level of control, gain in the feed-forward loop drifts away from its normal value; at the higher level, the cerebellum's adaptive role as a gain calibrator is suspended by acute loss of fuction of the vermis. Macrosaccadic oscillation results from gain fluctuation about the uncompensated high-gain value of 2.0. Similar control abnormality and the loss of vermis function also underlie the clinical phenomena of saccadic overshoot dysmetria.

5- VOLUNTARY NYSTAGMUS AND OSCILLOPSIA

5-1 Control models for eye movements

The motivation for presenting this section is to demonstrate control modelling in bioengineering. Current theories for eye movement control are most often embedded in such quantitive mathematical models that use simulation on digital computers as the preferred means to "crank" the model and to produce model behavioral output. Besides an explicit presentation of the theory, a model ensures consistency among the physical, physiological, anatomical components of the model. The behavior of the model can then be compared with known facts of eye movements and may even be used to discover new phenomena. Indeed, here we find clinical applications play a vital role in pure scientific research; often a puzzling clinical phenomenon can be used as a stringent clinical test of the model. The particular example this section provides us with was an exciting test for the reciprocal-innervation trajectory model that was developed over the years, first for arm movement (Stark 1968; Stark et al. 1961), and more recently for eye saccades by Cook and Stark (1967) and Clark and Stark (1974a; 1974b; 1974c).

The trajectory model is based upon time optimal control theory (Bellman 1957; Pontriagin et al. 1962; Clark and Stark 1975; Lehman and Stark 1979). It predicted higher-order controller signal switchings in the envelopes of nerve impulse firings that represent the neurological control signals for the eye saccade. These higher-order switchings account for the existence of dynamic overshoots in a majority of saccades- an important and successful prediction of the basic theory (Bahill, Clark and Stark, 1975a). It also demonstrated the mechanisms underlying the main sequence relationships studied experimentally since the early studies of Dodge in 1903. Simulation studies of the trajectory model clearly show that the saccade is not a "mechanically ballistic" movement, since muscular mechanical forces act during the entire saccadic trajectory. Contrariwise, a ballistic movement receives all of its inputs at the initiation of the trajectory, as is true for a baseball (Bahill and Stark 1979).

Neurological studies of movement are older than modern engineering control theory and are more intuitive than quantitative; they provide us with the concept of different levels in the Jacksonian sense of motor control. From this neurological point of view, the trajectory model is at the Jacksonian "lower level". A "higher level" control model for eye tracking movements using visual feedback was developed by Young and Stark (1963a, b). This sampled-data model (see preceding section and figure 5) captures important intermittent characteristics of saccades. After the neuronal signals for a saccade are preprogrammed, these signals are ordinarily not altered, and thus, we see the "neurologically ballistic" saccade eventuated. It may be helpful to use the term "neurologically ballistic" to clearly specify the intuitive understanding that neurophysiologists and neurologists have of the behavior results of this intermittant discontinuous control function. Finally, at the "highest level" of control, one might mention the scanpath model for visual recognition that incorporates saccadic movements along with sensory subfeatures as the internal components of memory traces of complex visual objects (Noton and Stark 1971). These "highest level" models, unfortunately, have not yet developed to the quantitative precision of the "higher level" sampled data model or the "lower level" trajectory model. They do, however, illustrate the role of multi-level control and of the necessarily different levels of models for different levels of control.

Those familiar with models in current scientific epistemology realize that models are not "absolutely true and forever". They are rather a tool for thinking and especially for suggesting new experiments (Stark 1977). Indeed, Wilkie has proposed that there is an optimal lifetime for a model or theory--- if too short, the model does not become well enough known to be useful; if too long the model has not succeeded in generating enough new experiments to require further modification and change. Thus, models are not put forward as arrogant or presumptuous final statements, but rather as entry vehicles to explore further and to expand our knowledge in their particular area.

5-2 Modelling the closely spaced saccades in voluntary nystagmus

In simulating voluntary nystagmus, we used the reciprocal innervation model of extraocular muscles, globe dynamics, and pulse-step innervation. The model translates a sequential train of pulse-step innervations into a sequential train of alternating saccades so constructed that the initial amplitudes (figure 8) produced velocities corresponding to representative peak velocities from our subjects' voluntary nystagmus traces.

Spacing between the saccades in the model was gradually collapsed by truncating the step portions of the controller signals. Behavior of these simulated trains of saccades (figure 8) was examined in terms of the acceleration time functions. As the pulse signals occurred closer together, the deceleration phase of one saccade approached the acceleration phase of the next, until close packing of these pulse signals produced superposition of successive decelerations and accelerations. At this point, the model reached "synchronization" frequency. At this frequency, saccades were overlapped and saccadic amplitudes truncated; peak accelerations, being superimposed, had values in excess of those for normal main sequence saccades (Figure 9).

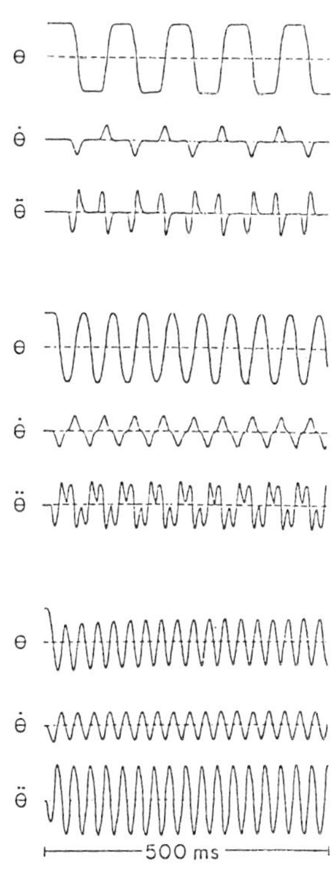

Figure 8. Simulation Studies:
Upper three traces show position, velocity and acceleration of simulated successive closely spaced, but not overlapping, saccades with 1 degree amplitude, 88 degrees/sec peak velocity and 11,300 degrees/sec/sec peak acceleration.
Middle three traces represent compression of successive saccades, but still without overlapping or amplitude attenuation. Peak velocity and peak acceleration values remain the same. Note absence of intersaccadic interval and also two distinct acceleration phases for each saccade.
Bottom three traces show further compression of successive alternating saccades to produce overlapping saccades and attenuation of saccadic amplitude to 0.66 degrees. Peak velocity remains approximately same value in center of saccade trajectory. Deceleratory phase synchronous with following acceleratory phase produces large summation acceleration of 17,000 degrees/sec/sec. (Stark, Hoyt, Cuiffreda, Kenyon and Hsu; 1980)

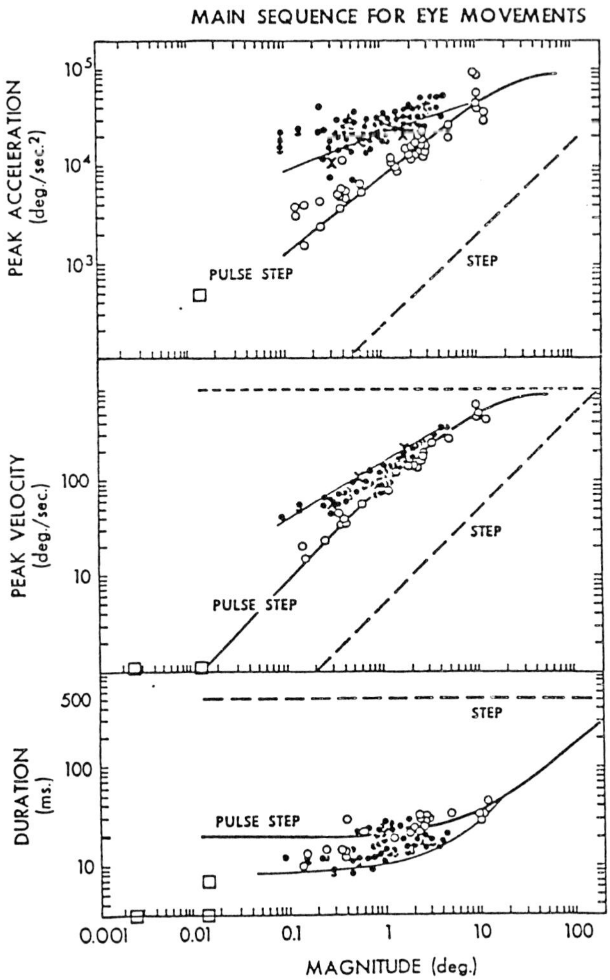

Figure 9. Main sequence of acceleration, velocity, and duration as functions of amplitude. Solid lines and x's represent simulation values for pulse-step controller and dashed lines values for step-controller. Refixation tracking saccades (open circles) of our subjects fit pulse-step controller lines, demonstrating normal controller signals, eye muscle contraction forces and patterns, and eyeball dynamics. Voluntary nystagmus saccades (solid circles) are clearly related to saccadic pulse-step controller lines, rather than to step-controller line for slower vergence and glissadic eye movements. Minor deviations with larger velocities and accelerations and shorter durations are understandable in terms of amplitude truncation produced by rapid succession of next alternating saccades seen in these high-frequency voluntary nystagmus saccadic trains and verified by simulations as in Figure 8. Peak velocities and accelerations of the saccades of voluntary nystagmus are somewhat higher and the durations somewhat shorter than normal main sequence values, suggesting that succession of alternating saccades is so rapid that full amplitude of saccades is not achieved. Thus, peak velocities found are appropriate for larger saccades than occur and are larger than normal for saccadic amplitudes measured. Also note six square boxes in small magnitude region of graphs. The two leftward boxes represent amplitude, duration, and velocity for physiological microtremor. The four rightward boxes are shifted to estimate unattenuated amplitude when fitted to main sequence velocity and acceleration curves for pulse-step control. (Stark, Hoyt, Ciuffreda, Kenyon and Hsu 1980)

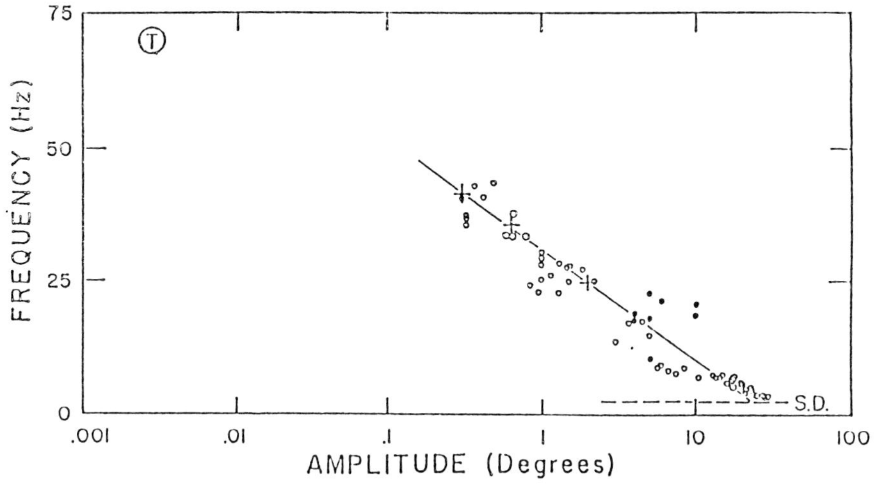

Figure 10. Frequency-amplitude diagram for voluntary nystagmus. Open circles are values derived by us from our subjects. Filled circles are data from literature. Crosses show results of simulations. Lowest frequency approaches 2.5 Hz sampled data frequency (S.D.). At high frequency region, point "T" represents the 0.0027 degree amplitude of 70 Hz physiological microtremor. Main sequence position of the microtremor values supports our novel suggestion that this microtremor is saccadic. Frequency-amplitude plot is determined both by dynamic and control characteristics of saccades as diagrammed on main sequence and also by overlapping of voluntary nystagmus saccades until synchronization and summation of successive acceleratory phases occurs (Shults, Stark, Hoyt and Ochs; 1977)

Peak velocity, because it occurs in mid-trajectory, is not altered by this close packing process. At synchronization frequency in our model, the data plots for peak acceleration, peak velocity, and duration closely fit plots from the parallel oculographic data of our subject's voluntary nystagmus. Also, at synchronization frequency, simulated voluntary nystagmus displayed the smooth pendular form documented in our oculographic recording and so often remarked upon by other investigators. For each amplitude, synchronization of the models' alternating opposed saccades (with superposition of acceleration phases) also determined a particular frequency. The frequency-amplitude relationship of the model nicely fits the frequency-amplitude relationship found in our oculographic recordings (figure 10).

Before starting these present oculographic and computer simulation studies, we knew that voluntary nystagmus is saccadic (Shults et al. 1977). The motor definition of saccades rests on the very high velocity of these extraordinary movements. All saccades--- schematic, refixational, nystagmic, corrective, and microfixational--- share the same defining velocity-amplitude relationship studied since the time of Dodge (1903).

An apparent discrepancy in the velocities of voluntary saccades is that they lie above the normal Main Sequence velocity amplitude relationship (figure 9). With our high resolution recordings, we established this apparent discrepancy. By means of our simulation studies (figure 8), we showed it to be a consequence of truncation of amplitudes of voluntary nystagmus saccades, while velocities remain normal. These simulations demonstrated the mechanism for truncation, namely, overlapping of closly packed saccadic trajectories. Peak velocity, occurring in the middle of the trajectory, is unaffected by overlapping and truncation. According to the model, the width of the pulse envelope of neural firing is much less than the duration of these small saccades, thus, the high frequency bursts of motoneural activity are also unaffected by overlapping and truncation. An alternative explanation explored was that voluntary nystagmus subjects might have unusually strong, fast ocular muscles. However, parametric data of normal refixation saccades from our voluntary nystagmus subjects lie correctly on the Main Sequence curves (figure 9); this alternate hypothesis was discarded.

Synchronization of acceleration phases with the preceding deceleration phases provides qualitative explanation for one of the striking features of voluntary nystagmus, its pendular form. The resulting summation of acceleration phases provides a quantitative explanation for the increased acceleration rates.

Synchronization frequency is analogous to the rhythmic rocking that a skilled driver produces by precisely timed shifting between first and reverse gears in working an automobile out of snow or sand. Apparently, subjects performing voluntary nystagmus pack saccades closely enough to obtain a similar synchronization.

This synchronization ties amplitude and frequency in an obligate relationship (figure 10). We have a wide enough range of amplitudes (0.4 to 30 degrees) and frequencies (42 to 3 Hz) from our six subjects and from data in the literature to confirm the validity and accuracy of the model. Our model of voluntary nystagmus successfully embodies both dynamics of normal saccades and close-packing to sychronization frequency of voluntary nystagmus saccades. Proposed neural models (Zee and Robinson 1979) should be tested to see if they can also predict these quantitative facts concerning voluntary nystagmus.

The wide range of amplitude and frequency evident in our measurements of voluntary nystagmus documents a clear and inverse relationship--- the smaller the amplitude, the higher the frequency. At the highest frequency, about 40 Hz, the nystagmus amplitude is less than 1/2 degree; at this level the shimmering of the eye is barely perceptible to the subject or to the clinician.

This voluntary ocular tremor at 40 Hz approaches the 50 to 80 Hz microtremor of 5 to 40 sec of arc recorded by optical lever techniques, during normal fixaton. We speculated that fixational microtremor lies at one extreme of the frequency-amplitude function for synchronized trains of alternating saccades. We calculated the velocity of the approximately sinusoidal 10 sec of arc, 70 Hz microtremor to be 1.2 degrees/sec, and the acceleration to be 50 degrees/sec/sec. By entering this data into the Main Sequence plot (figure 9), we found support for our speculation, since the values fitted reasonably at the low magnitude extreme of the curves identifying saccades. Simulation of the microtremor confirmed our analysis and demonstrated absence of mechanical limitations to oscillation at this high frequency and low amplitude.

5-3 Space Constancy; Corollary Discharge/Efferent Copy and Oscillopsia

Having dealt with the mechanical and motor control aspects of voluntary nystagmus, VN, (Stark, Hoyt, Ciuffreda, Keynon, and Hsu; 1980), we may now turn to its sensory consequences. First, is the outstanding symptom of oscillopsia, a shimmering, jiggling, illusory oscillating vision of the environment. Second, an after image placed on the retina of a VN subject yields no oscillopsia during VN (Nagle, Bridgeman and Stark, 1980). These observations have led to a series of experiments including sustained eye press (Stark and Bridgeman 1983) that clarify and explicate the sensory oscillation of oscillopsia (Stark 1985).

A block diagram (figure 11) is a useful device or tool to expose our understanding about a process and to coordinate different levels of information--- anatomical, behavioral (either physiological or psychological), and control theoretic. Lower and higher level feedforward motor controllers follow an error-processing sensory block and then control the eye muscle actuator and eyeball-orbit "plant" to produce output eye angle. Eye-angle information via the visual feedback path is differenced from target angle by a comparator. The higher level controller might include the sampled data mechanism of Young and Stark (1963a, 1963b) and be located in both frontal eye fields of the frontal cortex and superior colliculus. The superior colliculus has been shown, at least in part, to lie before the sampled-data operator (Sparks and Mays 1983) and also before the junction for corollary discharge (Guthrie, Porter and Sparks 1983). The lower level controller might include the brainstem pulse-shaping mechanism for time-optimal saccades (Clark and Stark 1975; Lehman and Stark 1979, 1983).

The highest level controller, the block named "Helmholtzian frame of reference comparator for space constancy", receives afferent signals (AFF) and efferent copy or corollary discharge (CD) information. When these angles are equal, the percept of space constancy is maintained. When these angles are almost equal, saccadic suppression (SS) and saccadic suppression of image displacement (SSID) provide tolerance for small errors, and space constancy is still maintained (Stark, Kong, Schwartz, Hendry and Bridgeman 1976). In an unstructured visual world with large errors, target or world motion occurs. With a structured visual field, visual capture of Matin (VCM) allows for visual space constancy, even for large discrepancies (Matin et al. 1982); Stark and Bridgeman (1983) suggested incomplete (90%) visual dominance; Shebilske (1976; and also personal communication, 1984) 50%, and Mittelstaedt (1985) exact summation of visual tilt and vestibular signals. A VN brainstem oscillator, accessible to 5% of the population, is a remarkable mechanism for producing "oscillopsia," a symptom of disruption of space constancy; VN controls eye movement after the corollary discharge has parted company from the efferent pathway.

It is hoped that the block diagram (figure 11) may serve as a framework for discussion and corrective modifications by workers in this evolving field of the rapid interaction of perceptual and motor processes.

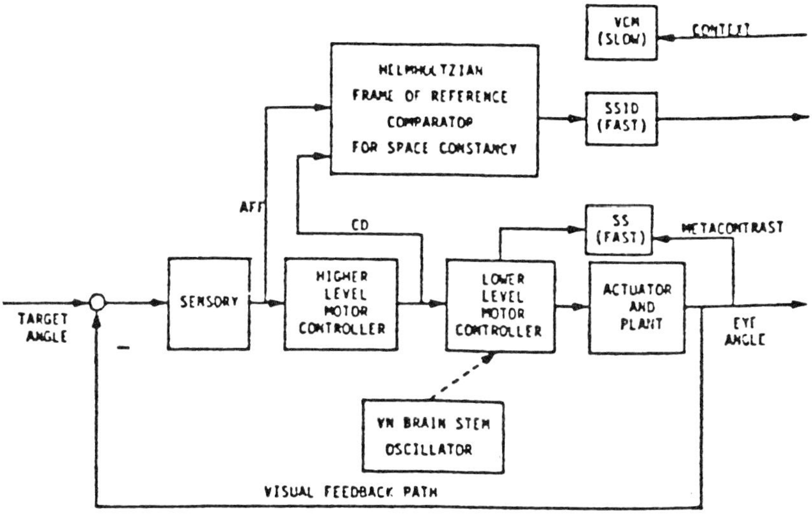

Figure 11. Hypothetical block diagram for space constancy

5-4 Classes of Space Constancy Experiments: Oscillopsia

Table 1 may serve to clarify the disparate protocol conditions and observations obtained in many space constancy experiments; it indicates the four different conditions of quantitative match of afferent and corollary discharge-efferent copy information.

6- NON-LINEAR OSCILLATIONS: STRANGE ATTRACTORS: POINCARE MAPS; BIFURCATION DIAGRAMS

Recently my colleages and I have applied strange attraction theory as a model for certain types of muscle tremor (Hannaford, Stark and Akumatsu 1985). A new model based on theory of non-linear dynamical systems was proposed for the intrinsic random or pseudo-random mechanism underlying certain types of muscular tremor. The active length-tension curve of the individual sarcomere, is a map from length to tension with an observed time delay between length change and resulting tension change. The series elastic passive length-tension relationship was assumed to instantaneously relate this tension change back to a change in length. The stability properties of this iterated interval (figure 12) map were investigated by means of computer simulation and computation of the Lyapunov exponent and the bifurcation tree (figure 13).

Table 1 Four Types of Space Consistancy Experiments: Match of Retinal Afferent (AFF) and Efferent (EFF) Signals (in different Protocol Conditions) and the resultant perceptions

Type	AFF REF	EFF COPY	Perception	Protocol Condition
I	+	+	No movement Space constancy	Normal saccade
II	+	0	Movement of target Movement of world Oscillopsia	Normal object motion Lightly and quickly jiggle eye Quick eyepress* Voluntary nystagmus or patients with deficient vestibular-ocular reflex
III	0	+	Movement of target Movement of world	Afterimage and saccade Slow eyepress** in restricted viewing Patients with fresh paralysis
IV	0	0	No movement Space constancy	Voluntary nystagmus with afterimage†

**Lightly and quickly jiggle eye; no eye muscle resistance (Descartes 1664/1972). **Sustained and resisted slow eye-press in restricted viewing conditions (Helmholtz, 1867; also Stark & Bridgeman, 1983). With structured visual field conditions, visual capture provides finally for space constancy. †Nagle, Bridgeman, and Stark (1980); also Grusser (1984).*

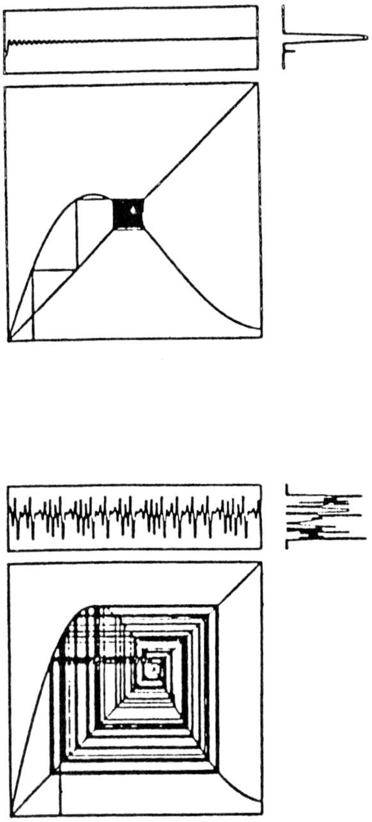

Figure 12. (left) Poincare Maps
Computer simulation of the time series resulting from iteration of the active length-tension curve at increasing levels of contraction (height of active length-tension curve and the passive series length-tension curve). Each panel contains: iterated function (large box), time function (oblong box) and density histogram (upper right of each panel)
Upper- marginally stable contraction (Note Lyapunov exponent, lambda approaches zero).
Lower- pseudo-random "chaotic" contradiction

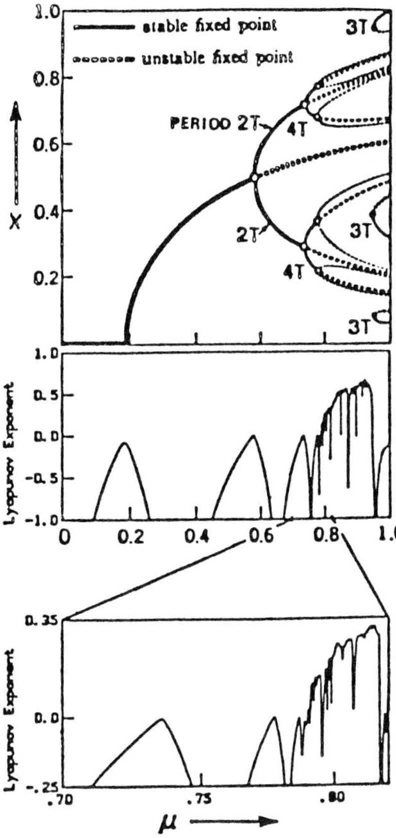

Figure 13. (right) Bifurcation diagram (top) and computation of Lyapunov exponent (middle and bottom).

Bifurcation diagram shows stable and unstable points of iterated map as a function of ordinate, 'x', initial length condition, and abscissa, 'mu', Poincare curve height, gain or muscle activation. Lyapunov exponent indicates rates of information creation [creation really means information received from the microscopic thermodynamic word (Shaw 1981)] or information destruction or loss [negative values: stable fixed point(s)] in bits per iteration. Zero crossings of Lyapunov exponent correspond to bifurcations.

Expanded plot: note strong similarity between expanded and full range curves; scales of expanded plot were chosen to emphasize fractal nature of the Lyapunov exponent as a function of gain, mu.

7- SUMMARY

This survey of neurological oscillations has reviewed the following: pupillary oscillations; gamma-B: a root distribution criterion; square-waved oscillations in a sampled-data control system; voluntary nystagmus and oscillopsia, and non-linear oscillations: strange attractors; Poincare maps; bifurcation diagrams.

In doing so we have emphasized bioengineering techniques of quantitative modeling, insights provided by control theory, understanding of the physiological and neurological bases of the particular systems studied, and the explanatory value especially for various clinical applications. The central beauty of the oscillatory phenomenon unites all these endeavors.

References

Aschoff, J.C, and Cohen, B., "Changes in Saccadic Eye Movements Produced by Cerebellar Cortical Lesions.", Experimental Neurology, 32: 123-133 (1971)

Aschoff, J.C., Becker, W., and Rettlebach, R., "Voluntary Nystagmus in Five Generations", J. Neurosurg. Psychiatr., 39: 300 (1976)

Bahill, T. A. and Stark, L., "Trajectories of Saccadic Eye Movements", Sci. Am. 240 (1979)

Bahill, T. A., Clark, M., and Stark, L., "Dynamic Overshoot in Saccadic Eye Movements is Caused by Neurological Control Signal Reversals", Exp. Neurol. 48: 107, (1975a)

Bahill, T. A., Clark, M., and Stark, L., "The Main Sequence, a Tool for Studying Human Eye Movements", Math. Biosci. 24: 191 (1975b)

Bellman, R., Dynamic Programming, Princeton University Press, Princeton (1957)

Clark, M. and Stark, L., "Control of Human Eye Movements: I. Modelling of Extraocular Plant", Math. Biosci., 20: 191-211 (1974a)

Clark , M. and Stark, L., "Control of Human Eye Movements: II. A Model for the Extraocular Plant", Math. Biosci. 20: 213, (1974b)

Clark, M. and Stark, L., "Control of Human Eye Movements. III. Dynamic Characteristics of the eye tracking mechanism." Math. Biosci., 20: 239 (1974c)

Clark, M. and Stark, L., "Time optimal behavior of human saccadic eye movement," IEEE Trans. on Automatic Control, AC-20: 345-348 (1975)

Clark, M., Jury, E. I. and Krishnan, V.V., "Glissades- eye movements generated by mismatched components of the saccadic motoneuronal control signal. Math. Biosci. 26: 303-318 (1975a)

Clark, M., Jury, E. I. and Krishnan, V.V., and Stark, L., "Computer Simulation of Biological Models using the Inners Approach", Comp. Prog. Biomed. 5: 263-282 (1975b)

Clark, M., Krishnan, V. V. and Stark, L., "Inners and biocontrol models," Bull. Math. Biol., 37: 161 (1975c)

Cook, G. and Stark, L., "Derivation of a model for the human eye-positioning mechanism," Bull. Math. Biophys., 29: 153 (1967)

Coren, S. and Komada, M. K., "Eye movement control in voluntary nystagmus," Am. J. Ophthalmol., 74: 1161 (1975)

Descartes, R., Treatise of Man, (T. S. Hall, Ed. and Trans.), Harvard University Press, Cambridge Mass (1972) (Original work published 1664)

Dodge, R., "Five types of eye movement in the horizontal meridian plane of the field of regard," Am. J. Physiol., 8: 307-329 (1903)

Grusser, O., "Time constant of pre- and post-saccadic recalibration of retinal spatial values as measured by a new after image method," Investigative Ophthalmology and Visual Science, 25: (Suppl.) 263 (1984)

Guthrie, B., Porter, J. and Sparks, D., "Corollary discharge provides accurate eye position information to the oculomotor system," Science, 221: 1193-1195 (1983)

H. von Helmholtz, H., Handbuch der physiologischen Optik, Leipzig: Voss (1867)

Hsu, F., Krishnan, V. V. and Stark, L., "Simulation of ocular dysmetria using a sampled data model of the human saccadic system," Annals of Biomedical Engineering, 4: 321-329 (1976)

Kalman, R. E., "When is a linear control system optimal?" Trans. ASME J. bal. Engng, 86D: 51-60 (1964)

Krishnan, V. V., Jury, E. I. and Stark, L., "Biological Optimality: Comparison of generalized feasibility and optimality conditions for linear, error-minimizing systems," Bull. of Math. Biology, 44: 777-791 (1982)

Lehman, S. and Stark, L., "Simulation of linear and nonlinear eye movement models: Sensitivity analyses and enumeration studies of time optimal control," J. of Cybernetics and Information Science, 2: 21-43 (1979)

Lehman, S. and Stark, L., "Multipulse controller signals: I. Pulse width and saccade duration; II. Time optimality; III. Dynamic overshoot," Biological Cybernetics, 48: 1-10 (1983)

Matin, L., Picoult, E., Stevens, J. K., Edwards, M. W., Young, D. and MacArthur, R., "Oculoparalytic illusion: Visual-field dependent spatial mislocalization by humans paralyzed with curare," Science, 216: 198-201 (1982)

Mittelstaedt, H., "The effect of visual on extraretinal information about the vertical: Suppression or superposition?" Proc. of the XXIII Intl. Cong. of Psychology, Acapulco, Mexico, 2-7 September 1984, Elsevier Science Publishers, Amsterdan (1985)

Nagle, M., Bridgeman, B. and Stark, L., "Voluntary nystagmus, saccadic suppression, and stabilization of the visual world," Vision Research, 20: 717-721 (1980)

Noton, D. and Stark, L., "Scanpaths in saccadic eye movements while viewing and recognizing patterns," Vision Res., 11: 929 (1971)

Optican, L. M. and Robinson, D. A., "Cerebellar-dependent adaptive control of primate saccadic system," J. Neurophysiol., 44: 1058-1076 (1980)

Pontriagin, L. S., Boltyanskii, V. C., Camkrendze, R. V. and Mischenki, E. F., The Mathematical Theory of Optimal Processes, Translation by K. N. Trirogoff, Interscience, N.Y., John Wiley & Sons, New York (1962)

Selhorst, J. B., Stark, L., Ochs, A. L. and Hoyt, W. F., "Disorders in cerebellar ocular motor control. I. Saccadic Overshoot Dysmetria: an oculographic, control system, and clinico-anatomic analysis; Brain, 99: 497-508 (1976a)

Selhorst, J. B., Stark, L., Ochs, A. L. and Hoyt, W. F., "Disorders in cerebellar ocular motor control. II. Macrosaccadic Oscillation: an oculographic, control system and clinico-anatomical analysis," Brain, 99: 509-522 (1976b)

Shaw, R., "Strange attractors, chaotic behavior, and information flow," A. Naturforsch, 36A: 80-112 (1981)

Shebilske, W., "Extraretinal information in corrective saccades in inflow vs. outflow theories of visual direction constancy," Vision Res., 16: 621-628 (1976)

Sparks, D. and Mays, L., "Spatial localization of saccade targets. I. Compensation for stimulation-induced perturbations in eye position; II. Activity of superior colliculus neurons preceding compensatory saccades," J. of Neurophysiology, 49: 45-74 (1983)

Shults, W., Stark, L., Hoyt, W., and Ochs, A. "Normal saccadic structure of voluntary nystagmus", Archives of Opthalmology 95: 1399- 1404 (1977)

Stark, L., "Stability, oscillations and noise in the human pupil servomechanism," Proc. IRE, 47: 1925-1939 (1959a)

Stark, L., "Vision: Servoanalysis of pupil reflex to light," Medical Physics, 3: 701-719 (1959b)

Stark, L., "Environmental clamping of biological systems: Pupil servomechanism," J. Opt. Soc. Amer., 52: 925-930 (1962)

Stark, L., Neurological Control Systems: Studies in Bioengineering, Plenum Press, New York (1968)

Stark, L., "Models of biocontrol systems," Clinic All-Round, 26: 9 (1977)

Stark, L., "The cerebellum as a calibrator organ", in Functional Basis Of Ocular Motility Disorders, Lennerstrand, G., Zee, D., and Keller, E., pp. 545-548, Stockholm (1982)

Stark, L., "Space constancy and corollary discharge," Perception & Psychophysics, 37: 272-273 (1985a)

Stark, L., "The pupil as a paradigm for neurological control systems," IEEE Trans. Biomed. Engr., BME-31: 919-924 (1985b)

Stark, L., and Baker, F., "Stability and oscillations in a neurological servomechanism," J. Neurophysiol., 22: 156-164 (1959)

Stark, L. and Bridgeman, B., "Role of corollary discharge in space constancy," Perception & Psychophysics, 34: 371-380 (1983)

Stark, L., and Cornsweet, T.N., "Testing a servoanalytic hypothesis for pupil oscillations," Science, 127: 588 (1958)

Stark, L. and Sherman, P., "A servoanalytic study of consensual pupil reflex to light", Journal of Neurophysiology, 20: 17-26 (1957)

Stark, L., Atwood, J., Elkind, J., Houk, J., King, M. and Willis, T., Prog. Rep., Res. Lab. Electr., 63: 215 (1961)

Stark, L., Vossius, G. and Young, L. R., "Predictive control of eye tracking movements," IRE Trans. on Human Factors in Electronics, HFE-3: 52-57 (1962)

Stark, L., Kong, R., Schwartz, S., Hendry, D. and Bridgeman, B., "Saccadic suppression of visual displacement," Vision Res., 16: 1185-1187 (1976)

Stark, L., Hoyt, W., Ciuffreda, K., Kenyon, R. and Hsu, F., "Time optimal saccadic trajectory model and voluntary nustagmus," in Models of Oculomotor Behavior and Control, B. L. Zuber, Ed., CRC Press, Boca Raton, Florida, pp. 75-89 (1980)

Stegemann, J., "Uber den einfluss sinusforminger leuchtdichteande-rungen auf die pupillenweite," Pfluger's Arch. fur die Gesamte Physiol. des Menschen und der Tiere, 264: 113-122 (1957)

Sun, F., Zhao, X., Dai, S., Liu, H. and Yang, R., "Dynamic characteristics of the pupillary control system: Measurement and mathematical model," Acta Automat. Sinica, 5, No. 2: 130-135 (1979)

Varju, D., "Der einfluss sinusfoermiger leuchtdichteanderungen auf die mittlere pupillenweite und auf die subjektive helligkeit," Kybernetik, 2, No. 2: 33-43 (1964)

Van der Tweel, L. H. and Van der Gon, J. S. D., "The light reflex of the normal pupil of man," Acta Physiol. Pharmacol. Neerlandica, 8: 69 (1959)

Wiener, N., _Cybernetics, or Control and Communication in the Animal and the Machine_, M.I.T. Press, Cambridge, Massachussetts (1948)

Young, L. R. and Stark, L., "A discrete model for eye tracking movements," _IEEE Trans. Mil. Electron., MIL-7_: 113 (1963a)

Young, L. R. and Stark, L., "Variable feedback experiments testing a sampled data model for eye tracking movements," _IEEE Trans. Hum. Factors Electron., HFE-4_: 38 (1963b)

Zee, D. S. and Robinson, D. A., "A hypothetical explanation of saccadic oscillations," _Ann. Neurol., 5_: 405 (1979)

Quantitative Theory of Changes in Oscillatory Hand Movements – Application of Methods of Synergetics

H. Bunz and H. Haken

Institute for Theoretical Physics and Synergetics, University of Stuttgart, Pfaffenwaldring 57/IV, D-7000 Stuttgart 80, Fed. Rep. of Germany

1. Introduction

One of the most characteristic features of life is the extremely high coordination between the different parts of a biological system. In higher animals we observe such a high coordination of neurons, muscles and other tissues which then leads to a well-pronounced heartbeat, breathing, blood circulation, coordination of movements up to perception. All these phenomena show a pronounced temporal order, or in pathological cases, pronounced disorders. It is therefore important to ask how to understand this so pronounced coordination. One possibility which is quite well known is based on the idea of a neuronal motorprogram. In such a case, a neuronal network similar to a computer determines the motion of the individual muscles or other tissues in order to produce a well-organized total action.

In our contribution, we wish to lend support to another paradigm which, in our opinion, plays a role at least as important as that of the motorprogram, namely the idea of self-organization. Over the past two decades, we have studied numerous systems in physics, chemistry and biology which can produce spatial or temporal structures without specific interference from organizing centres. Instead, the activity of these systems is organized by the interaction of the individual parts of the system itself. Upon changes of external conditions which are of a rather unspecific nature, these systems can undergo dramatic transitions between different modes of their activity.

As we could show, these specific transitions between different modes of activity are not determined by specific mechanisms of the interactions between the different parts of a system but depend on general principles which can be formulated mathematically. In order to reach a wide audience, we shall not dwell on the mathematical details here, but rather we shall report some general results and then elucidate these results by means of an explicit example taken from the transition from normal hand movements to "abnormal" ones. So, the question still to be discussed is, what is meant by normal and abnormal in this case?

Quite generally, the interdisciplinary field of synergetics [1, 2] deals with systems which are composed of many subsystems. In physics such a system can be a fluid which is composed of many individual molecules, or a laser which is composed of many individual atoms. In chemistry, a system may be composed of many individual molecules which may be the same or of different kinds. In biology, a system may be composed of neurons, muscles and perhaps other parts. Let us assume that such a system is at rest or performs some specific activity. Now let us assume that, for instance, an energy input is increased or chemicals are added to the system at an increased rate. Then, in a number of cases at critical values of these so-called control parameters the system may acquire the new state. For instance, a system which has been at rest may now start to oscillate, or a system which has been oscillating may start a different kind of oscillation or a more complicated one. For instance, one which eventually leads to deterministic chaos.

As has been revealed by synergetics, in systems close to such transition points specific phenomena will occur jointly. One of these phenomena is the occurrence of

critical fluctuations in which the values of observables such as the output of the laser light or the molecular concentration in a chemical reaction undergo large fluctuations. Another phenomenon consists in so-called **critical slowing down**. When a system is close to a transition point it reacts more slowly to external perturbations than in situations where the system is away from such a critical point. These phenomena are typical for processes of self-organization, where the system acquires its new state without specific interference from the outside, i.e. the control parameters do not anticipate the new state but rather indirectly force the system to acquire it. As is shown in synergetics, in situations where macroscopic patterns of behavior change qualitatively, the dynamics of even very many parts of a system is governed by one or a few order parameters.

In the following we present a specific example of such transitions of involuntary human hand movements, identify its order parameter and establish its equation. Excellent agreement with the experimental results is found. We believe that many more examples in biology can be found, for instance, in transitions of normal to abnormal heartbeats, breathing, blood circulation etc. which exhibit quite similar phenomena, but which have not been studied so far because of lack of an adequate theory. In the next section we shall describe the basic experiment and in the subsequent sections we shall discuss its theoretical treatment.

2. Phase Transitions in Human Hand Movement

While researching voluntary oscillatory motions of the two index fingers, KELSO [3] observed an interesting phenomenon. Under instructions to increase the frequency of out-of-phase, antisymmetrical motion (involving simultaneous flexor and extensor muscle activities), the subject's finger movements shifted abruptly to an in-phase symmetrical mode that involved simultaneous activation of homologous muscle groups. This finding was not restricted to finger movements. In later work [4, 5] that employed similar experimental manipulations, modal transitions in hand motions around the wrist were also observed: the antisymmetrical phase relationship between the hands was replaced by symmetrical phasing. Moreover, although the phase transition occurred at very different frequencies of hand motion for different subjects, it was nevertheless predictable.

The most dramatic aspect of these simple experiments is the sudden and completely involuntary change in the ordering or phasing among muscle groups that occurs at a critical, intrinsically defined frequency. In this feature, the hand movement data share a likeness to gait transitions in locomotion.

3. Initial Development of the Model: Order Parameters and the potential function

To summarize, the main features of the experiments described above are:

1) the presence of only two stable phase (or "attractor") states between the hands (which one is observed is a function of how the system is prepared, i.e. an instruction to move the hands in the out-of-phase or in-phase mode);

2) the abrupt transition from one attractor state to the other at a critical cycling frequency;

3) beyond the transition, only one mode (symmetrical in-phase) is observed;

4) when cycling frequency is reduced, the system stays in the symmetrical mode, i.e. it does not return to its initially prepared state - a result that suggests coexistence of the basins of attraction for the symmetrical and antisymmetrical modes and the depletion of one of them.

Taken together, these results as well as other findings in the motor control literature support the hypothesis that <u>phase</u> is a relevant macroscopic (or "essential") parameter of certain movement patterns. For example, the internal phasing structure of activities as widely varied as chewing, locomotion, handwriting, and speech remains invariant across scalar changes in force or rate [7 - 10]. Similarly, in the experiments described above, phase is preserved constant over a wide range of frequencies, even though the magnitudes and durations of muscle activities and other kinematic variables change considerably. Only when frequency is scaled beyong a critical value does a phase shift occur.

In the present paper it seems reasonable to propose phase as an order parameter for at least two reasons. First, unlike many other possible candidates, phase is an accurate reflection of the cooperativity among the components of the system. Thus, we can say, in a manner consistent with synergetics, that the configuration of the subsystems (in the present context defined as the individual hand motions) specifies their phase relation, and conversely, that the phase variable specifies the spatiotemporal ordering of the subsystems. Second, it is phase that remains invariant across transformations in many motor activities that involve very different anatomical substrates. This highlights an important further feature of the order parameter concept, namely, that the order parameter (by hypothesis here, the relative phase) changes much more slowly than the variables describing the behavior of the individual components (e.g. velocities of each hand motion).

Our first step in the development of the present model [6] is to provide a mathematically accurate description of the main qualitative features of the data. We therefore specify a potential function that corresponds to the layout of attractor states and how that layout is altered as a control parameter is changed. In a following section, we show how the model equations describing the potential function can be derived from the equations of motion of each hand and a (nonlinear) coupling between them.

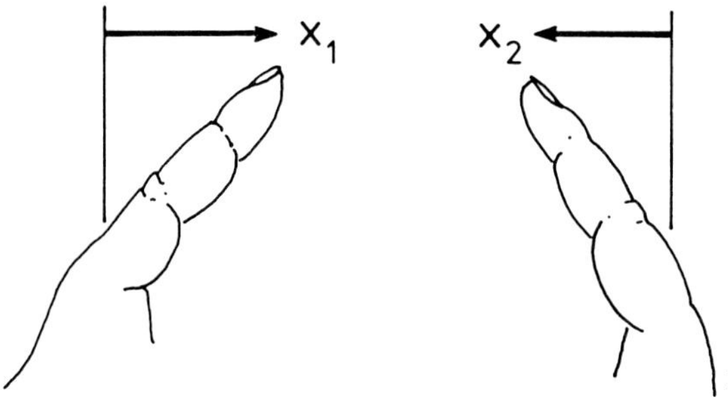

Fig. 1: Elongations of the finger tips

For the sake of clarity we introduce the elongations of the finger tips x_1 and x_2 as shown in Fig.1. In order to define the relative phase ϕ we assume that the motion of the hands is more or less harmonic, so we put

$$x_1 = r_1 \cos(\omega t + \phi_1) \quad , \tag{3.1}$$

$$x_2 = r_2 \cos(\omega t + \phi_2\ ) \quad , \tag{3.2}$$

where ω is the basic frequency of the hand movement while the amplitudes r_1, r_2 and the phases ϕ_1, ϕ_2 are time-dependent quantities whose time dependence is assumed to be much slower than that defined by the frequency ω. The relative phase is defined by

$$\phi = \phi_2 - \phi_1 \quad . \tag{3.3}$$

In order to describe the change of phase we adopt basic ideas from synergetics. As shown in synergetics, in many cases the equations for order parameters are of the form

$$\dot{\phi} = -\frac{\partial V}{\partial \phi} \quad , \tag{3.4}$$

where V is the so-called potential function. In our search for a model we make a few rather obvious assumptions about V. Since ϕ occurs under cosine or sine functions the properties of the physical system must not change when ϕ is replaced by $\phi + 2\pi$. Consequently, we shall postulate that the potential V is periodic:

$$V(\phi + 2\pi) = V(\phi) \quad . \tag{3.5}$$

We furthermore introduce the assumption that both hands play a symmetric role. In such a case the behavior of the system must not depend on the way we label the right hand and the left hand. This means that V must remain unchanged when we exchange the indices 1 and 2 in (3.3). This in turn means that the potential V is symmetric:

$$V(\phi) = V(-\phi). \tag{3.6}$$

We assume that V obeys the conditions (3.5) and (3.6) in the simplest form which explains the above-mentioned experimental results. To this end we write V as a superposition of two cosine functions:

$$V = -a \cos\phi - b \cos 2\phi \quad . \tag{3.7}$$

As is known from synergetics, the behavior of the system obeying (3.4) can be easily described by identifying ϕ with the coordinate of a particle which moves in an overdamped fashion in the potential V.

When we take the total superposition (3.7) but change the ratio b/a we run through a series of potential fields shown in Fig. 2. When we initially prepare the system in a state shown by the black ball and increase the frequency, and likewise assume that b/a decreases with increasing frequency, we obtain a critical value where the ball falls to the lower minimum belonging to $\phi = 0$. This means that the hand movement made a transition from the antisymmetric ($\phi = -\pi$ state) into the symmetric state with $\phi = 0$. The hand movement stays in that state when ω is

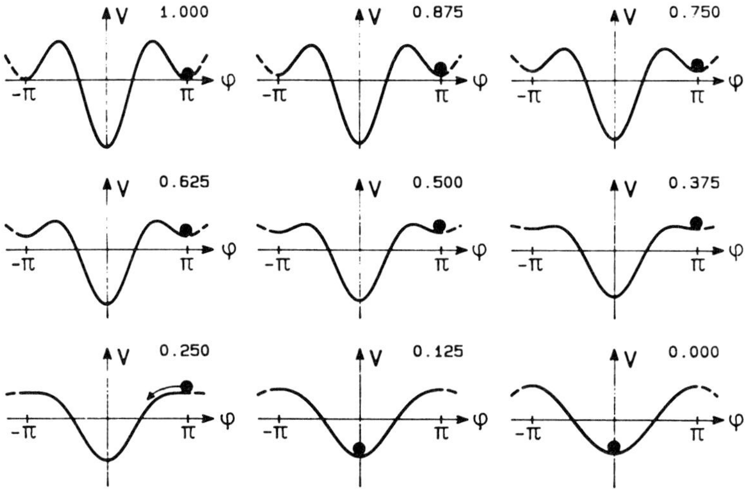

Fig. 2: The potential V for varying values of b/a. The numbers refer to the ratio b/a (after [6])

further increased. When we decrease b/a starting from high values, the system remains all the time in the $\phi = 0$ state even if ω drops below ω_o. This "hysteresis" phenomenon is well known in many physical and biological systems.

4. Formulation at the Next Lower Hierarchical Level

The order parameter equation for ϕ can be derived from equations at the next lower hierarchical level, namely at the individual hand movements [6]. We have studied the following type of equations

$$\ddot{x}_1 + f_1(\dot{x}_1, x_1) = K_{12}(x_1, x_2) \quad , \tag{4.1}$$

$$\ddot{x}_2 + f_2(\dot{x}_2, x_2) = K_{21}(x_1, x_2) \quad , \tag{4.2}$$

where the indices 1,2 refer to the right and left hand, respectively, and K_{12} is the coupling term brought about via the nervous system. For the sake of simplicity, the oscillators are assumed to have identical frequencies and damping constants, respectively, i.e. $f_1 = f_2$ and

$$K_{21}(x_1, x_2) = K_{12}(x_2, x_1) \quad . \tag{4.3}$$

In order to obtain (3.4) K_{12} must be a nonlinear function of (x_1-x_2) either via a time delay

$$K_{12} = \int e^{-\lambda(t-\tau)}[\alpha(x_1-x_2)_\tau + \beta(x_1-x_2)_\tau^3]\, d\tau \quad , \tag{4.4}$$

or by using time derivatives

$$K_{12} = (\dot{x}_1-\dot{x}_2)\,[\alpha + \beta(x_1-x_2)^2] \quad . \tag{4.5}$$

These coupling terms are not unique and a huge variety of other possibilities exists, but (4.4, 4.5) are the simplest representatives of the possible couplings. In order to achieve agreement with the experimental findings, we chose (4.5) in the following numerical simulations, but the other coupling terms show no qualitatively different behavior.

5. Numerical Results

In this section we present some numerical results that correspond to the analytical treatment provided above. HAKEN et.al. [6] solved the model of Sect. 4 on a digital computer using a fourth order Runge-Kutta method. To test the stability of a stationary solution small random fluctuations of finite amplitude were introduced. The resulting simulation shown in Fig. 3 compares quite favorably with the experimental data. In Fig. 3a the displacements x_1, x_2 are plotted against time and in Fig. 3b the corresponding phase difference between the oscillators is plotted for the same motions. As in the bimanual experiments, the coupled oscillation is prepared in the state $\phi=\pi$ and the frequency ω is increased monotonical. A transition from the out-of-phase mode to the in-phase mode is observed, when ω exceeds a critical value. However, the frequency of the oscillation changes rather quickly so that stationary oscillations are not reached. Thus the exact form of the curves depends strongly on the noise level and the rate of changing ω.

The steady state amplitudes for the in-phase mode and the out-of-phase mode are shown in Fig. 4. The unstable branch of the out-of-phase mode is shown by dotted lines. The ω^{-1} dependence of the amplitudes is quite clear. This feature rests on our special choice of f in (4.1, 4.2) and will be different for another choice of f. As shown in Fig. 4 for ω smaller than ω_c, the in-phase mode and the out-of-phase mode are both stable. Due to the coexistence of two basins of attraction, the particular mode observed depends on the initial conditions, i.e. which coordinative state is prepared.

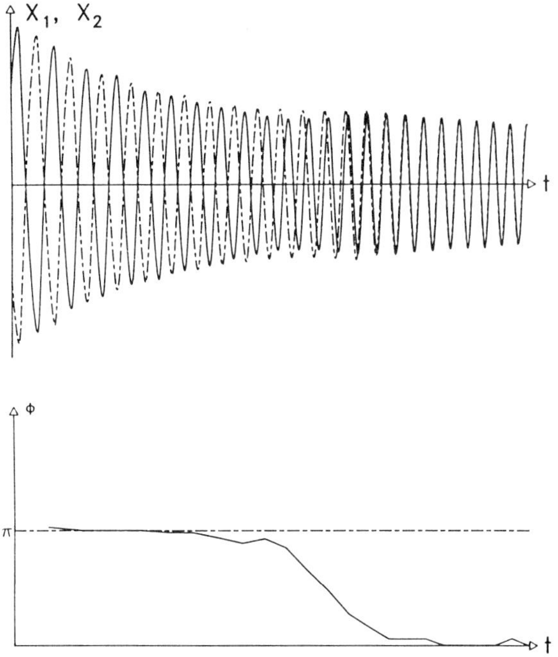

Fig. 3: In a the displacements and in b the corresponding phase difference between the oscillators is plotted (after [6])

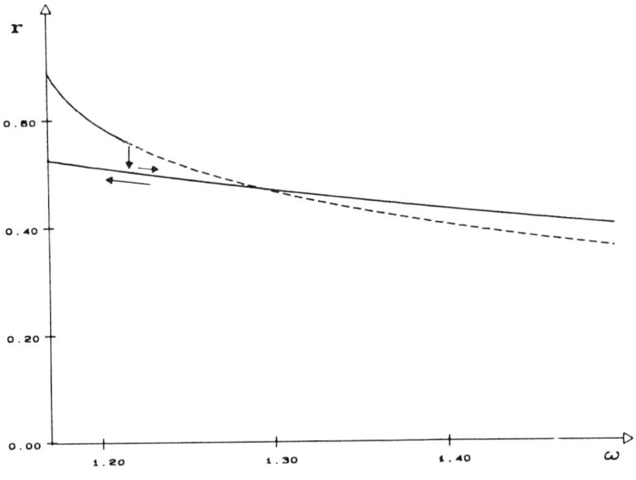

Fig. 4: The steady state amplitudes of the in-phase and the out-of-phase mode are shown as a function of ω

If one starts in the antisymmetric phase and increases ω slowly, the oscillation remains in this mode until the solution becomes unstable. At this point a jump in amplitude occurs and the only stable stationary solution revealed by the system corresponds to the in-phase mode. Such is the case when ω is increased further. On the other hand, if ω is decreased slowly the system stays within the basin of attraction of this solution even when ω drops below ω_c. As we mentioned earlier, this hysteresis phenomenon is typical for such bistable situations. To summarize, it is quite clear that the main features of the experimental data described at the beginning of Sect. 2 are captured by the present mathematical formulation as illustrated by these numerical results. But in addition to the main features which correspond to average values of ϕ or x_1, x_2, on the basis of synergetics we also expect a fine structure due to fluctuations close to the transition frequency.

6. Fluctuations and Their Significance

Looking at our above model and having in mind the typical critical fluctuations of synergetic systems close to their transition points, we suggested to Kelso that he look for such fluctuations. Figure 5 shows his experimental results (cf. e.g. [11]).

In this figure both the average phase and the phase fluctuations, or more precisely the root mean square of the phase fluctuations, are plotted. In the case of the transition from the antisymmetric to the symmetric hand motion large critical fluctuations indeed do occur. We have modelled this transition under the impact of fluctuations by means of adding a fluctuating force to (3.4), i.e. we have treated the equation [12]

$$\dot{\phi} = - \frac{\partial V}{\partial \phi} + F(t) \quad . \tag{6.1}$$

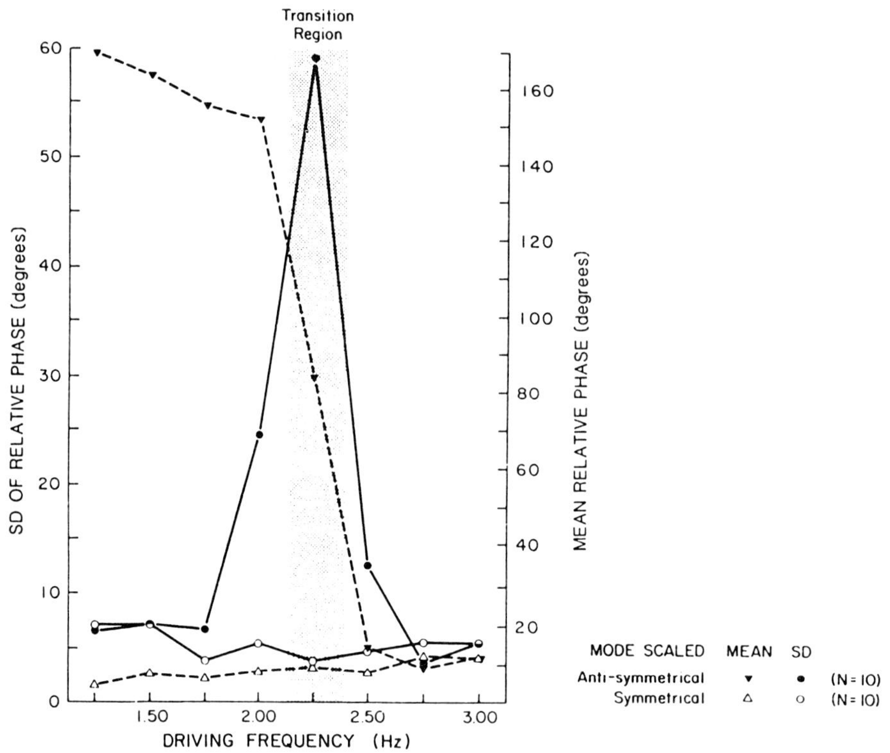

Fig. 5: The mean phase modulus $<\phi>$ (▼ AMS, Δ SMS) and its SD=$\{<\phi^2> - <\phi>^2\}$ (● AMS, o SMS) were determined in the stationary limit on each frequency plateau (i.e. for the last 3 s at each frequency). Each point on the graph represents an average from 10 runs of the experiment. AMS = antisymmetric mode scaled, SMS = symmetric mode

Using the Fokker-Planck equation, we have studied both the behavior of the root mean square as well as correlation functions and results are found in excellent agreement with the experiment.

What is most interesting and important, is the consequence of this treatment. Namely, when we first assume that the transition between one kind of hand movement to the other kind is caused by the change of a motorprogram of the neurons, it will be very hard to understand why any fluctuation should occur at all. Indeed a motorprogram is a fixed program and no fluctuations should be expected. The way the transition occurs in the hand movement rather indicates that we are dealing here with a typical act of self-organization. This system organizes itself, that means the individual neurons and muscles act jointly as if the whole system acts as a total autonomous system.

Quite clearly, this introduces an entirely new paradigm into biology and it can be hoped that similar mechanisms and models apply to more complicated motions, where the next step will be to study the change of gaits of horses. Other highly coordinated motions may most probably be treated very much the same way, for instance, rhythmic motions like breathing and heartbeat and their coordination.

References

1. H. Haken: Synergetics. An Introduction, 3rd ed., Springer Ser. Syn., Vol.1 (Springer, Berlin, Heidelberg, New York 1983)
2. H. Haken: Advanced Synergetics, Springer Ser. Syn., Vol.20 (Springer, Berlin, Heidelberg, New York 1983)
3. J.A.S. Kelso: Bull. Psychon. Soc. 18, 63 (1981)
4. J.A.S. Kelso: Invited paper presented at Kroc Foundation Conference on Nonlinear Mechanics in Brain Function, Santa Barbara, CA, March 1-5, 1982
5. J.A.S. Kelso: Am. J. Physiol. Reg.Integ.Comp. 15, R1000-R1004 (1984)
6. H. Haken, J.A.S. Kelso, H. Bunz: Biol. Cybern. 51, 347 (1985)
7. S. Grillner: In Speech Motor Control, ed. by S. Grillner, B. Lindblom, J. Lubker, A. Persson (Pergamon, Oxford 1982)
8. J.A.S. Kelso: In Attention and Performance (IX), ed. by J. Long, A. Baddeley (Erlbaum, Hillsdale, NJ 1981)
9. R.A. Schmidt: In Motor Control and Learning: A Behavioral Emphasis Champaign, IL: Human Kinetics (1982)
10. B. Tuller, J.A.S. Kelso, K.S. Harris: J. Exp. Psycholog. Hum. Percept. Perform 8, 460-472 (1982)
11. J.A.S. Kelso, J. Scholz: In Complex Systems - Operational Approaches, ed. by H. Haken, Springer Ser. Syn., Vol. 31 (Springer, Berlin, Heidelberg, New York 1985) p. 124
12. G. Schoener, H. Haken, J.A.S. Kelso: Biolog. Cybern. 53, 247 (1986)

Investigation of Agonistic/Antagonistic Movement in Parkinson's Disease from an Ergodic Point of View

P.H. Kraus[1,2], *H.R. Bittner*[3], *P. Klotz*[1], and *H. Przuntek*[1,2]

[1]Neurologische Universitäts- und Poliklinik, Josef-Schneider-Str. 11, D-8700 Würzburg, Fed. Rep. of Germany
[2]Present address: Neurologische Universitätsklinik, St. Josef-Hospital, Gudrunstraße 56, D-4630 Bochum 1, Fed. Rep. of Germany
[3]Permanent address: Institut für Biochemie, Frankfurter Straße 100, D-6300 Gießen, Fed. Rep. of Germany

The major symptoms of Parkinson's disease are motor deficiency (akinesia, bradykinesia, hypokinesia), rigidity and tremor. For assessment of motor symptoms we used a technical motor performance test developed by Schoppe [1].

This test consists of several subtests. One of them, "Tapping", is a good examination of fast agonist-antagonist movements. The person is required to tap on a contact board as fast as possible, using a contact pencil. In Schoppe's original version, the test compares only the number of contacts during the two halves of a selected time interval, providing only coarse information about performance speed and alterations of speed (e.g. caused by fatigue).

During the original tapping examinations we discovered, that some patients, suffering severe symptoms of Parkinsonism, tapped faster than the average of the healthy controls, unexpectedly. Also, there seemed to be a different acoustic impression of their tapping.

Therefore we used electrically conducting pen and board and recorded with a desktop computer the time intervals between two tapping contacts for 16 sec in units of 1 ms.

We found, that in fast tapping movements, the regularity was distinctly more disturbed than the speed [2] (Fig. 1) and so the question emerged, which of the Parkinsonian symptoms are pathophysiologically responsible for these changes.

Sensomotoric changes, found in many investigations (e.g. Horne [3] and Bowen *et al.* [4]), which influence every voluntary movement, could not be differentiated and evaluated in our investigations. It has not yet been clarified what effect tremor has on the regularity of tapping. We have seen patients who were able to make use of their tremor while tapping, as well as some whose performance was impaired. Fourier Transformation did not show different spectra for patients with tremor as main symptom.

Fast agonist-antagonist movements are to be described as a complex cybernetical model: Via afferent and efferent fibres, this system can perform damped oscillations, which additionally are influenced, e.g. by mechanical properties.

In contrast to slow complex movements, which are completely controlled by feed-back via afferent fibres, fast oscillating movements cannot be regulated by the same mechanism. Fast oscillations are a special case of voluntary movements and correspond to an external driven oscillator, modulated by complex feed-back

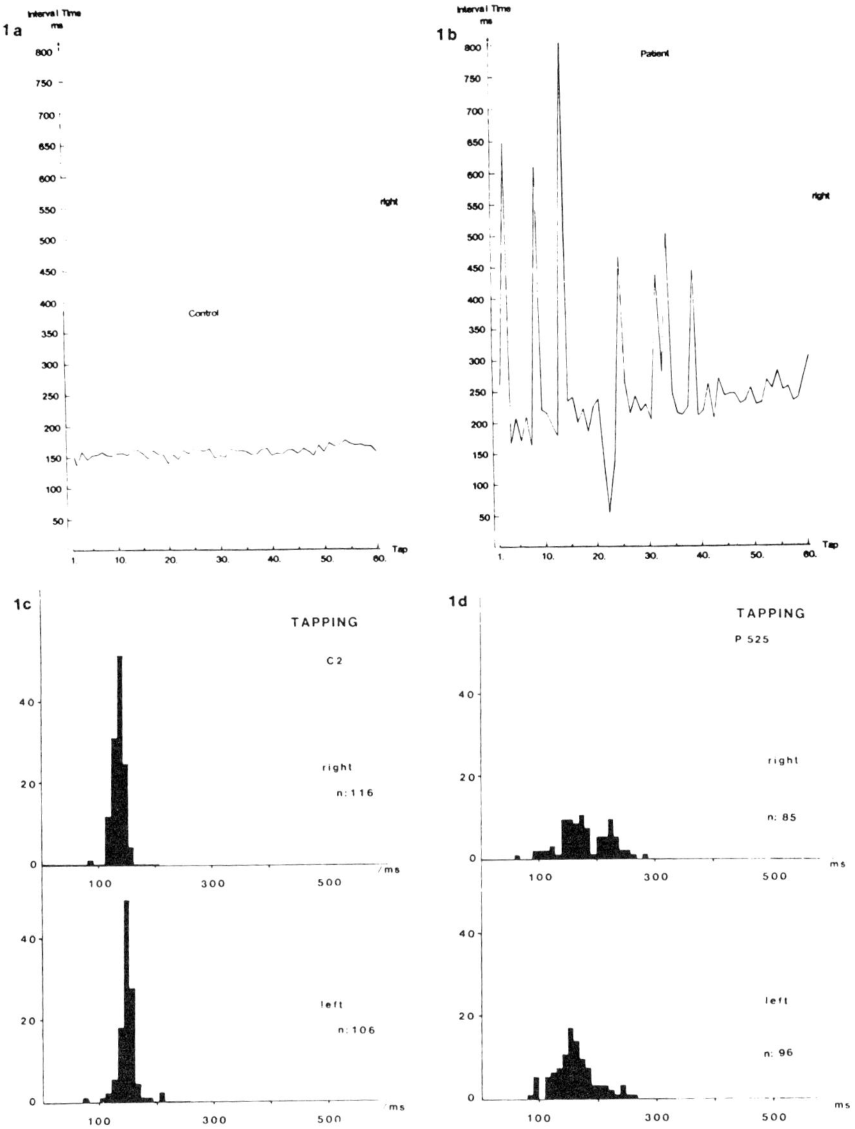

Fig. 1: Tapping results for single persons.
Variation of interval times (tapping intervals) during the first 60 taps of a healthy control (a) and a Parkinsonian patient (b).
For right-handed controls without clinically pathological findings, the relative performances of right and left hand are similar, showing a narrow distribution (Fig. 1c), whereas Parkinsonian patients show a distinct broadening of the distribution (Fig. 1d).

mechanisms. In analogy to the results of Haken [5], such movements could be described as non-linear oscillation: An increase of frequency leads to a decrease of the amplitude of the movement.

Therefore these fast movements meet the requirements for possible chaotic behaviour.

The diagrams of temporal spectra of the tapping intervals (Fig. 1a, b) raise the question, whether the difference of deviation between healthy controls and Parkinsonian patients is only quantitative or also qualititative, that means: is there a different state of order?

For investigating temporal order, the periods in which the patient is tapping fairly regularly are most interesting. Longer delays are caused by akinesia and represent an interruption of the oscillation.

Fast Fourier Transformation (FFT) over 64 intervals yielded no interpretable differences between patients and controls.

In order to apply the tools of "chaos-investigation", we interpolated the series of time intervals by using a cos(x) function and received the Poincaré-map with the states Y_i at the time $i \cdot \Delta t$ ($i = 1,2,3, \ldots, N$). To reconstruct phase portraits of the system's attractor, the embedding technique [6, 7] was used. After evaluating the correlation sum C_n for different distances ε in n-dimensional phase space, the attractor's dimension D_n is the limit slope of the linear region (if one exists) in the log-log-plot of $C_n(\varepsilon)$ vs. ε [8], if an increase of the number D_{emb} of phase space variables does not result in a considerable change of D_n (saturation).

$$C_n(\varepsilon) = \frac{1}{N_n} \cdot \sum_{j \neq k} \Theta(\varepsilon - \| Y_j - Y_k \|) \quad \text{with } \Theta(x) = \begin{cases} 0 & \text{for } x < 0 \\ 1 & \text{for } x > 0 \end{cases}$$

Two-dimensional ($n=2$; $Y_i | Y_{i+3}$) calculations with experimental data of 14 patients and 15 controls provide values for D_2 in the range of 0.85 . The values for the axial intercepts lie at 0.45, not significantly correlated to the slope D_2. The U-test (Wilcoxon/Mann/Whitney) revealed no significant differences between patients and controls.

This experiment does not provide a sufficient resolution of this problem, because the scanning frequency is only similar to the signal frequency. For obtaining further details of the observed phenomenon, we performed a more sophisticated experiment:

In test persons with fixed forearm, we assessed an oscillation of the hand, corresponding to a tapping movement, but without striking on a plate ("Pseudo-tapping"), to prevent effects of rebounds. The record was taken over 120 sec by using a one-dimensional accelerometer, fixed to the thumb (Fig. 2; 250 Hz scan frequency; 12 bit resolution), which provides data sets of about 500 periods.

In this way we assessed spontaneous and forced ("as fast as possible") pseudo-tapping as well as resting and postural tremor. Figure 3a displays the amplitudes in a two-dimensional, stroboscopic Poincaré-map. With the embedding tech-

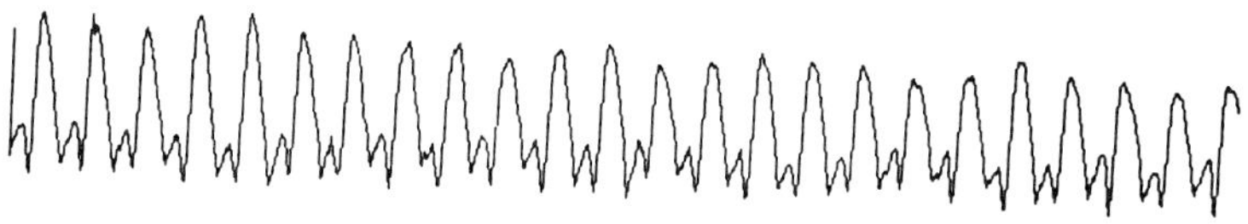

Fig. 2: Pseudo-tapping: Signal of a Parkinsonian patient, provided by the accelerometer

nique mentioned above, we looked for the Grassberger-Procaccia-dimension for different numbers of phase space variables (Fig. 3c), using the maximum norm. The resulting slope is very sensitive to the choice of the ε-interval, in which the linear region is assumed to be, so another method was used: In the linear region (if one exists), lg C_n and lg ε are proportional, so we chose a C_n-interval to describe the position of the linear region. This interval was set to the nearly constant region of the derivative function (Fig. 3b) and is indicated by bars in Figs. 3b and c. If the GP-dimension exists, the slopes should show a saturation effect with an increasing number D_{emb} of phase space variables (Fig. 3d). The results given below are based on 600 to 1200 points, in some cases different parts of the same set were evaluated and middled.

For scanning frequencies below 30 Hz, the scaling of the correlation sum shows random characteristics (no saturation). For testing our hypothesis, frequencies between 40 and 130 Hz seem to fit best, although no perfect saturation is reached. For the results described below, we used every fourth value (i.e. 62 Hz scanning).

Our hitherto results of four Parkinsonian patients and four healthy controls yield correlation exponents for controls ranging at 1.5 to 1.6 (spontaneous) and 1.5 to 1.8 (forced), resp. The values for spontaneous Pseudo-tapping of patients (1.5, 1.8, 3.2, 1.8) lie mostly above that of the controls. As expected, forced Pseudo-tapping (patients: 1.5, 1.75, 1.8 and 1.75 resp.) show nearly equal or more complex order in most cases. The result of 3.2 for spontaneous tapping of one of the patients cannot be explained yet, because other parameters provided no interpretable pecularities.

Resting and posturity tremor of controls (physiological tremor), whose frequency spectra look like that of noise, yield widely spread (maybe spurious) correlation exponents ranging above those of voluntary movements (between 3.4 and 6.4). For one Parkinsonian patient we found for resting tremor (5.8 Hz) a correlation dimension in the range of voluntary movements (1.6).

We are aware of difficulties in the interpretation of these kinds of data sets (too few data, spurious plateaus, etc. leading to too small dimensions, conf. [9]), but further experiments shall enable more precise statements about this kind of temporal disorder. The comparison of the dimensions of pathological tremor of different genesis (e.g. Parkinsonian, Essential tremor) which show overlapping frequency spectra will be our future subject of interest [10].

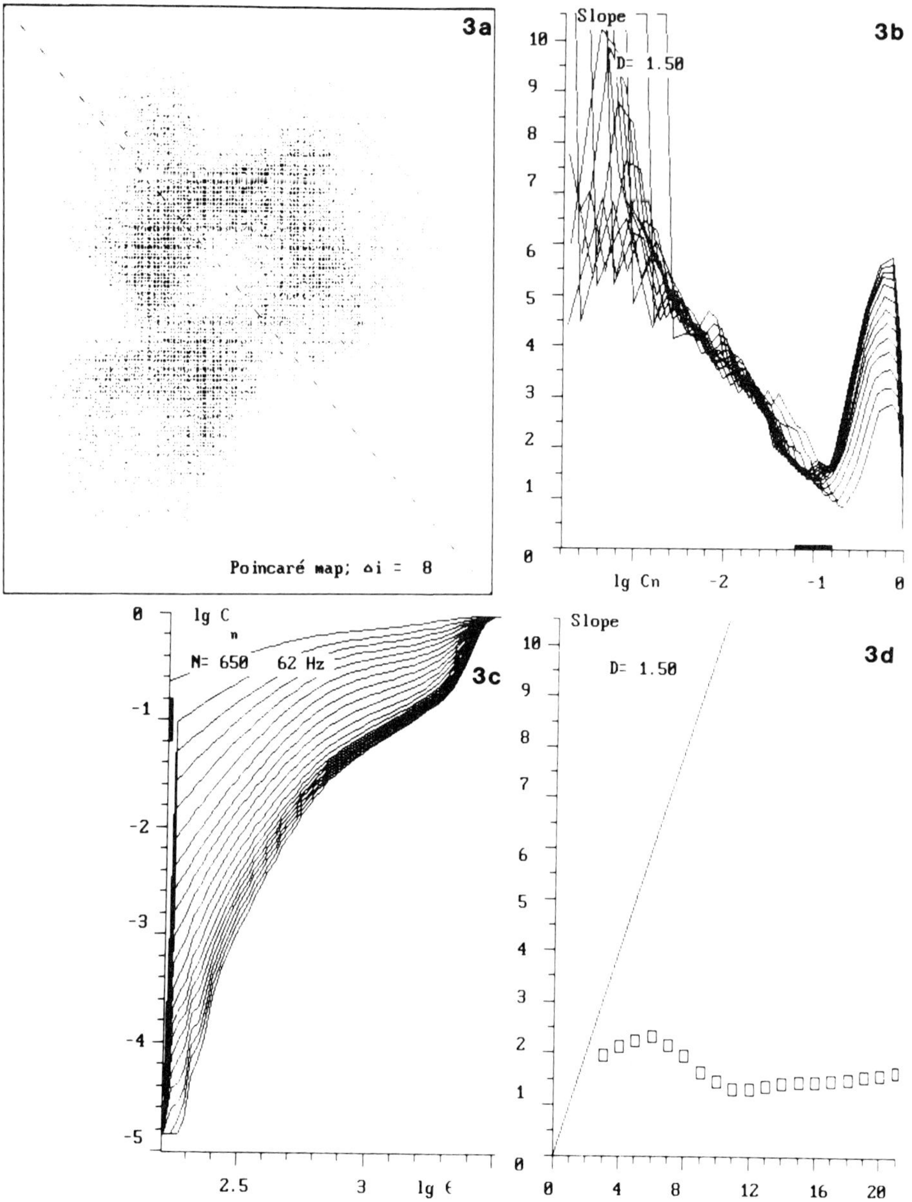

Fig. 3: a) Poincaré-map of Pseudo-tapping. (Equidistant time intervals)
b) Numerical derivative from Fig. 3c; the bar indicates the interval chosen for computation of the slope c) Scaling of the correlation sum C_n with phase space distance ε for different embedding dimensions (1...21) in a log-log-plot d) Dependence of the attractor's correlation dimension on the number of phase space variables in the marked region

References:

1. K.J. Schoppe: Das MLS-Gerät: Ein neuer Testapparat zur Messung feinmotorischer Leistungen. Diagnostica 20 (1974) 43-46.
2. P.H. Kraus, A. Fischer, P. Klotz and H. Przuntek: New aspects of assessment of Parkinson's disease. J of Neurology (to be published 1987)
3. D. Horne: Sensorimotor control in Parkinsonism. J of Neurology, Neurosurgery and Psychiatry 36 (1973) 742-746 .
4. F.P. Bowen, E. Brady, M. Yahr: Sensorimotor coordination in Parkinson's disease before and after Levodopa therapy. Neurology 23 (1973) 1101-1106 .
5. H. Haken, J.A.S. Kelso, H.A. Bunz: Theoretical Model of Phase Transitions in Human Hand Movements. Biological Cybernetics 51 (Springer, 1985) 347-356.
6. P. Grassberger: On the Hausdorff dimension of fractal attractors. Journal of Statistical Physics 26 (1981) 173-179 .
7. P. Grassberger, I. Procaccia: Measuring the strangeness of strange attractors. Physica 9D (1983) 189-208 ; and: Dimensions and entropies of strange attractors. Physica 13D (1984) 34-54 .
8. J.D. Farmer: Chaotic Attractors of an infinite-dimensional dynamical system. Physica 4D (1982) 366-393 .
9. P. Grassberger: Do climatic attractors exist? Nature 323 (1986) 609-612 .
10. H.R. Bittner, P.H. Kraus: (in preparation) .

Part III

Heart and Respiration

Nonlinear Dynamics, Fractals, Cardiac Physiology and Sudden Death

A.L. Goldberger

Cardiology Division, Beth Israel Hospital, Harvard Medical School, Boston, MA 02215, USA

1. Introduction

As implied by the commonly used term "clinical disorder," there is a tendency to equate healthy function with order and disease with chaos. This correlation is more than colloquial. The theory that fibrillation represents cardiac turbulence or chaos was proposed by MOE and colleagues [1] and more recently by SMITH and COHEN [2]. The latter investigators went a step further by suggesting that ventricular fibrillation, the dysrhythmia most commonly associated with sudden cardiac death, may occur at the end of a Feigenbaum-type period-doubling sequence.

The general notion that abstract mathematical models may be relevant to bedside clinical medicine has generated considerable interest. However, the precise applicability of these models is a subject of ongoing debate. With regard to the question of sudden death and chaos, for example, we [3-5] have proposed a diametrically opposite viewpoint to that just described: namely, that certain features of dynamical chaos related to fractal structure and fractal dynamics may be important organizing principles in normal physiology and that certain pathologies, including ventricular fibrillation, represent a class of "pathological periodicities." The dynamics of certain diseases, therefore, may reflect a type of re-ordering rather than dis-ordering.

This essay will briefly review some of the work from our laboratory bearing on the relation of nonlinear phenomena and nonlinear analysis to physiological and pathophysiological data. It should be emphasized from the outset that all the theories and models described here are tentative and that key questions (e.g. what is the mechanism of ventricular fibrillation?) remain unanswered. At the same time, we face the intriguing prospect that the application of nonlinear analysis to cardiovascular dynamics and indeed to physiology in general may provide new approaches to a class of problems that have been refractory to conventional analysis [5].

2. Fractals and Normal Physiology

MANDELBROT's concept of fractals [6] and the development of related concepts of strange attractors, chaotic dynamics and critical phase transitions (renormalization group theory) have been major tools in the approach to complex physical systems. The geometric fractal defines a class of irregular structures that 1) have no characteristic scale of length; 2) have a myriad of layers of structural detail, and 3) demonstrate self-similarity such that the small-scale structure is reminiscent of the larger-scale form. Mandelbrot [6] pointed out the ubiquity of fractal architecture in nature, from wrinkly coastlines to branching trees and blood vessels, to turbulent flows. Furthermore, fractal concepts can be applied more generally to dynamical function, particularly in the context of complex processes that are governed by self-similar scaling mechanisms [6,7]. Such processes, which lack a characteristic scale of time, are associated with spectra having a broadband frequency profile with <u>inverse power-law</u> (1/f-like) distributions.

Over the last few years in collaboration with B. WEST and others [3,5,8-10] we have tried to apply fractal concepts to both physiological structure and function. On a structural level, fractal anatomy appears in multiple organ systems, as revealed by inspection of the bronchial and vascular trees, hepatic-biliary network, urinary collecting ducts and so forth [5,8-11]. From a teleological viewpoint, fractal morphogenesis offers an attractive way of generating complex structures which combine variability and order. The absence of a characteristic scale leads to interesting anatomic consequences perhaps best appreciated in the lung where detailed measurements of bronchial tube dimensions have been made by a number of previous investigators.

The classic model of the bronchial tree is that of WEIBEL and GOMEZ [12] who proposed an exponential fit to the data from the 20 plus generations of bronchial branchings in a normal human lung cast on which they had performed detailed morphometric measurements. Using the Weibel-Gomez numbering system, "generation one" is comprised of the left and right mainstem bronchi, "generation two" of the four daughter branches, and so forth. According to the exponential model, the mean bronchial diameter $\overline{d(z)}$ at the (z)th generation scales as $d(0)e^{-az}$ where a= (ln2)/3 and d(0) is the tracheal diameter. This single exponential, however, only successfully accounts for the scaling pattern of the mean bronchial diameters in the first 10 generations [Fig. 1A]. After generation 10, there is a systematic deviation of the data points away from the exponential regression line, a discrepancy Weibel and Gomez attributed to a change in the nature of airway conduction as one advances to progressively smaller tubes [12].

A new model of scaling in the bronchial tree is suggested by the fractal concept [6,9]. If the lung is indeed a fractal tree, then there should be no single characteristic scaling factor. Instead, bronchial dimensions should be governed by a multiplicity of different scales, each contributing with a different probability of occurrence. The mathematics underlying this scaling process is provided by renormalization group theory and leads to the prediction that bronchial dimensions should follow a type of inverse power-law distribution rather than the exponential scaling relationship previously proposed [9]. In particular, the fractal (renormalization group) model of WEST, BHARGAVA, and GOLDBERGER [9] predicts a harmonically-modulated inverse power-law relationship:

$$\overline{d(z)} = [A_1 + A_2 \cos (2 \pi \ln z/\ln \lambda)]/z^{\mu}$$

where A_1, A_2, μ, and λ are independent parameters. The cosine term in the numerator leads to a harmonic modulation of the inverse power-law in the logarithm of generation number with a period of ln λ. When the data from Weibel and Gomez are replotted in a log-log format the observed scaling is consistent with this model [Fig. 1B]. Similarly, bronchial data from other mammalian species follow a remarkably similar pattern [9] [Fig. 1C].

The fractal (renormalization) model is of interest from several perspectives [3,6,9,10]. First, this model provides a new mechanism for biological variability: instead of a single characteristic scale, there are multiple contributing scales. Second, the fractal model gives some underlying order to the chaos of multiple tube sizes, an order which is reflected in the harmonically-modulated inverse power-law scaling. Third, this model is consistent with the notion that bronchial morphogenesis is a type of critical phenomenon evolving over time. Fourth, the fractal model affords a mechanism for generating highly complex and irregular structures based on a simple governing principle--self similarity--which should minimize constructional error.

A number of key questions remain unanswered and may serve as a focus for future nonlinear biological research [3,5,10,11,13]. How is this fractal scaling information encoded and processed? What are the functional consequences of this type of scaling for airflow down the fractal tubes toward the alveoli where gas exchange actually occurs? What are the analogies between flow down the fractal lung tubes and flow in the fractal vascular network?

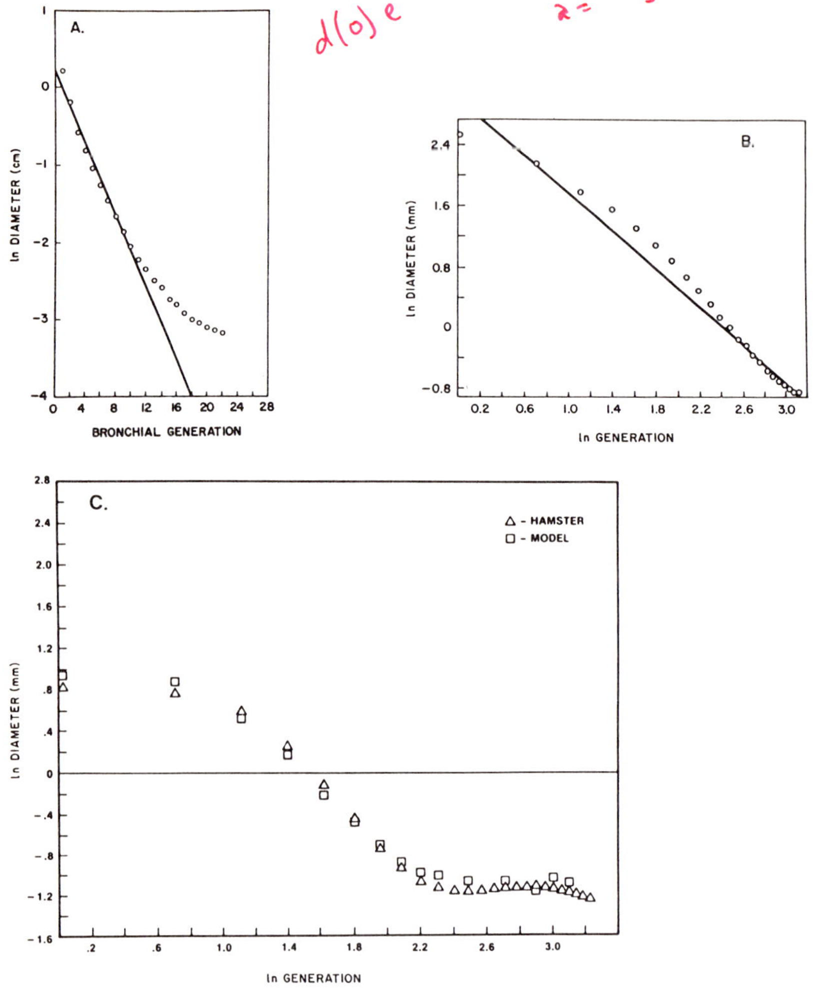

Fig. 1 Mean bronchial diameters for successive bronchial generations are traditionally assumed to follow exponential scaling. However when data [12] from a single human lung cast are plotted on a log-linear graph (A), systematic deviation of data points for higher bronchial generations is observed, where a straight line gives exponential fit for generations 1-10. Replotting the same data points on log-log graph (B), reveals an inverse power-law relationship with apparent harmonic modulation. This pattern is consistent with the prediction of renormalization group theory for a fractal morphogenetic process in which there is no single characteristic scale. Similar scaling is noted for hamster lung (C) with excellent fit between measurements and model. (Adapted from reference 9.)

We have also been interested in a related question of fractal structure-function relationships: namely, the implications of a fractal-like conduction network found in the heart [8] . Under normal circumstances cardiac electrical conduction is initiated by pacemaker cells in the sinus node. The impulse then spreads through the atria and down toward the AV node. Following depolarization of the AV node, the impulses spread rapidly down an irregular, but self-similar, branching network of fibers called the His-Purkinje system into the ventricles [Fig 2A]. Spread of current through the fractal His-Purkinje network, therefore, is the electrophysiological basis of stable ventricular activation [8].

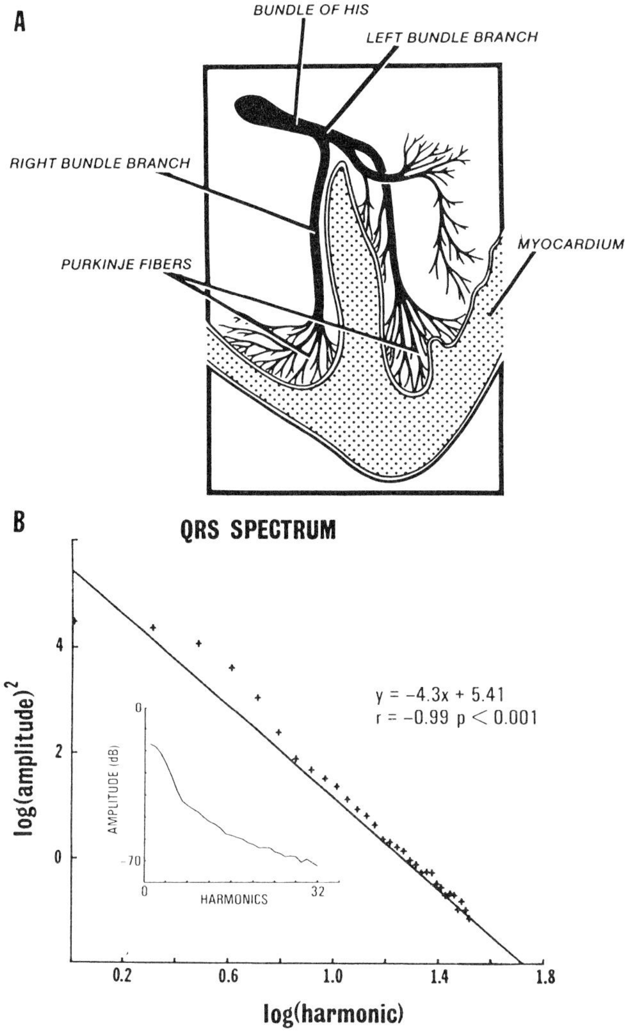

Fig. 2 Fractal conduction system (A) may serve as the anatomic substrate for the broadband inverse power-law spectrum of the normal ventricular depolarization waveform (QRS complex) of the electrocardiogram (B). Fundamental frequency = 7.8 Hz. (Adapted from reference 8.)

What are the dynamical consequences of this fractal depolarization process? One effect of this fractal conduction tree will be to shatter a cardiac impulse starting at the top of the tree into a myriad of stimuli [8]. These stimuli will not arrive at the myocardial interface simultaneously. Instead, owing to the irregular branching structure, the impulses will become decorrelated. However, because of the fractal nature of the process, this decorrelation cascade cannot be characterized by a single term. Instead, an infinite series of decorrelation rates should contribute to this process, each with a different probability or weighting, analogous to the reasoning underlying the multiplicity of scales in bronchial tree. In the case of fractal cardiac conduction, the renormalization procedure leads to the prediction that the voltage-time pulses which represent the output of the entire ventricular activation sequence should have an inverse power-law frequency spectrum. Spectral analysis of normal EKG waveforms representing ventricular depolarization (the QRS complex) does show this type of scaling pattern [Fig 2B]. We [8] have conjectured, therefore, that the broadband spectrum of the ventricular depolarization waveform is related at least in part to the fractal conduction system and that fractal dynamics may be an important mechanism underlying cardiac electrical stability.

In the heart, fractal scaling is not limited to the ventricular conduction system. The coronary arterial network is a self-similar branching tree. In addition, the mitral and tricuspid valves are anchored to the underlying ventricular muscle by fractal canopies referred to as the chordae tendineae.

Is there evidence for fractal dynamics elsewhere in physiological control systems? A marker of fractal scaling is a broadband spectrum with an inverse power-law distribution. Such spectra appear to be widespread in physiology [14-16]. For example, heart rate variability in healthy subjects is characterized by a 1/f-like spectrum [15]. Such spectra appear to reflect a kind of "constrained randomness" [5,17] necessary for physiological adaptiveness. That is to say, a "well-tuned" physiological system requires a wide repertory of frequency responses to cope with an unpredictable, changing environment. At the same time, there must be some structure or order to this physiological variability, reflected in the scaling patterns [18]. As a corollary, a variety of perturbations leads to a narrowing of this physiologically broadband spectrum. We have termed this frequency-narrowing phenomenon the loss of spectral reserve [3,5]. In the case of the most severe pathologies, loss of spectral reserve may manifest itself in at least two major ways: by a virtually complete loss of variability or by the emergence of a relatively low frequency oscillation which appears to "slave" the entire system such that the system becomes dominated by one major mode [18,19].

We are currently studying these pathological patterns through the analysis of heart rate data from subjects with severe congestive heart failure at the Arrhythmia Laboratory of Boston's Beth Israel Hospital, Harvard Medical School [20]. Figure 3 contrasts a normal heart rate time series and its associated broadband, 1/f-like power spectrum with data from two patients with severe heart failure. The striking loss of variability (panel A) observed at times in these patients may be related to impaired autonomic function [21-23] observed in the setting of advanced cardiac decompensation. The relatively low frequency (about 0.02 Hz) oscillations at other times (panel B) are congruent in frequency with the periodic breathing pattern observed in this setting (Cheyne-Stokes respirations) [18]. Detection of such loss of variability and pathological periodicities in heart rate time series may provide a new means of monitoring patients at high risk of sudden death before the onset of fatal cardiac dysrhythmias, including ventricular fibrillation [3,5,18].

3. The Nature of Fibrillation: Order vs Chaos

By appearance, the fibrillating heart with its agonal, squirming gyrations appears completely erratic. Indeed, as mentioned earlier, the prevailing viewpoint is that fibrillation is a chaotic or turbulent process [1,2]. The surface EKG during fibrillation seems to confirm this impression by showing apparently chaotic oscillations. The hypothesis that fibrillation represents nonlinear chaos has been formally proposed [2]. As noted, a countervailing hypothesis has also been advanced [4]: namely, that fibrillation is not chaos, but rather represents another type of pathological periodicity (or periodicities). This viewpoint is supported by several lines of evidence:

1. Power spectrum analysis of epicardial and body surface EKG recordings (Fig. 4) during ventricular fibrillation from animals and man reveals a narrowband rather than a broadband pattern [4,24,25]. Furthermore, with time this spectrum may become even narrower [24,25]. Autocorrelation studies of atrial fibrillation have revealed similar patterns [26].

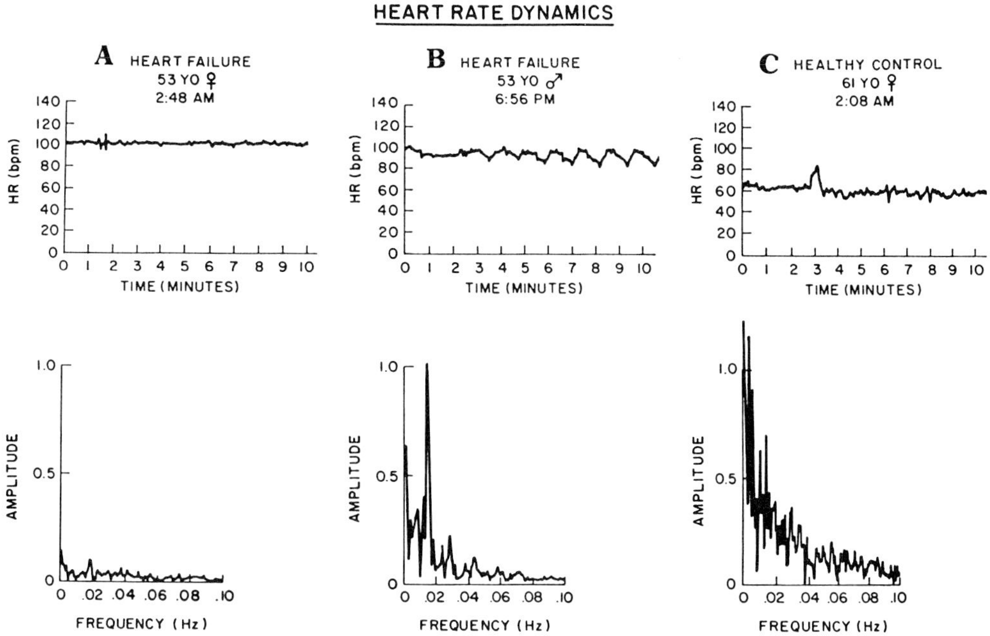

Fig. 3 Patients with severe heart failure (panels A and B) may show a striking alteration in the normal heart rate variability which is characterized by a physiological 1/f-like spectrum (panel C). Pathological dynamics in congestive heart failure may be associated with a marked reduction in variability (A) and at other times with relatively low frequency fluctuations which "slave" the system (B). These oscillations at about 0.02 Hz correlate with Cheyne-Stokes breathing patterns. These time series were processed with an algorithm designed to filter out non-sinus beats (extrasystoles). HR (bpm)= heart rate in beats/min.

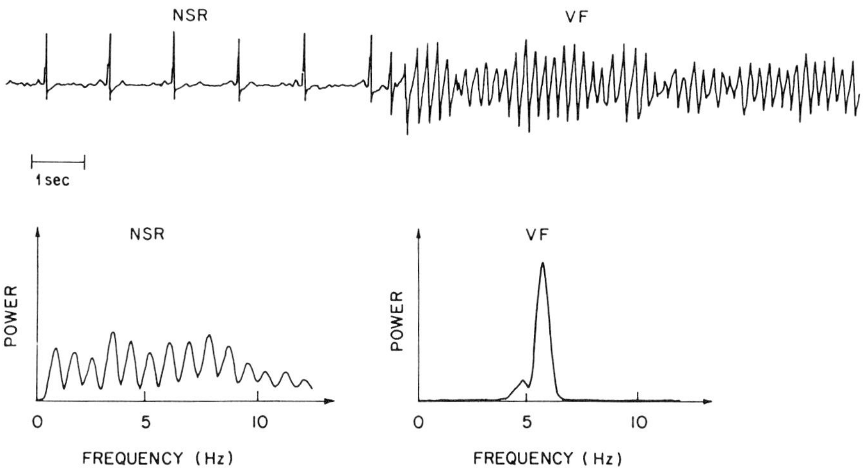

Fig. 4 Transition from normal sinus rhythm (NSR) to ventricular fibrillation (VF) is associated with a bifurcation from a process with a broadband spectrum to one with a narrowband pattern (inverse bifurcation). Amplitude is in arbitrary units. (Adapted from Nygards and Hulting, reference 24.)

2. Epicardial mapping studies during the onset of canine ventricular fibrillation have shown unexpectedly periodic, organized wave-fronts [27].

3. Endocardial recordings during ventricular fibrillation have shown a highly regular, monotonous pattern of activation [28].

While these findings do not address the underlying mechanism of ventricular fibrillation, they do suggest some type of relatively organized, periodic process(es) rather than the chaotic dynamics generally believed to occur [1,2]. Highly periodic behavior is also characteristic of a related type of potentially fatal ventricular dysrhythmia called torsades de pointes [29]. An intriguing possibility is that these lethal arrhythmias may be related to a spiral type wave mechanism of the kind suggested by KRINSKY [30] and by WINFREE and STROGATZ [31]. Better understanding of life-threatening electrical disturbances may suggest novel ways of preventing or interrupting them using pharmacological or other techniques.

4. Nonlinear Pharmacology

The effects of drugs on the frequency response of different systems is of considerable interest. If pathology is marked in a wide class of disturbances by a narrowing of the frequency response of the system, then successful pharmacological intervention should broaden this response and, ideally, restore the scaling associated with physiological dynamics. Digitalis is of considerable interest in this regard in light of data showing an increase in heart rate variability in atrial fibrillation after therapeutic doses of digitalis [32]. Toxic doses of digitalis, in contrast, may lead to highly periodic cardiac electrical behavior evidenced by regularization of the ventricular rate, bigeminal patterns or by so-called bidirectional ventricular tachycardia. Other drugs such as atropine, a parasympathetic blocking agent, may also narrow the frequency response of the cardiovascular system [33].

5. Epilog: Order, Reorder, and Disorder in Physiology

A wide class of pathologies is characterized by increased order (excessive mode-locking) rather than chaos. Pathological periodicities, rather than being noteworthy curiosities (34) may be more the rule than the exception. Such pathologies represent a reordering rather than a disordering. In contrast, physiological function appears to be characterized under normal circumstances by a constrained type of randomness which may be related to fractal structure/function interactions and which is represented by broadband, inverse power-law spectra. In physiology, therefore, the (1/f-like) "noise" may be the "signal" (Fig. 3, panel C) and successful pharmacological therapy in certain circumstances may relate to prevention of excessive mode-locking and the restoration of spectral reserve. The detection of pathological periodicities and the loss variability may also offer new approaches to designing early warning monitoring systems (3,16) and suggest new ways of assessing pharmacological interventions.

Acknowledgement

This work was supported by a grant from NASA-AMES Research Center, Moffett Field, California.

References

1. G.R. Moe, W.C. Reinboldt, J.A. Abildskov: Am. Heart J. 67, 200 (1964)
2. J.M. Smith, R.J. Cohen: Proc. Natl. Acad. Sci. USA. 81,233 (1984)
3. A.L. Goldberger, B.J. West, V. Bhargava: In Proc. 11th IMACS World Congress Oslo, Norway, ed. by B. Walstrom, R. Henriksen, N.P. Sundby, Vol.2 (North-Holland Publishing Company 1985). p.239

4. A.L. Goldberger, V. Bhargava, B.J. West, A.J. Mandell. Physica 19D, 282 (1986)
5. A.L. Goldberger, B.J. West: Ann. N.Y. Acad. Sci. In press.
6. B.B. Mandelbrot: The Fractal Geometry of Nature (W.H. Freeman and Company, New York 1982)
7. E.W. Montroll, M.F.Shlesinger: Proc. Natl. Acad. Sci. USA 79, 3380 (1983)
8. A.L. Goldberger, B.J. West: Biophys. J. 48, 525 (1985)
9. B.J. West, V. Bhargava, A.L. Goldberger: J. Appl. Physiol. 60, 1089 (1986)
10. B. West, A.L. Goldberger: Am. Scientist. In press.
11. J. Lefèvre: J. Theor. Biol. 102, 225 (1983)
12. E.R. Weibel, D.M. Gomez: Science 137, 577 (1962)
13. M. Sernetz, B. Gelléri, J. Hofmann: J. Theor. Biol. 117, 209 (1985)
14. T. Musha: In Proc. 6th Int. Conf. Noise in Physical Syst. (NBS Special Publ. 614, 1982) p. 143
15. M. Kobayashi, T. Musha; IEEE Trans. Biomed. Eng. 29, 456 (1982)
16. A.L. Goldberger, K. Kobalter, V. Bhargava: IEEE Trans. Biomed. Eng. 33, 874 (1986)
17. A.J. Mandell, S. Knapp, C.L. Ehlers, P.V. Russo: In Neurobiology of the Mood Disorders, ed. by R. M. Post, J.C. Ballenger (Williams & Wilkins, Baltimore MD, 1983)
18. A.L. Goldberger, L. Findley, M.J. Blackburn, A.J. Mandell: Am. Heart J. 107, 612 (1984)
19. H. Haken: Synergetics. (Springer-Verlag, New York, 1978)
20. G. Moody, J. Weinstein, A. Berman, R. Mark, W.R. Jarisch, R.C. Pasternak, A.L. Goldberger: Unpublished observations
21. D.L. Eckberg, M. Drabinsky, E. Braunwald: N. Engl. J. Med. 285, 877 (1971)
22. G.S. Francis, S.R. Goldsmith, S. Ziesche, H. Nakajima, J.N. Cohn: J.Am. Coll. Cardiol. 5, 832 (1985)
23. W.N. Leimbach, Jr., G. Wallin, R.G. Victor, et al.: Circulation 73, 913 (1986)
24. M.E. Nygards, J. Hulting: In Computers in Cardiology. (IEEE Computer Society, Long Beach, California, 1978) p.393
25. J.N. Herbschleb, R.M. Heethaar, I. van der Tweel, et al.: In Computers in Cardiology. (IEEE Computer Society, Long Beach, California 1979) p.49
26. E.J. Battersby: Circ. Res. 17, 296 (1965)
27. R.E. Ideker, G.J.Klein, L. Harrison, et al.: Circulation 63, 1371 (1981)
28. S.J. Worley, J.L. Swain, P.G. Colavita, et al.: Am. J. Cardiol. 55, 813, (1985)
29. V. Bhargava, A.L. Goldberger, D. Ward, S. Ahnve: IEEE Trans. Biomed. Eng. 33 894 (1986) In press
30. V.I. Krinsky: Pharm. Ther. 83, 539 (1978)
31. A.T. Winfree, S.H. Strogatz: Nature 311, 611 (1984)
32. B.K. Bootsma, A.J. Hoelen, J. Stackee, F.L. Meijler: Circulation 41, 738 (1970)
33. A.L. Goldberger, D. Goldwater, V. Bhargava: J. Appl. Physiol. In press
34. H.A. Reimann: Periodic Diseases (F.A. Davis, Philadelphia 1963)

Afterpotentials and Pacemaker Oscillations in an Ionic Model of Cardiac Purkinje Fibres

M.R. Guevara

Department of Physiology, McGill University, 3655 Drummond Street, Montreal, H3G 1Y6, Quebec, Canada

1. INTRODUCTION

Cardiac Purkinje fibres run along the inner surface of the ventricles of mammalian and avian hearts. These weakly contracting cells form the terminal part of the specialized electrical system that conducts the cardiac impulse from the point where it is generated (the sinoatrial node lying in the right atrium) to the working myocardium of the walls of the ventricles. When Purkinje fibres are removed from the heart, they are sometimes found to be spontaneously beating, othertimes not. Quiescent Purkinje fibres can be made to begin beating by a variety of interventions (e.g. by decreasing the K^+ concentration in the solution bathing the fibre [1]). Conversely, it is quite easy to abolish activity in a spontaneously beating Purkinje fibre (e.g. by elevating the external K^+ concentration).

When the normal periodic input to the ventricles from the sinoatrial node is removed, a subsidiary focus often emerges and takes over as pacemaker for the ventricles. This subsidiary pacemaker is often thought to be located in the Purkinje fibre network. The emergence of this subsidiary pacemaker can be life-preserving, since ventricular muscle does not usually beat on its own, and, without contraction of the ventricles, cardiac output falls to zero and life comes to an end. In fact, in the days before the invention of the artificial electronic pacemaker, many human beings owed their continued existence to the presence of such a subsidiary ventricular pacemaker. In contrast, abnormally enhanced automaticity in Purkinje fibres can lead to a life-threatening situation. This occurs when an abnormally located or "ectopic" ventricular focus begins to fire in competition with the normal input provided by the sinoatrial node to the ventricles. A premature ventricular beat falling at a critical phase of the sinoatrial cycle can provoke an episode of ventricular tachycardia or fibrillation [2]. The latter arrhythmia almost invariably results in death in human beings if not treated. Note however that ectopic activity can presumably result in benign ventricular parasystole; in addition, the extent to which malignant premature beats arise as a result of enhanced automaticity - in contrast to a reentrant mechanism - is presently unknown. It is thus important from a clinical point of view to understand how repetitive activity in individual cells of the Purkinje fibre network can be initiated or terminated. To this end, numerical simulations of an ionic model of cardiac Purkinje fibre were carried out on a digital computer. The findings described below are mentioned in passing in GUEVARA [3].

Numerical simulation of activity in a single Purkinje cell has the following practical advantages over experimental work: (i) once the model is implemented on the computer, it is more straightforward to carry out numerical experiments than animal experiments; (ii) parameters can be tuned more finely than in experimental work; (iii) drifts, fluctuations, and electrical membrane noise intrinsic to experimental work are not as pronounced in the numerical counterpart; (iv) the interpretation of experimental results obtained from strands of Purkinje fibre can be clouded by complicating effects due to propagation: it is only very recently that techniques for isolating and recording from single Purkinje cells have been perfected. In addition, the ionic mechanisms underlying particular behaviours can be investigated in the model. Finally, comparison of the output of a model with that of experiment can demonstrate where the model breaks down; such a comparison can also, at times, even suggest further experimental work.

The ionic model of Purkinje fibre studied is that of McALLISTER, NOBLE, and TSIEN [4], generally called the MNT model. There are nine different ionic currents incorporated in the MNT model. Ionic currents flow through specific channels in the cell membrane: in some channels, it is thought that a single ionic species (e.g. Na^+) flows through that channel; in other instances, a channel can be permeable to more than one species of ion. The flow of current through channels in the cell membrane - an insulating lipid bilayer - charges and discharges the capacitance of the cell, and so changes the transmembrane potential, V, which is habitually expressed in millivolts. The equations describing a given current are deduced from data obtained in voltage-clamp experiments, in which the transmembrane potential V is clamped to a fixed value using an electronic servomechanism and the current injected into the cell to maintain that voltage measured. In the MNT model, the value of a given current at a particular point in time t is determined by V(t) and, in most instances, by auxiliary variables called activation and inactivation variables. The MNT model is a ten-dimensional system of nonlinear ordinary differential equations: the variables are the transmembrane potential V and the activation and inactivation variables m, h, d, f, x_1, x_2, q, r, and s. Note that this model describes a patch of isopotential membrane - conduction does not occur.

2. NUMERICAL METHODS

Numerical integration was carried out in single precision (approximately 6.4-6.9 significant decimal digits) on a Hewlett-Packard computer (model 1000F), using an efficient variable-time-step algorithm, the convergence of which can be analytically proven [5]. The maximum change in the transmembrane potential ΔV allowed in iterating from time t to time $t+\Delta t$ was 0.4 mV. When a value of ΔV larger than this upper limit resulted, the integration time step Δt was successively halved and the calculations redone until ΔV was less than 0.4 mV. When ΔV was less than 0.2 mV, Δt was doubled for the following iteration. Allowing Δt to lie in the range 0.002 msec $\leqslant \Delta t \leqslant$ 8.192 msec permits ΔV to lie in the range 0.2 mV $\leqslant \Delta V \leqslant$ 0.4 mV. Under these conditions, the voltage waveform during spontaneous activity is within a few percent of that obtained using a very accurate Runge-Kutta fourth-order integration scheme employing a fixed Δt of 0.005 msec [5]. In advancing from time t to time $t+\Delta t$, the contribution of the membrane current to ΔV was calculated using the formula appearing in footnote (2) of VICTORRI et al. [5]. Initial conditions, unless otherwise stated, were as follows: V = -80.00 mV, m = 0.01946, h = 0.8591, d= 0.002089, f = 0.7725, x_1 = 0.02694, x_2 = 0.01986, q = 2.156 x 10^{-6}, r = 0.1190, and s = 0.7791. The initial value of Δt was 0.512 msec. L'Hôpital's rule was applied when necessary in calculating the rate constants α_m, α_d, α_q, and α_s as well as the current I_{K1}. We have used equations (25) and (26) rather than (27) and (28) of McALLISTER et al. [4] to describe α_r and β_r, and (16) rather than the equation appearing in Table 1A to describe α_f.

3. RESULTS

Figure 1 shows the transmembrane potential V as a function of time in the MNT model. Note that action potentials are spontaneously generated, indicating the

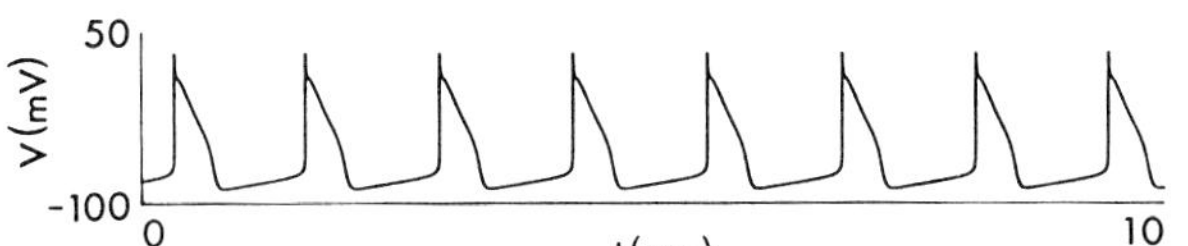

Fig. 1 Spontaneous activity in the MNT model. Initial conditions given in Methods

presence of a limit cycle in the phase space of the system. The other nine variables in the system (not shown) are, of course, also periodic in time. The initial conditions (see Methods above) were chosen so as to closely approximate a point on the limit cycle. The period of the oscillation or the time interval between action potentials ("interbeat interval") is about 1307 msec, and the action potential is several hundred milliseconds in duration, which is characteristic of ungulate Purkinje fibre. The waveform seen in response to decreasing the ranges of ΔV and Δt allowed by a factor of 10 is essentially superimposable with that shown in Fig. 1, with the interbeat interval decreasing slightly to 1304 msec.

The effect of changing, one at a time, many of the parameters appearing in the MNT equations was investigated. Spontaneous activity ceased in several instances when the parameter was altered so as to be sufficiently different from its normal value. Figure 2 shows an example, in which a constant hyperpolarizing bias current I_0 is injected into the cell. The polarity of the bias current is hyperpolarizing, in that it tends to hyperpolarize (i.e. make more negative) the transmembrane potential. As I_0 is increased, the interbeat interval gradually increases: at $I_0 = 3.3\ \mu A/cm^2$, the interbeat interval has increased from its normal value of 1307 msec to 2839 msec (Fig. 2A). As I_0 is increased beyond this point, the morphology of the waveform changes: subthreshold events or skipped beats (termed "delayed afterdepolarizations" in the cardiac electrophysiology literature [6]) begin to appear (Fig. 2B). As I_0 is increased still further the frequency of occurrence of these skipped beats relative to action potentials gradually increases (Figs. 2C-2E). Eventually, one sees a maintained subthreshold small-amplitude or "pacemaker" oscillation (Fig. 2F). Finally, if I_0 is

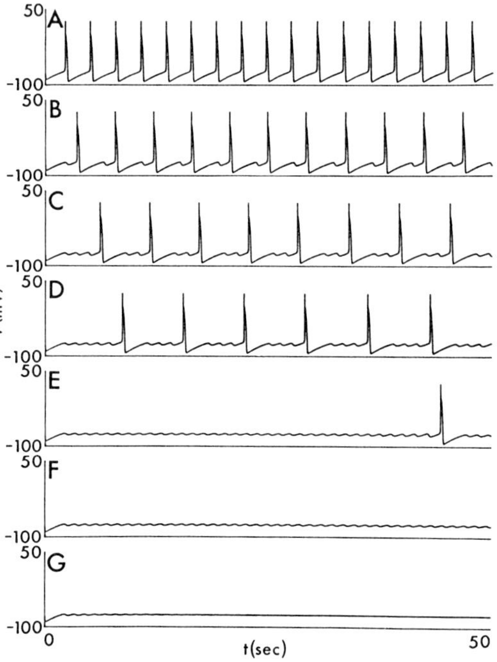

Fig. 2 The effect of injecting a constant hyperpolarizing current I_0 in the MNT model. I_0 ($\mu A/cm^2$) = 3.3 (A), 3.34 (B), 3.36 (C), 3.37 (D), 3.3785 (E), 3.3787 (F), 3.4 (G). Transients attributable to initial conditions can be seen in some traces. Note the appearance of skipped-beat runs in (B)-(E), a pacemaker oscillation in (F), and damped subthreshold oscillatory activity followed by quiescence in (G). Same initial conditions as in Fig. 1

increased sufficiently, one finds that all spontaneous activity is extinguished - the cell becomes quiescent (Fig. 2G). Note that when quiescence occurs, the membrane is still excitable: injection of a suprathreshold depolarizing current pulse results in an action potential. However, unlike the case in Figs. 2B-2E, the action potential is then followed by afterpotentials that decrement in amplitude, with a waveform very similar to that shown in Fig. 2G.

We refer to a cycle consisting of N action potentials followed by M skipped beats as an N_M cycle; a periodic pattern consisting of repeating N_M cycles will be called an $\{N_M\}$ pattern. We will use the symbol ρ to denote the number of action potentials divided by the sum of the number of action potentials plus the number of skipped beats. For a periodic $\{N_M\}$ pattern, $\rho = N/(N+M)$. The usual activity of the MNT model (Figs. 1,2A) is thus a $\{1_0\}$ pattern with $\rho = 1$. Figure 2 would seem to suggest that, as I_0 is increased, one sees simple $\{1_M\}$ patterns with increasing M until the $\{0_1\}$ pattern ($\rho = 0$) of a maintained pacemaker oscillation results (Fig. 2F). However, more complex periodic patterns consisting of combinations of 1_M cycles with differing M can also be seen. For example, a $\{1_0 \bullet 1_1\}$ pattern can be seen (Fig. 3A) at values of I_0 intermediate to those at which $\{1_0\}$ and $\{1_1\}$ patterns exist (Figs. 2A, 2B); this pattern can also be referred to as a $\{2_1\}$ pattern. Similarly, a $\{1_1 \bullet 1_2\}$ pattern can be observed (Fig. 3B) at values of I_0 intermediate to those at which $\{1_1\}$ and $\{1_2\}$ patterns occur (Figs. 2B, 2C). Note that a $\{1_1 \bullet 1_2\}$ pattern is not the same as a $\{2_3\}$ pattern, which would consist of repeating cycles each made up of two action potentials followed by three skipped beats. We have not seen such $\{N_M\}$ patterns with $N \neq 1$ as I_0 is increased in these simulations. However, they can be seen in the MNT model when other parameters are changed.

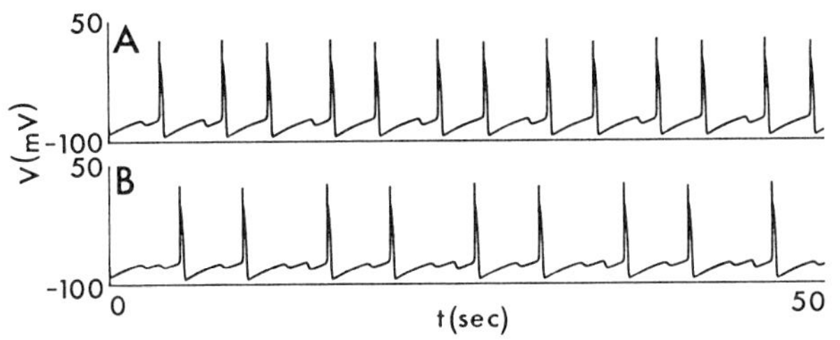

Fig. 3 Complex periodic patterns seen at values of I_0 intermediate to those used in Fig. 2: a $\{1_0 \bullet 1_1\}$ pattern (A), a $\{1_1 \bullet 1_2\}$ pattern (B). I_0 ($\mu A/cm^2$) = 3.338 (A), 3.358 (B). Same initial conditions as in Figs. 1 and 2

4. DISCUSSION

While there are several reports of skipped-beat runs in experimental work on Purkinje fibre (e.g. in response to changing the external K^+ concentration [1], during the recovery period following driving the fibre at a very rapid rate [7]), we are not aware of any reports showing the existence of a maintained small-amplitude subthreshold pacemaker oscillation. This fact fits in well with the modelling work detailed above, since the subthreshold oscillation is seen only over an exceedingly narrow range of the control parameter (Fig. 2F). More particularly, this finding in the model also suggests that it would be unlikely that the maintained subthreshold oscillation of Fig. 2F would be seen if the experiment of injecting a hyperpolarizing bias current into a spontaneously firing Purkinje fibre were to be actually carried out. However, in the presence of membrane voltage noise, $\{1_N\}$ patterns with N very large (e.g. Fig. 2E) might convert into a noisy $\{1_0\}$ pattern, thus effectively widening the range of I_0 over which $\{1_0\}$ pattern would be seen.

Patterns of activity similar to one or other of the $\{1_N\}$ patterns ($N \geq 1$) shown in Fig. 2 have been described in experiments on other spontaneously active cardiac tissues (e.g. the sinoatrial node [8], embryonic chick heart cell aggregates [9]).

A maintained pacemaker oscillation has also been described in both experimental [9] and modelling [10] work on heart cell aggregates. In fact, the entire sequence shown in Fig. 2 has recently been observed in experimental and modelling work on the sinoatrial node [11]. Skipped-beat runs can also be seen in other biological membrane-based oscillators (e.g. neuronal axons [12] and smooth muscle [13]). A sequence of patterns complementary to that shown in Fig. 2, in which the skipped beats ("early afterdepolarizations" [6]) are the result of abortive attempts at repolarization and not depolarization, can be seen in Purkinje fibre [6] and ventricular muscle [14], as well as in ionic models of both of these tissues [15-18]. It is not clear at the present time whether the sequence of patterns in these cases is strictly analogous to the sequence of patterns shown in Fig. 2.

Patterns of activity resembling those shown in Figs. 2 and 3 have been described in experimental [19-25] and modelling [21,23,26-31] studies on a number of chemical and physical systems; in fact, our notation $\{N_M\}$ is adapted from that used in some of these other studies [23,31,32]. In the majority of these instances, chaotic dynamics is said to exist. One of the features of chaotic dynamics is the appearance of deterministically aperiodic temporal patterns. In both experimental and modelling work on these other systems, chaotic dynamics can come about via a cascade of period-doubling bifurcations. Period-doubled patterns or irregular temporal patterns were not observed in the work described above, even when I_0 was changed in the sixth decimal place. However, the possibility that period-doubling bifurcations and chaotic dynamics might be seen if double-precision computation were to be used has not been ruled out. Should that be the case, the matter would be somewhat academic: it would be exceedingly unlikely that the corresponding behaviour would be found in experimental work, since it would be impossible to tune the value of I_0 sufficiently finely. In addition, there is significant voltage noise present in Purkinje fibre (~ hundreds of microvolts). It is of some interest to note that in a very recent experimental study of an oscillating chemical reaction, patterns of activity similar to those shown in Fig. 2 were seen, but with no evidence of period-doubling or chaotic behaviour [32]. This indicates that, at least at the present time, caution should be exercised in claiming that chaotic dynamics exists simply based on the fact that a sequence of patterns analogous to the one shown in Fig. 2 is seen [e.g. 17,18].

We have attempted to determine whether or not a description of the system in terms of a one-dimensional map could be made by plotting successive maxima of the waveforms of Fig. 2 as a function of the immediately preceding maximum, in a fashion similar to that carried out in other studies [19,22,24,25,27,30]. However, these maxima occur in our simulations only within two very narrow ranges of the transmembrane potential, one lying at about -75 mV, and the other at about +25 mV; maxima at intermediate values of V have not been encountered. Since there appear to be no saddle points in the phase space of the system in the range of bias current used in Fig. 2, one would expect that such data points should exist [33,34]. These data are absent in our numerical work probably as a result of the presence of a virtually all-or-none depolarization threshold in cardiac models such as the MNT that possess the fast sodium current [3,34]. Thus, a first-return map that is undefined over most of the range of transmembrane potential results. To determine a continuous first-return map would therefore involve carrying out computations at a much greater degree of precision than that presently available to us (see [35] for an analogous situation in a neural ionic model). Nevertheless, one can say at the present time that the return map must have at least one extremum, since a large-amplitude action potential is followed by a low-amplitude afterpotential, and consecutive afterpotentials increment in amplitude (Fig. 2).

We have not yet completely worked out the bifurcations responsible for producing the sequence of patterns shown in Fig. 2. However, as bias current is decreased, the small-amplitude subthreshold oscillation (Fig. 2F) appears to arise out of quiescence (Fig. 2G) via a Hopf bifurcation. The pattern shown in

Fig. 2E is suggestive of the presence of a homoclinic orbit [36-39]. We have not attempted to track down this orbit numerically. As the bias current is increased in Fig. 2, ρ gradually decreases from 1 to 0. One possibility consistent with our simulations is that the sequence shown in Fig. 2 is part of a periodic-quasiperiodic sequence, with all rational values of ρ ($0 \leqslant \rho \leqslant 1$) appearing and being maintained over an interval of the control parameter. Irrational values of ρ would then thoeretically - but, of course, not numerically - be found at isolated values of the bias current. In that case, saddle-node bifurcations of periodic orbits would be responsible for the appearance and disappearance of the periodic orbits corresponding to various $\{N_M\}$ skipped-beat patterns as the control parameter is increased. Periodic-quasiperiodic sequences have been described recently in heart cell aggregates periodically stimulated with a train of hyperpolarizing current pulses [3]. In the limit of the time interval between current pulses approaching the pulse duration, the case of periodic stimulation with a pulse train reduces to that of a constant bias current. Thus, it is not unreasonable to expect that, by continuity, the periodic-quasiperiodic sequence seen in response to periodic stimulation might be carried over into the case of injection of a constant current. However, the fact that the first-return map has at least one extremum is not consistent with the existence of the simple periodic-quasiperiodic sequence expected with invertible maps of the circle.

Alternatively, the period-doubling bifurcations and chaotic dynamics expected at intermediate pulse amplitudes in a periodically stimulated limit-cycle oscillator [3,40,41] might carry over into the case of a steadily applied stimulus. Analysis of the one-dimensional return maps resulting in these cases involving periodic stimulation [3,40-42] shows that two extrema exist: again by continuity, one would expect that the return map would also possess two extrema in the case where periodic stimulation is not applied. In fact, two-extremum maps have been found in at least two systems, not involving periodic stimulation, in which behaviour similar to that shown in Fig. 2 has been described [22,30,38]. Bistability is expected to exist in cases where return maps have two extrema [38,40,42]: we have not searched for evidence of bistability in Fig. 2. In some systems (periodically stimulated and not) homoclinic orbits [36-39] and cusp catastrophes [42] have been shown to be intimately involved in generating bistability, period-doubling bifurcations, and chaotic behaviour. However, the existence of these organizing features only emerges if one considers the dynamics as a function of two parameters [38-42]. It might be worthwhile to carry out such a two-parameter analysis for the MNT equations, changing some other parameter as well as the bias current.

We have not reported above upon the ionic basis of the behaviours shown in Figs. 2 and 3. However, the pacemaker oscillation of Fig. 2F is essentially due to two contributions: the time-dependent pacemaker current I_{K2} and the time-dependent ("background") currents. A small negative-slope steady-state ("window") contribution from either the fast sodium current (I_{Na}) or the slow inward current (I_{si}) is also necessary. However, the MNT model is very close to the point where a pacemaker oscillation would occur in the absence of both I_{Na} and I_{si}. In fact, slight modification of either I_{K2} or the background currents in the MNT model can lead to a situation where the pacemaker oscillation arises in a two-dimensional model consisting only of the pacemaker and background currents (variables V and s). In that case, it is quite easy to show that the pacemaker oscillation arises out of quiescence via a Hopf bifurcation as the bias current is decreased. The existence of a pacemaker oscillation has also been documented in numerical simulations carried out on a reduced two-dimensional model of ventricular heart cell aggregates [10]. A damped oscillation similar to that shown in Fig. 2G was seen in early experimental work on Purkinje fibre [43]; it can also be seen in the reduced Purkinje fibre model. Note that one does not have to invoke the existence of the oscillatory current I_{ti} [44] to account for the presence of such oscillatory behaviour in the pacemaker range of potentials. It is simply accounted for by the presence of the pacemaker and background currents and is due to the existence of an equilibrium point in the pacemaker range of potentials that posesses a pair of complex eigenvalues with negative real parts.

The MNT model - which is now more than a decade old - is presently becoming replaced by other models of Purkinje fibre incorporating more recent experimental results [e.g. 45]. In particular, the pacemaker current I_{K2}, activated upon depolarization, has been re-interpreted as a hyperpolarization-activated current, I_f [46]. A simple algebraic argument shows that, insofar as the voltage waveform is concerned, identical activity is to be seen in models using either the I_{K2} or the I_f description [46]. However, more recent models also have changes in other currents. While we have seen behaviour similar to that shown in Fig. 2 in one of the replacements of the MNT model [45], an investigation of the ionic basis of this behaviour is not yet complete.

As mentioned earlier, automaticity in the Purkinje network can be either life-sustaining or life-threatening: a subsidiary pacemaker can ensure that the ventricles continue to be paced at a rate sufficiently fast to maintain life when the normal input to the ventricles fails; an ectopic ventricular focus can generate a premature contraction that initiates a terminal episode of ventricular fibrillation. The modelling work described above indicates that the way in which a fully-established rhythm (Fig. 2A) arises out of quiescence (Fig. 2G) is not abrupt, but involves a complex sequence of temporal patterns (only a few of which are shown in Figs. 2 and 3). In particular, Figs. 2D and 2E provide a novel mechanism for the production of very long interbeat intervals, and indicate that such long intervals might not necessarily be a manifestation of periodic exit block out of a parasystolic focus, as is generally assumed. Finally, we wish to stress once again that determination of the complete sequence of bifurcations (part of which is shown in Figs. 2 and 3) remains an open problem; indeed, experimental confirmation of even the partial sequence predicted to exist in Fig. 2 is yet to be made in Purkinje fibre.

5. ACKNOWLEDGEMENTS

The author wishes to thank J. Bélair, L.N. Bouman, J.R. Clay, L. Glass, J. Grasman, H.J. Jongsma, A. Shrier, and A. van Ginneken for helpful discussions, Sandra James and Christine Pamplin for typing the manuscript, Robert Lamarche for photographing the figures, and the Canadian Heart Foundation and the Natural Sciences and Engineering Research Council of Canada for fellowship support during the time this work was carried out. Supported in part by a grant from the Medical Research Council of Canada.

REFERENCES

1. M. Vassale: Am. J. Physiol. 208, 770 (1965)
2. F.H. Smirk: Br. Heart J. 11, 23 (1949)
3. M.R. Guevara: Chaotic Cardiac Dynamics, Ph.D. Thesis (McGill University, Montreal 1984)
4. R.E. McAllister, D. Noble, R.W. Tsien: J. Physiol. (Lond.) 251, 1 (1975)
5. B. Victorri, A. Vinet, F.A. Roberge, J.-P. Drouhard: Comp. Biomed. Res. 18, 10 (1985)
6. P.F. Cranefield: Circ. Res. 41, 415 (1977)
7. R.L. Vick: Am. J. Physiol. 217, 451 (1969)
8. E. Bozler: Am. J. Physiol. 138, 273 (1943)
9. T.F. McDonald, H.G. Sachs: Pflüg. Arch. 354, 165 (1975)
10. J.R. Clay, A. Shrier: unpublished
11. M.R. Guevara, T. Op't Hof, H.J. Jongsma: unpublished
12. R. Guttman, R. Barnhill: J. Gen. Physiol. 55, 104 (1970)
13. J.A. Connor, C.L. Prosser, W.A. Weems: J. Physiol. (Lond.) 240, 671 (1974)
14. K. Matsuda, T. Hoshi, S. Kameyama: Jap. J. Physiol. 9, 419 (1959)
15. Y.M. Kokoz, V.I. Krinskii, O.A. Mornev: Biophysics 19, 502 (1974)
16. A. Coulombe, E. Coraboeuf, E. Deroubaix: J. Physiol. (Paris) 76, 107 (1980)
17. T.R. Chay, Y.S. Lee: Biophys. J. 45, 841 (1984)
18. T.R. Chay, Y.S. Lee: Biophys. J. 47, 641 (1985)

19. L.F. Olsen, H. Degn: Nature (Lond.) 267, 177 (1977)
20. R.A. Schmitz, K.R. Graziani, J.L. Hudson: J. Chem. Phys. 67, 3040 (1977)
21. O.E. Rössler, K. Wegmann: Nature (Lond.), 271, 89 (1978)
22. A.S. Pikovsky, M.I. Rabinovich: Physica 2D, 8 (1981)
23. J.S. Turner, J.-C. Roux, W.D. McCormick, H.L. Swinney: Phys. Lett. 85A, 9 (1981)
24. R.H. Simoyi, A. Wolf, H.L. Swinney: Phys. Rev. Lett. 49, 245 (1982)
25. J.-C. Roux, R.H. Simoyi, H.L. Swinney: Physica 8D, 257 (1983)
26. O.E. Rössler: Z. Naturforsch. 31a, 1168 (1976).
27. A.S. Pikovskii, M.I. Rabinovich: Sov. Phys. Dokl. 213, 183 (1978)
28. J.J. Tyson: J. Math. Biol. 5, 351 (1978)
29. K. Tomita, I. Tsuda: Phys. Lett. 71A, 489 (1979)
30. A.S. Pikovsky: Phys. Lett. 85A, 13 (1981)
31. R. Lozi: C. R. Acad. Sc. Paris, 294, 21 (1982)
32. J. Maselko, H.L. Swinney: Physica Scripta T9, 35 (1985)
33. R. FitzHugh: J. Gen. Physiol. 43, 867 (1960)
34. J.R. Clay, M.R. Guevara, A. Shrier: Biophys. J. 45, 699 (1984)
35. J.R. Clay: J. theor. Biol. 64, 671 (1977)
36. L.P. Sil'nikov: Math. USSR Sbornik 10, 91 (1970)
37. A. Arnéodo, P. Coullet, C. Tresser: J. Stat. Phys. 27, 171 (1982)
38. P. Gaspard, R. Kapral, G. Nicolis: J. Stat. Phys. 35, 697 (1984)
39. P. Glendinning, C. Sparrow: J. Stat. Phys. 35, 645 (1984)
40. L. Glass, M.R. Guevara, J. Belair, A. Shrier: Phys. Rev. 29A, 1348 (1984)
41. M.R. Guevara, L. Glass: J. Math. Biol. 14, 1 (1982)
42. M. Schell, S. Fraser, R. Kapral: Phys. Rev. 28A, 373 (1983)
43. W. Trautwein, D.G. Kassebaum: J. Gen. Physiol. 45, 317 (1961)
44. M. Vassale, A. Mugelli: Cir. Res. 48, 618 (1981)
45. D. DiFrancesco, D. Noble: Phil. Trans. Roy. Soc. Lond. 307B, 353 (1985)
46. D. DiFrancesco: J. Physiol. (Lond.) 314, 359 (1981)

Causes of Propagation Failure in Excitable Media

J.P. Keener

Department of Mathematics, University of Utah,
Salt Lake City, UT 84112, USA

§1. Introduction

In the cardiac conduction system, temporal order is related to spatial order and temporal disorder may very well be due to spatial disorder. For example, the normal heartbeat is initiated by a wave of excitation generated by the SA node which propagates across the atrium, through the AV node, down the His-Purkinje system and finally across the ventricles. However, if there is some disruption of the way action potentials propagate, it is possible that the normal sequence of events can change and lead to a disorder of the EKG, that is, to a temporal disorder.

One of the principal forms of spatial disorder is propagation failure. As is well known, propagation failure in the cardiac conduction system can be disastrous. For example, conduction failure in the SA node or Purkinje network has direct physical consequences, and it is also believed that propagation failure in the myocardium plays an important role in the initiation of fibrillation [4].

Propagation failure occurs in two ways as either geometric block or functional block. Geometric block is a permanent condition of the conducting medium that disallows propagation, whereas functional block occurs when the dynamic state of the medium causes propagation to fail although a fully recovered medium would allow normal propagation. From the viewpoint of clinical diagnosis, functional blocks are much more difficult to detect, since they depend on dynamic, rather than static, properties of the medium.

In this paper we give a summary of the mathematical analysis of the problem of propagation failure. The majority of results relate to geometric block, because, quite simply, it is an easier problem to study than functional block. We will discuss propagation failure due to weak coupling between cells, slight inhomogeneities in a weakly conducting fiber, and rapid spatial changes in physical properties such as cable diameter or recovery properties. Included in our discussion will be aspects of the cause of one-way block and functional block.

Our study is based on the FitzHugh-Nagumo equations [11,25] for propagation in excitable media, and their simplifications. We find these model equations to be acceptable because they give excellent qualitative agreement with cardiac conduction properties, and, in all honesty, more complicated and realistic equations, [2, 12, 21, 26, 33] are much too difficult to analyse at present. In fact, it is already a formidable task to obtain reliable numerical computations for these models [15].

Our starting point, then, is the system of equations

$$\frac{\partial u}{\partial t} = \nabla\cdot(D\nabla u) + f(u,v)$$

$$\frac{\partial v}{\partial t} = \varepsilon\, g(u,v). \tag{1.1}$$

The variable u represents the voltage potential, v represents a recovery variable, and ε is a small positive number, indicating that recovery processes are much slower than excitation. The function $f(u,v)$ is the typical "cubic" function. That is, there are numbers v_* and v^* so that for each v with $v_* < v < v^*$ there are three solutions of $f(u,v) = 0$ while for $v > v^*$ or $v < v_*$, there is only one solution of $f(u,v) = 0$. The isocline $g(u,v) = 0$ has a unique intersection (usually taken to be $(u,v) = (0,0)$ with $f(u,v) = 0$. The function $f(u,v)$ is negative above and positive below the isocline $f(u,v) = 0$ and the function $g(u,v) = 0$ is negative above and positive below the isocline $g(u,v) = 0$. Typical examples of f and g are

$$f(u,v) = u(1-u)(u-\alpha) - v \qquad 0 < \alpha < 1/2$$
$$g(u,v) = u-v, \tag{1.2}$$

although we will use these only for illustrative purposes.

We identify the smallest solution $u = u_-(v)$ of $f(u,v) = 0$ as the recovered, or polarized, state and the largest solution $u = u_+(v)$ of $f(u,v) = 0$ as the excited state. In order that the medium be excitable, we require that $\int_{u_-}^{u_+} f(u,v)du > 0$ when v is at rest. By a wave of excitation we mean a front that changes the value of u from $u = u_-(v)$ to $u = u_+(v)$ as the front passes a point in space.

To study propagation of waves of excitation we will assume that, since $0 < \varepsilon \ll 1$, the recovery variable v does not change substantially during excitation and therefore, for most of this paper, we shall be interested in the simplified equation

$$\frac{\partial u}{\partial t} = \nabla\cdot(D\nabla u) + f(u,v_0) \tag{1.3}$$

with v_0 a constant.

§2. Weak Coupling

An excitable medium, such as myocardium, is not really a continuous medium, but rather it is a massive array of discrete coupled cells. The usual model for studying propagation in a uniform one-dimensional continuous medium is the Nagumo equation

$$\frac{\partial u}{\partial t} = D\frac{\partial^2 u}{\partial x^2} + f(u). \tag{2.1}$$

One derivation of equation (2.1) is to assume that there is a large array of linearly coupled cells, and the potential of the nth cell, assumed to be at equipotential, satisfies

$$\frac{du_n}{dt} = d(u_{n+1} - 2u_n + u_{n-1}) + f(u_n) \tag{2.2}$$

where d is the intercellular resistance, u_n is the potential of the nth cell in a doubly infinite string of cells. To get equation (2.1) from (2.2), one takes $u_n = u(x+n\Delta x)$, $D = d(\Delta x)^2$ and then lets Δx go to zero. Of course, since cells are discrete, the approximation $\Delta x \to 0$ need not be valid and, as we shall see, leads to erroneous conclusions.

The equation (2.1) supports propagation for all values of $D > 0$. We suppose that $f(u)$ has the typical "cubic" structure, that is,

$$f(0) = f(\alpha) = f(1) = 0 \qquad 0 < \alpha < 1$$

with $f'(0) < 0$, $f'(1) < 0$, $f'(\alpha) > 0$ and $f(u)$ is nonzero elsewhere. It is well known [1,9] that (2.1) has stable traveling wave solutions of the form

$$u(x,t) = U_0\left(\frac{x - c_0\sqrt{D}t}{\sqrt{D}}\right) \tag{2.3}$$

where U_0 satisfies the nonlinear eigenvalue problem

$$U_0'' + c_0 U_0' + f(u_0) = 0, \tag{2.4}$$

with $\lim_{x\to\infty} U_0(x) = 1$, $\lim_{x\to-\infty} U_0(x) = 0$. The value c_0 is uniquely determined and has the opposite sign of $\int_0^1 f(u)du$.

The same is not true for equation (2.2). That is, for all $d > 0$, there need not be a traveling (translation invariant) solution. Indeed, for $d > 0$ sufficiently small, no initial data can lead to propagation, and there are an infinite number of stable, standing solutions which block propagation.

Theorem [18]: Suppose $f(x)$ is continuously differentiable for $0 \le x \le 1$ and $f(0) = f(\alpha) = f(1) = 0$. Suppose there are values $\hat{x}_0$, $\hat{x}_1$ so that

$$2(\hat{x}_0 - 1) - f(\hat{x}_0)/d = 0 \qquad \text{i)}$$

$$2\hat{x}_1 - f(\hat{x}_1)/d = 0 \qquad \text{ii)}$$

$$f'(x) < 2d \quad \text{on} \quad 0 \le x \le \hat{x}_0, \quad \hat{x}_1 \le x \le 1. \qquad \text{iii)}$$

To every doubly infinite sequence $\{s_n\}$ with $s_n \varepsilon \{0,1\}$ there corresponds at least one stable steady solution of (2.2) with $u_n \varepsilon [0,\alpha)$ when $s_n = 0$ and $u_n \varepsilon (\alpha,1]$ when $s_n = 1$.

In addition, let $\bar{x}_0$, $\bar{x}_1$ be such that

$$2(\bar{x}_0 - 1) - f(\bar{x}_0)/d = 0, \quad 2\bar{x}_1 - f(\bar{x}_1)/d = 0 \qquad \text{iv)}$$

$$f(x)/d - 2(x-1) < 0 \quad \text{for} \quad \hat{x}_0 < x < \bar{x}_0$$

$$f(x)/d - 2x > 0 \quad \text{for} \quad \bar{x}_1 < x < \hat{x}_1 . \qquad \text{v)}$$

If $u_k \varepsilon [0,\bar{x}_0)$ at $t = 0$ for some k, then $u_k(t) \varepsilon [0,\bar{x}_0)$ for all $t \ge 0$, and if $u_k \varepsilon (\bar{x}_1,1]$ at $t = 0$ for some k, then $u_k(t) \varepsilon (\bar{x}_1,1]$ for all $t \ge 0$.

In simple words, if d is small enough, there are an infinite number of stable standing solutions of (2.2) and propagation is impossible. The proof of this theorem makes use of a theorem of Moser [24] on maps of the plane and simple comparison arguments for differential equations, and is given in detail in [18].

§3. Weak Inhomogeneity in Weakly Propagating Medium

The invariant solutions of (2.1) have $c_0 = 0$ if $\int_0^1 f(u)du = 0$, and if $\int_0^1 f(u)du$ is small then the medium is only weakly propagating. We inquire if inhomogeneities can cause propagation failure in a weakly propagating medium. For an inhomogeneous axonal cable, the equation (2.1) takes the form [30]

$$\frac{\partial u}{\partial t} = \frac{1}{2r}\frac{\partial}{\partial x}\left(\frac{r^2}{R}\frac{\partial u}{\partial x}\right) + f(u,x) \tag{3.1}$$

where r is the radius of the cable, R is the resistance (in ohm-cm) of the intracellular medium and $f(u,x)$ is the ionic current per unit area of the membrane at position x. For example, we could have weak variations in cable radius r, resistivity R, or ionic currents.

We seek a standing solution of equation (3.1) with weak inhomogeneities. If a standing solution exists, then comparison arguments preclude the possibility of propagation [1]. Upon setting $\frac{\partial u}{\partial t} = 0$ and making the change of spatial variable $x = (r_\infty/R_\infty)^{1/2}\xi$, where $r_\infty = \lim_{x\to\infty} r$, $R_\infty = \lim_{x\to\infty} R$, we have the equation

$$0 = \frac{\partial}{\partial \xi}\left(\frac{R_\infty}{R}\frac{r^2}{r_\infty^2}\frac{\partial u}{\partial \xi}\right) + 2\frac{r}{r_\infty} f(u,\xi). \tag{3.2}$$

We suppose that $\frac{2r}{r_\infty} f(u,\xi) = f_0(u) + \varepsilon f_1(u,\xi)$ where $\int_0^1 f_0(u)du = 0$ and that $\frac{R_\infty}{R}\frac{r^2}{r_\infty^2} = 1 + \varepsilon p(x)$, with $0 < \varepsilon \ll 1$.

We use perturbation arguments to find a solution of (3.2) with $\lim_{\xi\to\infty} u(\xi) = 1$, $\lim_{\xi\to-\infty} u(\xi) = 0$. We seek a solution of the form

$$u(\xi,t) = U_0(\xi) + \varepsilon U_1(\xi) + \dots$$

and we must therefore require

$$U_0'' + f_0(U_0) = 0,$$

$$U_1'' + f_0'(U_0)U_1 + (p(\xi)U_0')' + f_1(U_0,\xi) = 0, \tag{3.3}$$

and so forth.

It is easy to show that U_0 exists. If we take ϕ_0 to satisfy $\phi_0'' + f_0(\phi_0) = 0$, $\lim_{\xi\to\infty}\phi_0(\xi) = 1$, $\lim_{\xi\to-\infty}\phi_0(\xi) = 0$, then $U_0(\xi) = \phi_0(\xi+\eta)$ for any fixed η. Next we observe [3] that $u_1'' + f_0'(U_0)u_1 = g(\xi)$ has a bounded solution if and only if $\int_0^1 g(x)U_0'(x)dx = 0$. Thus, to obtain a standing solution, we require

$$\int_{-\infty}^{\infty} [(p(\xi)U_0')' + f_1(U_0,\xi)]U_0'(\xi)d\xi = 0.$$

Shifting the ξ axis and integrating by parts, we require

$$\int_{-\infty}^{\infty} p'(\xi-\eta)F_0(\phi_0(\xi))d\xi = \int_{-\infty}^{\infty} f_1(\phi_0(\xi),\xi-\eta)\phi_0'(\xi)d\xi \tag{3.4}$$

for some η, where $F_0'(u) = f_0(u)$. In the special case that f_1 is independent of the spatial variable, we require

$$\int_{-\infty}^{\infty} p'(\xi-\eta)F_0(\phi(\xi))d\xi = \int_0^1 f_1(u)du. \tag{3.5}$$

This last expression requires some interpretation. For fixed functions $p(x)$, and $f_1(u,x)$, if a value η can be found so that (3.5) holds then propagation from right to left can be blocked. On the other hand if we replace $p(x)$ by $p(-x)$ and $f_1(u,x)$ by $f_1(u,-x)$ in (3.5) and find a value of η for which the revised version of (3.5) holds, then propagation from left to right can be blocked. If, however, for a given pair $p(x)$, $f_1(u,x)$, one, but not both, of these conditions hold, it suggests (but does not prove) that there is a one-way block in the medium.

From this analysis, what kinds of spatial inhomogeneities produce one-way block? In equation (3.5) we take $\int_0^1 f_1(u)du > 0$ so that the medium is excitable, if only weakly so. Since $f_0(u) = \frac{d}{du} F_0(u)$ and $\int_0^1 f_0(u)du = 0$ we have that $F_0(u) < 0$ on $0 < u < 1$. Thus, there can be block only if $p'(\xi)$ is somewhere sufficiently negative. One-way block occurs if $p'(\xi)$ is somewhere large and negative, but never particularly large positive. If this occurs, then fronts moving from right to left are blocked, but fronts moving from left to right are not. In terms of cable resistivity, this means that a rapid decrease in resistivity in the direction of proposed propagation may be responsible for block but rapid increases in resistivity do not cause block. Similarly, one can use (3.5) to show that rapid increases in the cable radius in the direction of proposed propagation may cause propagation failure, but rapid decreases in radius do not block propagation. Thus a rapid increase followed by gradual decrease in radius may produce one-way block. The reciprocal is true for resistivity, namely a rapid decrease of resistivity followed by a gradual increase may produce one-way block.

Block of waves due to rapid changes of cable radius or other cable properties have been studied numerically [13,14,22] and via phase plane arguments assuming the medium has piecewise constant properties [17,27,28]. The results of these studies give the same qualitative picture as that just given, namely, that assymmetrical increases in radius, and assymetrical decreases in resistivity, as well as other asymmetrical variations of local cell properties, can produce one way block.

§4. Rate Dependent Block

It is certainly more difficult to study functional block because of the necessity to include effects of recovery. In this section we will discuss a simplified model for propagation that exhibits one-way functional (rate dependent) block.

We suppose that we have a tube of excitable medium with uniform interior. Thus, we are thinking of a tubal collection of many axons, say, and we assume that propagation in the tube is governed by the equations (1.1) with D a constant using three-dimensional spatial gradients. We also rescale space and time by ε so that the tube is assumed long compared to the thickness of a typical front of excitation.

We idealize the wave front of excitation to be a two-dimensional surface moving through the three-dimensional tube, that is, we ignore the thickness of the wave front along the axial direction. Then, using singular perturbation arguments [19, 20] one can show that the normal velocity N of a wavefront is given by $N = c_0 - DK$ where c_0 is the velocity of a plane wave, K is the sum of principal curvatures of the wavefront, and D is the diffusion.

The velocity of plane wave propagation depends on how long the medium has been at rest. In particular, since excitable medium is always dispersive, (ie. waves of different period travel with different speed) we take c_0 to depend on T, the temporal period of the stimulus. Typically $c_0 = c_0(T)$ is an increasing function of period T with maximum $c^* = c_0(\infty)$ corresponding to the speed of a solitary pulse [7, 23, 29, 31, 32].

Next we suppose that, since we have a tubular medium, the wavefront propagates as a spherical surface which is always normal to the boundary of the tube. Thus, the radius of curvature of a wavefront is

$$R = \frac{r(x)}{r'(x)} \left(1+r'(x)^2\right)^{1/2}$$

and the curvature term K is

$$K = \frac{2r'(x)}{r(x)\left(1+r'^2(x)\right)^{1/2}}$$

where $r(x)$ is the radius of the tube at position x. It follows that the speed of propagation of this spherical wavefront is

$$\frac{dx}{dt} = c_0(T) - \frac{2Dr'(x)}{r(x)\left(1+r'^2(x)\right)^{1/2}} \qquad (4.1)$$

if propagation is from left to right and

$$\frac{dx}{dt} = -\left(c_0(T) + \frac{2Dr'(x)}{r(x)\left(1+r'^2(x)\right)^{1/2}}\right) \qquad (4.2)$$

if propagation is from right to left.

From this we see the potential for rate dependent block, and if $r(x)$ is not symmetric (ie $r(x) \neq r(\eta-x)$ for any fixed η) we see that rate dependent one way block may occur. For example, if

$$c^* = c_0(\infty) > \max_x \frac{2D|r'(x)|}{r(x)\left(1+r'^2(x)\right)^{1/2}}$$

solitary pulses traveling in either direction are not blocked. However, if $r(x)$ has a rapid increase and a gradual decrease, moving left to right, say, then a sufficient decrease of stimulus period T will reveal a block of right moving waves, while left moving waves of the same frequency are not blocked. Sufficient decrease of period may, however, induce propagation failure in both directions. For a known dispersion relation $c = c_0(T)$, the precise values of temporal period T for which one-way block and two-way block occur can be determined by setting $\frac{dx}{dt} = 0$ in equations (4.1) and (4.2).

Although this model of one-way functional block is simple to describe and understand, its main disadvantage is that it predicts "all or nothing" block while it is often the case that rate dependent blocks reveal a Wenckebach phenomena [16] and in some situations are hysteretic in the period T [6,10]. It is possible to rectify these shortcomings, but only with a significantly more complicated singular perturbation analysis which is beyond the scope of this presentation. A more detailed study of functional block will be presented in a forthcoming publication.

This research was supported in part by NSF grant 8601134.

1. E. G. Aronson, H. F. Weinberger: In Lecture Notes in Mathematics 446 5 (Springer, Berlin 1975)
2. G. E. Beeler, H. Reuter: J. Physiol. 268 177 (1977)
3. S. N. Chow, J. K. Hale, J. Mallet-Paret: J. Diff. Eqn. 37 351 (1980)
4. P. F. Cranefield, The Conduction of the Cardiac Impulse (Futura Publ., New York 1975)
5. P. F. Cranefield, H. O. Klein B. F. Hoffmann: Circ. Res. 28 199 (1971)
6. P. Denes, D. Wu, R. C. Dhingra, F. Mat-y-Leon, C. Wyndham, K. M. Rosen: Circ. 51 244 (1975)
7. J. D. Dockery, J. P. Keener, J. J. Tyson: (to appear)
8. N. El-Sherif, R. R. Hope, B. J. Scherlag, R. Lazzara: Circ. 55 702 (1977)
9. P. C. Fife, J. B. McLeod: Arch. Rat. Mech. Anal. 65 333 (1977)
10. C. Fisch, D. P. Zipes, P. L. McHenry: Circ. 48 714 (1973)
11. R. FitzHugh: Biophys. J. 1 445 (1961)
12. A. L. Hodgkin, A. F. Huxley: J. Physiol. 177 500 (1952)
13. R. W. Joyner: Biophys. J. 35 113 (1981)
14. R. W. Joyner, J. Picone, R. Veenstra, D. Rawling: Circ. Res. 53 526 (1983)
15. M. Kawato, A. Yamanaka, S. Urushibara: J. Theor. Biol. (to appaer)
16. J. P. Keener: J. Math. Biol. 12 215 (1981)
17. J. P. Keener: In Modelling of Patterns in Space and Time, ed. W. Jager and J. D. Murray (Springer, Berlin 1984)
18. J. P. Keener: SIAM J. Appl. Math. (to appear)
19. J. P. Keener: SIAM J. Appl. Math. (to appear)
20. J. P. Keener, J. J. Tyson: Physica D. (to appear)
21. R. E. McAllister, D. Noble, R. W. Tsien: J. Physiol. 251 1 (1975)
22. R. N. Miller: J. Math. Biol. 7 385 (1979)
23. R. N. Miller, J. Rinzel: Biophys. J. 34 227 (1981)
24. J. Moser: Stable and Random Motion in Dynamical Systems (Princeton University Press, Princeton 1973)
25. J. Nagumo, S. Arimoto, S. Yoshizawa: Proc. IRE 50 2061 (1962)
26. D. Noble, S. J. Noble: Proc. Roy. Soc. Lond. B 222 295 (1984)
27. J. Pauwelussen: J. Math. Biol. 15 151 (1982)
28. J. P. Pauwelussen: Physica 4D, 67088 (1981)
29. J. Peon, G. R. Ferrier, G. K. Moe: Circ. Res. 43 125 (1978)
30. W. Rall: N. Y. Acad. Sci. 96 1071 (1952)
31. J. Rinzel: In Nonlinear Diffusion, ed. by W. E. Fitzgibbon and H. F. Walker (Pitman, 1977)
32. M. S. Spach, P. C. Dolber: In Cardiac Electrophysiology and Arrhythmias, ed. by D. P. Zipes and J. Jalife, (Grune and Stratton 1984)
33. K. Yanagihara, A. Noma, H. Irisawa: Japanese J. Phys. 30 841 (1980)

Ultradian Oscillations in Human Blood Pressure: Effects of Age

L.A. Benton, S.J. Berry, and F.E. Yates

Crump Institute for Medical Engineering, 6417 Boelter Hall, University of California, Los Angeles, CA90024, USA

1. ABSTRACT

We postulated that normative aging is a progressive loss of dynamic stability that might manifest itself through spectral changes in cardiovascular processes. Using ambulatory monitoring we obtained 24 h time-series data on systolic pressure, diastolic pressure and heart rate in 13 subjects younger than 50 years and 25 subjects age 50 or older. All were in good health without history of cardiovascular disease. The two groups did not differ in heart rate or diastolic pressure with respect to means, variances, or power spectral profiles; but they differed significantly in systolic pressures. Overall, the old had higher 24 h mean systolic pressure than the young. In 15 of the old systolic pressures during sleep were at the same levels as those of the young during sleep, but in 10 it was approximately 25 mm Hg higher. We therefore subcategorized the old as sleep-normotensive systolic old (NTO) or sleep-elevated systolic old (ESO). In both subgroups systolic pressure during wakefulness was the same and averaged 15-20 mm Hg higher than that for the young. Although systolic 24 h variance was higher overall in the old than in the young, the NTO group provided most of that increase; their systolic pressure was low during sleep but elevated during wakefulness. Power spectral profiles showed that the variance of the systolic pressure spectrum of the young was evenly distributed over ultradian period ranges. In contrast, both subgroups of the old showed concentration of systolic variance at periods of approximately 40 min and 3 h. We concluded that with respect to systolic pressure dynamics, the two subgroups of old may represent different physiological states: those normotensive during sleep but with slightly elevated pressures during wakefulness may reveal a normative aging process; those with elevated systolic pressures during sleep as well as during the day may represent early stages of impending isolated systolic hypertension. In both cases the appearance of ultradian rhythms with periods of about 40 min and 3 h may be a manifestation of intrinsic aging, independent of disease.

2. INTRODUCTION

We assume that there is an intrinsic aging process, not itself a disease, that is part of the normal trajectory of human life, and that its chief macroscopic feature is progressive loss of dynamic stability. According to one interpretation of thermodynamic theory for open systems, stability of persistent systems involves multiple, near-periodic processes that are weakly coupled [1] [2] [3]. If such theory is applicable to the human cardiovascular system, normative aging might reveal itself by changes both in levels and in power spectral profiles of arterial pressure - the macroscopic thermodynamic potential that drives that physiological system.

3. METHODS

3.1 Subjects and Protocol

We carried out non-invasive ambulatory monitoring of blood pressure and heart rate in 38 subjects divided into two groups: (1) young - 8 men and 5 women, age 24 to 44 years; and (2) old - 13 men and 12 women, 50 to 95 years of age. All were healthy by self-report, without history of cardiovascular disease, and were active community dwellers of middle level socioeconomic background. All were Caucasian except for one black woman (age 65). None was significantly obese, but few engaged in regular, strenuous exercise. One (male, age 62) was a current cigarette smoker.

Subjects were monitored during their routine activities for 24 hours using an automatic recorder (Del Mar Avionics Pressurometer III, Model 1978) set to measure blood pressure (indirect method) and heart rate every 7.5 minutes. Measured values were stored in digital memory. The accuracy of the recorder was verified to be within 5 mm Hg of comparison readings by mercury sphygmomanometer before and after each monitoring session. Subjects annotated their activities and posture in a diary at 30-min intervals while awake. The diary was used to edit and to denote sleep and wake portions of the record.

3.2 Data Analysis

Data on blood pressures and heart rates were downloaded from the recorder using an Apple IIe microcomputer [4], then transferred to an IBM PC/AT for analyses. The record was edited by hand for missing values and measurements judged to be artifact because of noise and vibration accompanying arm movement, walking, and driving or riding in an automobile. Readings were rejected according to the following criteria: pulse pressure < 10 mm Hg; diastolic values higher than systolic; zero values; or isolated very high or low readings. Rejected data were replaced by linearly interpolated values across four or fewer consecutive samples. If editing was required across more than four samples, or if the record length was not 23-25 hours, the record was not accepted.

Values measured during nighttime sleep were flagged using the diary. Because sleep onset could not be determined exactly, the next measurement after a subject recorded "lights out" was marked as the beginning of sleep. End of sleep was marked as the value displayed on the monitor at morning awakening. Subjects were asked to note if they awoke during the night and arose from bed, but the sleep portion of record was defined to be the whole period from lights out to morning arising, whether or not it was interrupted. Daytime naps were noted, but not included as part of the "sleep" portion of record.

Quality of sleep could not be accurately assessed, but most subjects did not consider that the monitor had interfered with it. Some reported that they usually awoke during the night, usually to go to the toilet, and that they had arisen briefly during the monitoring night.

3.3 Outlier Criterion and Statistical Significance of Differences

To maintain the homogeneity of our cohorts, we did not accept the record of any subject whose 24 h mean systolic or diastolic pressures or heart rate were greater than three standard deviations from the cohort mean calculated after excluding his value. In all computations we did not regard any differences to be statistically significant values unless $p \leq 0.01$.

3.4 Spectral Analysis

We used standard Fourier analysis, dividing the spectrum into 11 bins (harmonic windows) - ten for ultradian (shorter than 24 hour) periods, plus one bin for the approximately "circadian" component. To highlight and separate components of the higher spectral frequencies from the larger amplitude lower ones, we developed a filter that divided the raw data into two domains: (1) "fast", for periodicities ranging from approximately 40-275 minutes; and (2) "slow", for periodicities from approximately 275-1440 minutes (one cycle/24 h). The filter operates on the Fourier transform of the raw data and uses a taper to reduce end-effects during spectral analysis. The approximately 24-hour record was padded to 32 hours by adding four fictional hours of data collection to the beginning and to the end of the real record. The padded values were assigned after calculating the mean of the first and last real data measurements; values then were faded up or down to that mean by straight line interpolation between the first and last real points.

Components of the Fourier transform of the padded data were calculated from number 1 (the mean) to number 7 (representing six cycles/24 hours) to generate a low-frequency component that served as a low pass filter for the original data. The low-frequency component carries the data mean and the circadian variation amplitude. We subtracted it from the original data to give a high pass residue which had zero mean value.

We calculated a power spectral density function (PSDF) separately for the high pass and the low pass extracts using the fast Fourier transform (FFT) and standard methods. Because we did not consider any supposed near-periodic variation as a possible oscillation unless it was sampled at least five times per putative cycle, the fastest periodicity we could have detected (sampling every 7.5 minutes) was one cycle per 38 minutes. We considered then only the spectrum between one cycle per 38 minutes and one cycle per 24 hours and divided those 50 Fourier coefficients into 11 bins.

4. RESULTS

4.1 Blood Pressures and Heart Rate in the Young

Figure 1 shows a typical 24 hour ambulatory monitoring record of the three primary variables from a 33-year old woman. Table 1 (top) presents the average values ($\pm$S.D.) of five aspects of each of those variables for all 13 young subjects. The blood pressures and heart rates of the young were lower during sleep than during wakefulness ($p < 0.01$). The 24 h "circadian" rhythm is conveyed both by the difference between the means during sleep and wakefulness and by the amplitude of the low-frequency extract. The fraction of the total, 24 h variance that was accounted for by low-frequency variations was nearly the same for all three variables.

4.2 Blood Pressures and Heart Rates in the Old

Data from the 25 subjects aged 50-95 years are shown in Table 1 (bottom). Systolic pressures of the old during sleep were significantly lower than during

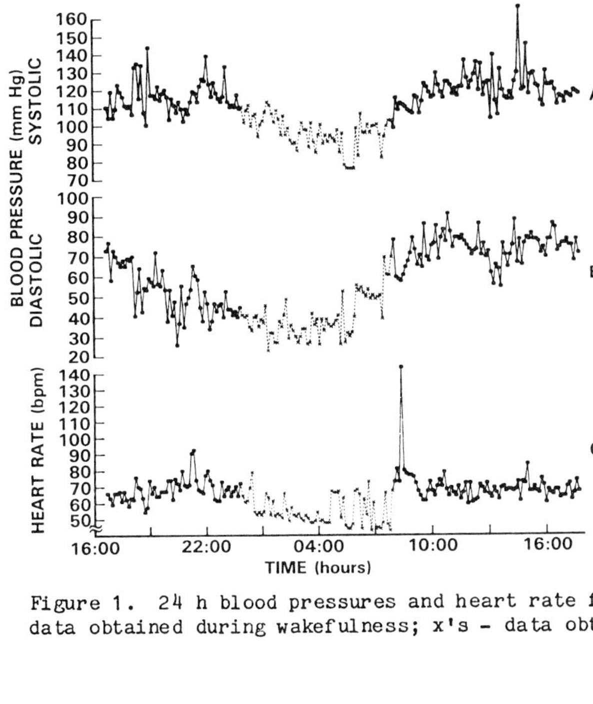

Figure 1. 24 h blood pressures and heart rate from 33-year old woman. Dots - data obtained during wakefulness; x's - data obtained during sleep.

TABLE 1

Average 24 Hour Monitoring Values for Young and Old Groups

Variable*	Group Mean 24 h	Group Mean Sleep	Group Mean Wake	Amplitude of Low Frequency Extract (peak/trough)	% Total Variance in Low Frequency Extract
YOUNG (n=13)					
Systolic (mm Hg)	110 ± 5.2	97 ± 7.5	115 ± 4.9	35 ± 8.6	57 ±12.4
Diastolic (mm Hg)	63 ± 6.4	53 ± 9.2	68 ± 5.6	31 ± 7.9	58 ±18.0
Heart Rate** (bpm)	72 ± 7.5	60 ± 6.2	76 ± 8.5	30 ±12.1	53 ±15.5
OLD (n=25)					
Systolic (mm Hg)	125★ ±12.1	110★ ±13.3	132★ ±13.1	49★ ±15.7	55 ±14.9
Diastolic (mm Hg)	69 ± 8.2	59 ± 9.5	74 ± 9.1	30 ±10.1	51 ±17.3
Heart Rate*** (bpm)	72 ±10.2	63 ±10.2	76 ±10.5	33 ±12.8	58 ±12.6

* = approx. 190-200 samples/record　　** = 12 records for heart rate

*** = 23 records for heart rate　　★ old>young : p<0.01

wakefulness ($p < 0.01$). The only significant differences between the old and the young were in systolic pressures: the 24 h mean, the mean during sleep, the mean during wakefulness, and the amplitude of the low-frequency extract were all higher ($p < 0.01$) in the old. The old were indistinguishable from the young with respect to diastolic pressure and heart rate.

The 24 h mean systolic pressure for each of the 38 subjects plotted against his age is shown in Figure 2A. Figure 2B shows the average systolic pressure value for the same individuals <u>during sleep</u>. We thought that sleep data might more closely represent fundamental hydrodynamic properties of the cardiovascular system than data obtained during wakefulness because variations in arousal, activity or affect might contribute to systolic pressure fluctuations during wakefulness. Nevertheless, the two sets of data resembled each other closely, except that the sleep measurements were slightly lower.

4.3 Comparison of Blood Pressures and Heart Rate between Men and Women

In the old group, women had higher average diastolic pressures and heart rates during sleep than the men, but the difference ($p < 0.02$) did not reach our criterion for claims of statistical significance. When all women, young and old, were compared to all men, however, they showed significantly higher mean 24 h heart rate ($p < 0.01$) and heart rate during sleep ($p < 0.003$).

4.4 Four Interpretations of the Relationship of Systolic Pressure to Age

Figure 3 shows four interpretations of the data of Figure 2B. Panel A expresses the assumption that there is a monotonic-increasing function relating systolic

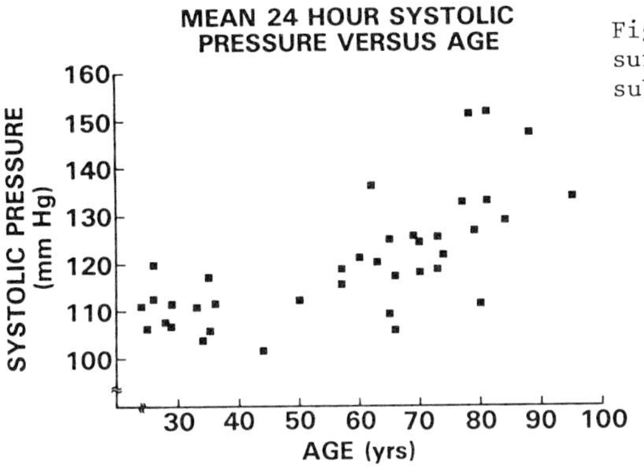

Figure 2(A). 24 h mean systolic pressure vs. age, all young and old subjects.

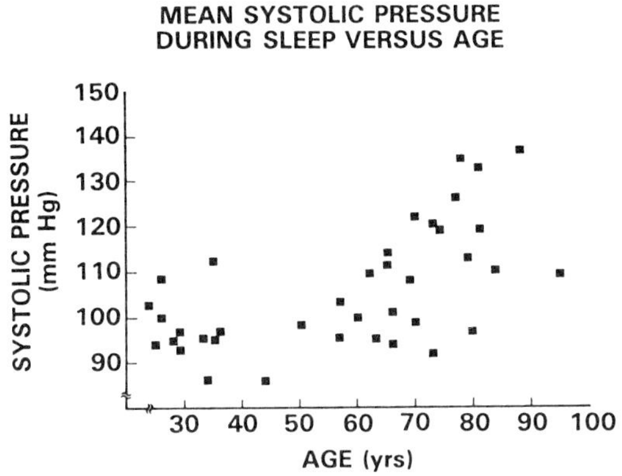

Figure 2(B). Mean systolic pressure during sleep only for all young and old subjects.

pressure to age. In Panel B the hypothesis is that the subjects older than 50 years have wider variation in systolic pressure than the younger group. The vertical line through age 50 divides the two populations. In Panel C the hypothesis is that systolic pressure does not increase intrinsically as a function of age, but that the likelihood that an individual will manifest the early stages

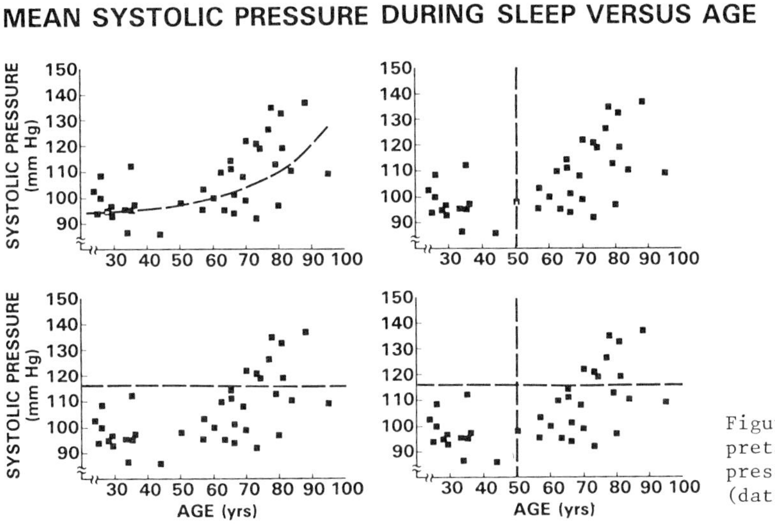

Figure 3. Four interpretations of systolic pressure during sleep (data of Figure 2B).

of isolated systolic hypertension increases with age. Thus, the data are seen as representing two populations, here separated by the horizontal line through 113 mm Hg, just above the highest mean value during sleep seen in the young. On the basis of this hypothesis we submitted the systolic sleep mean data from all 38 subjects to cluster analysis (BMDPKM), nominating a priori the possibility that there were two clusters. The same division of the population (at 112 mm Hg) was confirmed.

Panel D combines the hypotheses represented by B and C and suggests that there may be some differences in systolic pressure (not seen in the mean values during sleep) between sleep-normotensive old and normotensive young, and that there is indeed a separate group among the old who may be pre(systolic)-hypertensive. This three-group image of the data is the one we tested further (and confirmed) by spectral methods. In the subsequent analysis we assumed that there might be three clusters of the systolic pressure data: (1) the pressures obtained in the young, (2) those of the sleep-normotensive old (NTO), and (3) those from the old with elevated systolic pressures during sleep (ESO). Specifically, the ESO group had sleep mean systolic pressures above 112 mm Hg; members of the NTO group and the young all had systolic sleep means equal to or less than 112. Of the 25 subjects 50 years and older whom we studied, 10 fell into the ESO group and 15 into the NTO group.

Table 2 shows the data from the 25 subjects aged 50 years and older divided into NTO and ESO groups. With respect to diastolic pressure and heart rate there were no significant differences between the data of the two groups. Similarly, they showed no statistical difference in their average systolic pressures during wakefulness. By construction, however, values obtained during sleep were significantly higher in the ESO group than in the NTO group ($p < 0.001$): the average sleep value for the ESO was 124 mm Hg, compared to 102 for the NTO.

TABLE 2

24 Hour Monitoring Values for Sleep-Normotensive Old (NTO) and for Sleep-Elevated Systolic Old (ESO)

Variable*	Group Mean			Amplitude of Low Frequency Extract (peak/trough)	% Total Variance in Low Frequency Extract
	24 h	Sleep	Wake		
NTO (n=15)					
Systolic (mm Hg)	121 ± 8.3	102 ± 6.6	129 ± 9.4	53 ±16.2	62 ±13.0
Diastolic (mm Hg)	68 ± 7.2	57 ± 8.8	73 ± 8.0	33 ±10.9	55 ±18.3
Heart Rate** (bpm)	69 ± 9.5	59 ± 8.8	73 ± 9.8	36 ±13.6	59 ±12.4
ESO (n=10)					
Systolic (mm Hg)	133 ±13.9	124★ ± 8.4	136 ±16.7	42 ±13.2	43 ±10.0
Diastolic (mm Hg)	70 ± 9.9	63 ± 9.8	74 ±10.9	27 ± 8.3	44 ±13.7
Heart Rate*** (bpm)	78 ± 9.2	69 ± 9.0	81 ± 9.4	27 ± 9.5	57 ±13.6

* = approx. 190-200 samples/record ** = 14 records for heart rate
*** = 9 records for heart rate ★ ESO>NTO $p<0.01$

The average systolic pressure during sleep for the young was 97 mm Hg, not different from the NTO group (again, by definition of the NTO group). During wakefulness, however, the average value for the young (115 mm Hg) was significantly lower than the values for the older groups (129; 136) ($p < 0.001$, each case). Thus, there are two aspects to the question of whether or not systolic pressure increases with age: (1) <u>during sleep</u> systolic pressure is not necessarily a function of age, although there is an increasing likelihood of a pre-hypertensive state manifested by elevated systolic pressure during sleep; (2) <u>during wakefulness</u> there is some tendency for systolic pressure to be elevated in individuals aged 50 years and older, compared to younger persons, even in those whose systolic pressures during sleep decline to the same level shown by the young. The mean age of the NTO group was 68 years (range 50-95; median age 66), whereas that of the ESO group was 76 years (range 65-88; median age 78); this was not a significant difference ($p < 0.04$).

The amplitude of the low-frequency extract (roughly, that of the circadian variation) in systolic pressure was significantly higher in the NTO group (53 mm Hg) than in the young (35 mm Hg), whereas that for the ESO group (42 mm Hg) was not significantly different from that of the young. This result was a consequence of the fact that in the NTO group the sleep minimum values for systolic pressure were the same as those of the young, while the pressures during wakefulness were greater. Thus, compared to the young, the NTO group demonstrated "amplitude hypertension" around a nearly normal mean operating point, whereas the ESO group showed "elevated operating point" hypertension, with normal amplitude of excursion.

4.5 Spectral Analysis of Cardiovascular Variables

There were no differences in the variance spectra between the young and the group of 25 old for diastolic pressure and heart rate. In contrast, the total variance for the older subjects for systolic pressure (336 $(mm\ Hg)^2$) was significantly greater ($p < 0.001$) than that for the young, (168 $(mm\ Hg)^2$). Furthermore, the spectra for systolic pressure in the old showed significantly more concentration of the variance in the bins with center periods of approximately 40 min and 3 h (ANOVA, $p < 0.01$). The low-frequency (circadian) amplitudes were also significantly higher in the older subjects (Table 1).

Figure 4 shows the ultradian systolic pressure power spectra for the NTO and ESO groups separately, compared to the spectra for the young. By ANOVA the spectra of the two groups of old did not differ from each other. However, they <u>both</u> differed from the young in showing a tendency to concentrate variance at periods of 40 min and 3 h ($p < 0.01$ for both periods). In addition, the NTO group also showed a concentration of variance at a period of 7 h that was significantly greater than that of the young ($p < 0.01$). Thus, the spectral changes we have

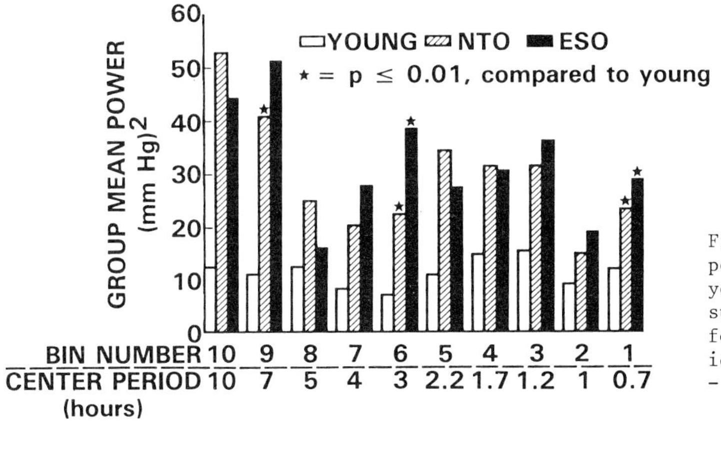

Figure 4. Systolic power spectra for young and NTO, ESO subgroups of old for ultradian periodicities (40 min - 10 h).

observed, with heightened emphasis on variations with periods of approximately 40 min and 3 h, particularly, seem to be partly a function of age and not only of systolic pressure levels; they are present in the sleep-normotensive old as well as in the old with elevated systolic pressure during sleep.

5. DISCUSSION

It is well known from population and longitudinal studies that systolic pressure tends to be elevated in older persons [5] [6] [7] [8] [9] [10] [11] [12]. The prevalence of isolated systolic hypertension, defined as systolic pressure above 160 mm Hg with associated diastolic pressure less than 90-95 mm Hg (according to single, casual measurement), increases with age and is about 30% in people older than 65 years. Prevalence varies with race and sex [13] [14] [15]. In order to assess systolic pressure changes with age in the present study, we first characterized its variations and levels in a group of 13 young normotensive subjects to establish those values as a reference "gold standard". We then compared those reference data with the data from 25 well older subjects.

We confirmed that systolic blood pressure is generally elevated in the old compared to the young (we noted a mean increase during waking hours of approximately 17 mm Hg), but our chief finding was that during sleep the old seemed to fall into two groups: a subgroup (15/25 subjects) whose systolic pressures during sleep were the same as those of the young (about 100 mm Hg), and another subgroup (10/25 subjects) whose pressures remained elevated during sleep - approximately 25 mm Hg higher than seen in the young. We called these two groups "sleep-normotensive old (NTO)" and "sleep-elevated systolic old (ESO)." Our decision to divide the population of old into these subgroups was supported by cluster analysis applied to the systolic sleep data for all 38 subjects (young and old), nominating *a priori* a possibility of two clusters. This analysis separated a group of "sleep hypertensives" from normotensive subjects at 112 mm Hg.

We conclude that there are two different ways in which systolic pressure differed in our older group, compared to the young. In the first pattern (NTO group), systolic pressure was higher than that of the young during wakefulness but not during sleep, with a resultant increase in the amplitude of the low-frequency (circadian) systolic variation. These changes were associated with an altered spectral profile indicating an increased concentration of variance at periods of approximately 40 min, 3 h, and 7 h. The total, 24 h variance of systolic pressure in this subgroup of the old also was substantially greater than that of the young. The second pattern of systolic pressure change in the old (ESO group) manifested an elevation during wakefulness similar to that of the NTO group, but with the continuing systolic elevation during sleep - even though a circadian rhythm decrease during sleep was preserved. Because the systolic pressure of the ESO group during wakefulness was at approximately the same level as that of the NTO, the amplitude of their systolic variation over the 24 hours was slightly less than that of the NTO group and their low-frequency variance on systolic pressure was between that of the NTO and the young.

All old subjects, whether or not they showed elevated systolic pressures during sleep, did show changed systolic pressure spectra, compared to the young. Thus, this spectral change appears to be related to age, not just to pressure levels, and may be a manifestation of an intrinsic aging process in the cardiovascular system.

6. ACKNOWLEDGMENTS

Supported by the John Hartford Foundation (Grant No. 84079-IG) and the Crump Institute for Medical Engineering, UCLA. These results have been reported in fuller detail elsewhere (L.A. Benton, S.J. Berry, D.O. Walter, F.E. Yates: "Two Patterns of Systolic Pressure Dynamics in Human Aging." Circulation -- Submitted Sept., 1986).

7. REFERENCES

1. F.E. Yates: Can. J. of Physiol. and Pharmacol. 60, 217 (1982)
2. F.E. Yates: In Biological Regulation and Development, ed. by R.F. Goldberger and K.R. Yamamoto, Vol. III, Hormone Action (Plenum Press, New York 1982) p. 25
3. H. Soodak, A.S. Iberall: Science 201, 579 (1978)
4. K. Bolen, G.L. Ramsey, R.W. Gifford, Jr.: In Ambulatory Blood Pressure Monitoring, ed. by M.A. Weber and J.I.M. Drayer (Springer-Verlag, New York 1984), p. 35
5. W.E. Miall, H.G. Lovell: Br. Med. J. 3, 660 (1967)
6. T. Gordon, D. Shurtleff: Means at Each Examination and Inter-examination Variation of Specified Characteristics: The Framingham Study, ed. by W.B. Kannel and T. Gordon (DHEW Publ. No. (NIH) 74-478. Government Printing Office, Washington, DC. 1974)
7. E.W. Lew: Build and Blood Pressure Study, (Society of Actuaries, Chicago 1959)
8. S.W. Rabkin, M.B. Mathewson, R.B. Tate: Circulation 65, 291 (1982)
9. P. Froom, M. Bar-David, J. Ribak, et al.: Circulation 68, 467 (1983)
10. A. Oberman, N.E. Lane, W. R. Harlan, et al.: Circulation 36, 812 (1967)
11. National Center for Health Statistics: Blood Pressure Levels of Persons 6-74 Years of Age in the United States, Series II, No. 203 (Government Printing Office, Rockville, MD 1977)
12. A.M. Master, R.P. Lasser: In Hypertension. Recent Advances, ed. by A.N. Brest and J.H. Moyer (Lea and Fibiger, Philadelphia 1961)
13. R. W. Gifford, Jr.: JAMA 247, 781 (1982)
14. W.B. Kannel, J.R. Dawber, D.L. McGee: Circulation 61, 1179 (1980)
15. W.B. Applegate: In Geriatric Medicine Annual 1986, ed. by R.J. Ham (Medical Economics Books, Oradell, NJ (1986) p. 40

New Aspects of the Dynamics of Acute Myocardial Infarction

R.N.A. Gasser[1], *F. Dienstl*[1], *S. Hauptlorenz*[2], *and B. Puschendorf*[2]

[1;*]Department of Cardiology, University Clinic, A-6020 Innsbruck, Austria
[2]Institute of Biochemistry, University of Innsbruck, A-6020 Innsbruck, Austria
*Present address: Institute of Physiology, University of Freiburg, Hermann-Herder-Str. 7, D-7800 Freiburg, Fed. Rep. of Germany

Until recently, acute myocardial infarction (AMI) has been regarded as a single event. Only the latest results have indicated that AMI can be considered as an oscillating event based on a series of heavy coronary spasms (1-4). Alonso et al. (5) first described the course of AMI as an "episodic extension" in 1973. Then Kagen et al. (6) described the oscillating course of the serum curve of the biochemical marker myoglobin (Mb) (Fig.1) and were the first to ask: "Is AMI in man an intermittent event?"(6).

We ascribed this phasic behavior to a discontinuous release from the area of infarction (7). The infarction-typical ST-segment elevation, which we have measured and evaluated using a computerized system, also defines the dynamics of AMI as an oscillating system by showing a rise and fall in height (8) (Fig.1). A further parameter, the creatinekinase isoenzyme MB, shows an undulating behavior in its time course as well, especially when measured at short intervals (3) (Fig.1). We attributed this phase-like behavior of the various parameters to a series of reperfusion waves which follow several heavy coronary spasms (8).

All the infarction markers mentioned are well known. However, only close-meshed measurements of their time course have led to the recognition of the phase-like character of AMI. We have developed a biochemical model that takes the basic mechanism of AMI into account (1).

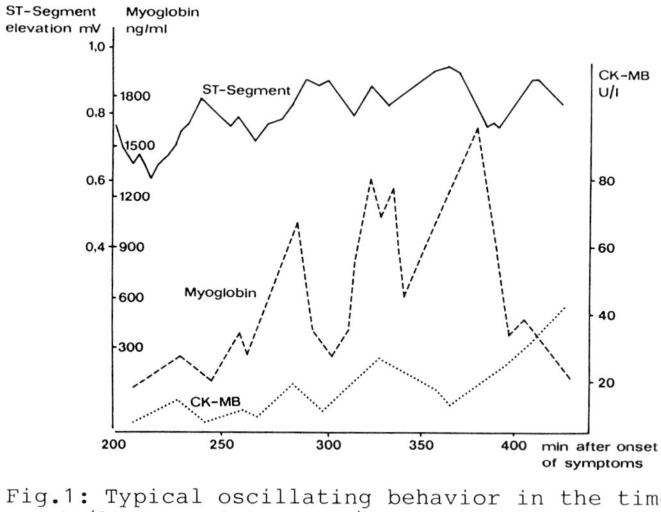

Fig.1: Typical oscillating behavior in the time course of serum CK-MB (U/l), myoglobin (ng/ml) and ST-segment elevation (mV) during the early phase of AMI.

The thrombo-ischemic re-entry mechanism (TRM): Platelets aggregate in areas with atherosclerotic lesions and release strongly vasoconstrictive substances (thromboxan A_2, serotonin, histamine ...) (9). These lead to strong spasms of the coronary vessel at sites of damaged endothelium, ending up in ischemia. During ischemia vasodilative metabolites appear locally (lactate, pyruvate, ADP, H^+-ions....). These are effective in counteracting thrombogenic factors, as known from the physiological phenomenon "autoregulation of the coronary blood flow", and thereby lead to a dilatation of the vessel, followed by spontaneous reperfusion. However, the components effective in dilatation are also washed out and the vasoconstrictive forces become predominant again. In this manner the vicious circle is re-entered.

After 3 - 4 phases, the oscillation becomes exhausted for reasons so far unknown and the pathological serum levels of CK-MB and Mb return to normal values. The myocardium in the area affected is destroyed for the most part. The dependence of the TRM upon the presence of platelet aggregates has been proven by us, on the one hand, by autopsy findings, and, on the other, by the fact that early intravenous infusion of thrombolytic substances can interrupt the TRM so that only 1 peak instead of several can be seen in the course of time (9,10). Quite recently the dependence of peak height upon coronary blood flow has also been established (2).

The results presented here are especially important since AMI, an event that has always been considered as a single catastrophe, could be shown to be phasic in character with oscillating behavior due to changes in a complex biochemical system.

Conclusion: When one regards coronary perfusion as an oscillating system with increasing and decreasing blood flow which is directly dependent on myocardial pumping function, AMI can be considered as the following: A change in period and oscillation width of coronary perfusion pressure induced by the action of platelet-born factors, in which the intervals of low perfusion are excessively long.

References:

1. R. Gasser, F. Dienstl: Angiology 37, 417 (1986)
2. R. Gasser, F. Dienstl: Pflüg. Arch. 406, R32 (1986)
3. R. Gasser, S.Hauptlorenz, M.Moll, M.Kahler, F. Dienstl, B.Puschendorf: J. Cell. Mol. Cardiol. (revision submitted) (1987)
4. R. Gasser, F. Dienstl: Clin. Physiol. 6, 397 (1986)
5. D. Alonso, S. Scheidt, M. Post, T. Killip: Circulation 48, 588 (1973)
6. L. Kagen, S. Scheidt, A. Butt: Am. J. Med. 62, 86 (1977)
7. H. Drexel, E. Dworzak, W. Kirchmair, M. Milz, B. Puschendorf, F. Dienstl: Am. Heart J. 105, 642 (1983)
8. H. Drexel, F. Dienstl: New Engl. J. Med. 309, 1457 (1983)
9. R. Gasser, F. Dienstl: Angiology 37, December issue (1986)
10. R. Gasser, F. Dienstl, B. Puschendorf: Proc. X World Congress of Cardiology, abstr. (1986)

Coordination in the Circulatory and Respiratory Systems

F. Raschke

Institut für Arbeitsphysiologie und Rehabilitationsforschung, Phillips-Universität Marburg, Robert-Koch-Str. 7a, D-3550 Marburg/Lahn, Fed. Rep. of Germany

Temporal coordination of various physiological and biochemical processes is an obvious prerequisite of functional efficiency and regulation.

In the circulatory system, coordinated activity is found in diverse functions: Cardiac cycle and arterial pressure oscillation (dicrotic wave), originated in pulse wave reflexions through arterial bifurcations, reveal integer ratios of their period length /1, 2/. These integer ratios increase early at night, if diurnal assessment was applied /3/. Spontaneous muscle blood flow change frequently prefers a period length of 30 sec and 1 min /4/. Fluctuations in cardiac interval times due to respiration, blood pressure, and muscle blood flow change exhibit integer ratios in their period length too, if undisturbed night sleep was considered /5/. Maternal and foetal heart rate in humans prefer a ratio of 2:1 /6/.

In the respiratory system we find basic rhythmicity at rest which can be superimposed by modulations in tidal volume (often called Cheyne-Stokes-, or Biot-breathing), which frequently show periods of about 30 sec and 1 min /7/.

Additionally to these investigations concerning specific properties of the respective system, manifold interactions exist by means of coordinated activity. Three functional levels are known to be responsible for coordination: central neural activity, reflexogenic, and mechanical coupling /8/.

With respect to the central origin issue, e.g. KOEPCHEN and THURAU /9/, in their experiments in rabbits, used pharmacological blocking of respiratory mechanics and vagal cooling. Nevertheless aortic pressure changes and phrenic nerve activity were coordinated by integer ratios 1:1, 2:1, 3:1, and sometimes 4:1 in a very strict way.

The reflexogenic origin of cardiovascular-respiratory coordination has been derived from cardiac afferents /10/, and systemic arterial baroreceptor reflexes /11/, linked in the common brainstem neurons enabling coupling /12/.

Even mechanical effects may contribute to coupling phenomena between respiratory and cardiac movement /13/.

In humans, cardiovascular-respiratory coordination has been found to be enhanced during resting and recuperative conditions, whereas it can be easily disturbed by even low levels of strain /8/. Experiments run during undisturbed night sleep therefore should reveal the highest degree of coordination.

The relationship between frequency ratio and phase tuning, i.e. frequency (integer ratios), and phase (distinct phase preference) coordination between these rhythms has not yet been studied simultaneously. The following experiment therefore was designed to check the temporal relationship of different modes of coordination and to clarify the mechanisms involved.

Methods

The assessment of coordination with respect to phase and frequency reference is compiled in Fig. 1. The lower line gives trigger pulses of R-wave (ECG) and inspiratory (I) as well as expiratory onset (E). Onsets have been calculated from the respiratory curve (nasal thermistor record, dotted line) by use of a computerised pattern recognition system /14/, which takes into account cardiac-respiratory artifact detection (cardiac-pneumatic pulses), apneas, and biasing of respiratory records during long-term measurement. The step function indicates instantaneous heart rate as converted from RR-interval times. Two modes of coupling are obvious: respiratory heart rate modulation as assessed by its magnitude $\hat{x}$, and interval time between preceding R-wave and inspiratory onset (RI_i). Inspiratory phase was calculated with reference to the RR_i-interval using the formula $(RI_i/RR_i)*100$. This yields a phase reference for standardized cardiac cycle length, which has been divided into 20 classes à 5%. Polar coordinate system was not used for reasons of comparison with the literarure /15/. Because phase coordination varies with time, a large number of inspiratory events ($n \geq 100$) is necessary for calculation of preferred phases. We therefore used histograms, and plotted these as joint interval histogram, which gave the change in phase position from one inspiratory onset to the next. Additionally to the evaluation of phase coordination, frequency coordinating mechanisms were cal-

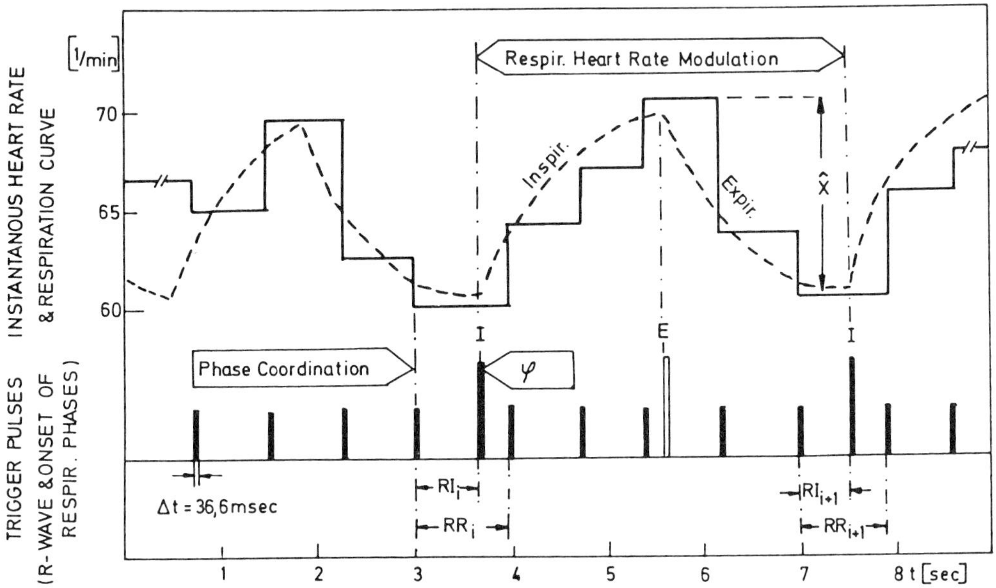

Fig. 1 Respiratory curve (dotted line) and ECG trigger pulses (below) converted into instantaneous heart rate (step function). Two modes of cardiorespiratory coupling are assessed: (1) respiratory heart rate modulation (magnitude $\hat{x}$), and (2) phase coordination RI_i calculated as phase reference between preceding R-wave signal and inspiratory onset (I)

culated, using four different joint interval histograms. The actual number of heart beats (2-5) served as a parameter, which appeared during each respiratory cycle. The subjects in this study on undisturbed night sleep were 16 healthy men (age: 19-37 years), half untrained, half high performance athletes /15/. Their sleep behavior was polygraphically recorded until spontaneously waking up in the morning. For computerized sleep stage recording /16/, we used the criteria of RECHTSCHAFFEN and KALES /17/.

Results

A typical pattern of joint interval histograms from an untrained subject is shown in Fig. 2, another subject (well-trained athlete) in Fig. 3. The histograms are compiled in a three-dimensional plot with preceding RI_i interval on the x-axis, and RI_{i+1} on the y-axis. Standardized cardiac cycles are divided into 20 classes totalling a matrix of 400 elements. On the z-axis the number of events is counted. Whole number ratios (WNR) include 2 to 5 heart beats per respiratory cycle, whereas numbers beyond these parameters have been neglected.

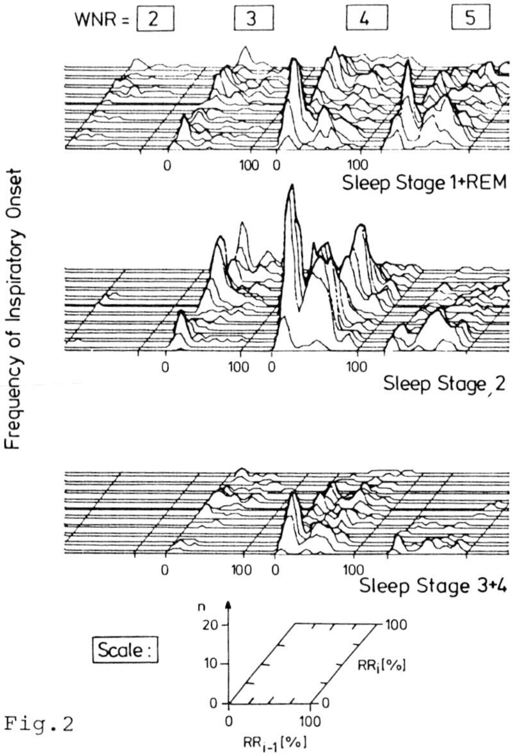

Fig.2

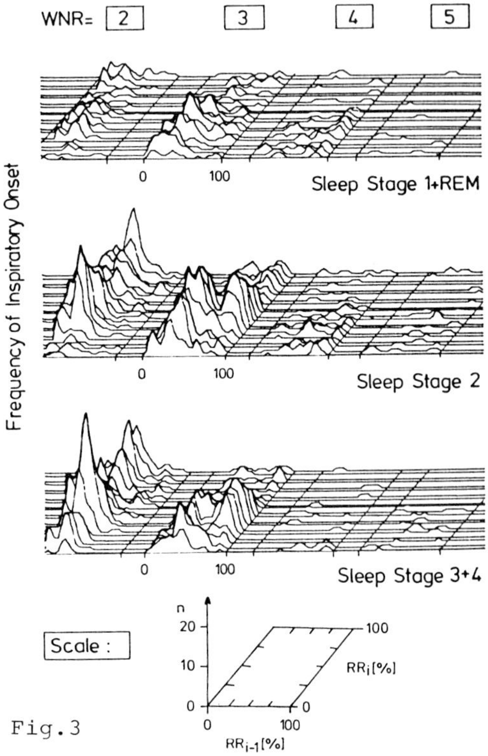

Fig.3

Fig. 2 Joint interval histograms for two inspiratory onsets following each other. Onsets are determined with reference to standardized cardiac cycles (scale below). In each histogram a matrix with 20*20 elements is used. 4 different histograms in each row, according to the number (WNR = whole number ratio) of heart beats per respiratory cycle. Sleep stages 1 and REM, 2, and 3 and 4 are separated. Untrained subject, total sleep time

Fig. 3 Same methods as used in Fig.2. Diagram of a well-trained athlete; total sleep time

Three panels are used for a distinction made between various sleep stages. Very light sleep (stage 1) and rapid eye movement sleep (REM) are combined. Stage 2 (light sleep) stands in the middle, deep sleep (stages 3 and 4) below. Analysis comprises total sleep time of each subject, yielding 6319 respiratory cycles in Fig. 2, 7218 cycles in Fig. 3.

The data are characterized by a number of rationales: (1) The untrained subject mainly shows 4 heart beats per respiratory cycle, whereas 3 and 5 occur much less. In the athlete the ratio of 2:1 and 3:1 is most dominant. (2) The preferred number of heart beats per respiratory cycle changes with the depth of sleep leading to higher values during stages 1 and REM, and lowered ratios during deep sleep. (3) Very high peaks in several histograms indicate constant phase reference from one inspiratory onset to the next. A phase coordination therefore exists for at least one respiratory cycle. Bimodal, or multimodal distributions indicate, that several modes of phase reference are preferred. (4) The position of the peaks varies with the depth of sleep, the training status, and the pulse-respiration-ratio. (5) Height and shape of the peaks indicate both, a varying probability and strictness of phase coordination.

These observations can be generalized after some modifications: (1) A biasing of the density of probability is produced through normal distributions of pulse-respiration-ratios, which must be taken into account. The parameters of these normal distributions have been calculated, followed by subtracting the normal distributions from the histograms. (2) The time spent in each sleep stage, and the number of inspiratory onsets should be normalized if one compares different subjects. We therefore used the relative frequency of inspiratory onsets in each subject and sleep stage, and pooled the data after these corrections. Additionally the joint interval histograms have been reduced to a two-dimensional plot. This enables clear phase estimation with respect to the cardiac cycle.

The result is shown in Fig. 4. From this diagram it is quite evident, that the phase position changes mainly with the number of heart

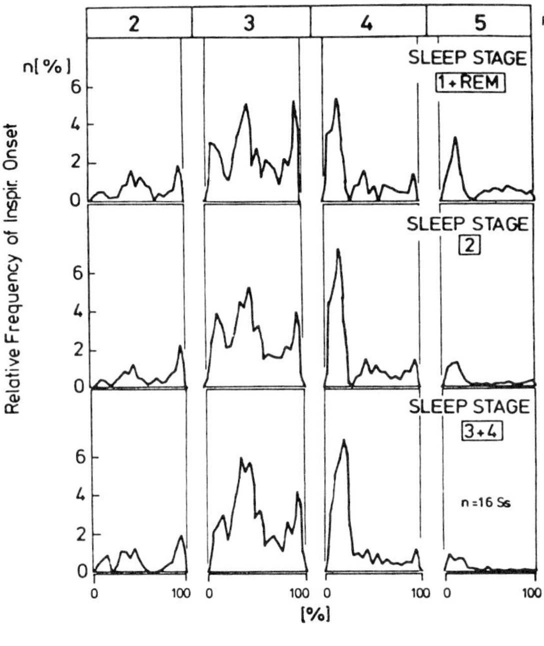

RI/RR [%] According to the Number of Heart Beats (2-5) per Respiratory Cycle; Corrected for Probability

Fig. 4 Histograms of relative frequency of inspiratory onset, each divided into 20 classes of normalized cardiac cycle (%). From top to bottom different sleep stages (1 and REM, 2, 3 and 4). From left to right 4 different histograms, each according to the actual number of heart beats per respiratory cycle. Total sleep time of 16 subjects, eight untrained, eight well-trained athletes. For position of the peaks and interpretation see text beats per respiratory cycle due to the subject's training status. Trained subjects, who have a ratio of 2:1 or 3:1, exhibit a mid cardiac cycle peak. Those histograms using 4 and 5 heart beats as a parameter exhibit a very pronounced peak early within cardiac cycle. In this case the mid-cycle peak disappears. Sleep stage-dependent changes show that the early peak is more dominant during stage 1 and REM as compared to stages 3 and 4.

With respect to the functional meaning of preferred phases we have distinguished between systolic (0-35%, 90-100%), and diastolic (36-89%) phases of normalized cardiac cycles of sleeping subjects /15/. A distinction therefore can be established that systolic phase coordination is primarily found for normal /7/ or increased pulse-respiration ratios, whereas lowered ratios (3:1) exhibit both, systolic and diastolic coordination. Extremely low ratios (2:1) exhibit only diastolic coordination, as found in top performance athletes.

Discussion

Our results have shown that during sleep there is a statistically evaluated, strong phase coordination between cardiovascular and respiratory systems. The mechanisms responsible for this phenomenon have been discussed in detail elsewhere /8/. They can be summarized by means of afferent neural inputs from the cardiovascular system (baro- and volume reception in the right atrium of the myocard, baroreception from arteries in carotide bifurcations, and aortic arch) as well as central coordinated neurogenic cardiovascular-respiratory activity. In this paper the discussion is restricted to the distinction made between phase and frequency coordination, i.e. the temporal order as measured during sleep and repose. These functional states are compared with others having shown break down of coordinating mechanisms.

Phase coordination, as described in this study, is dependent on both, the intensity of coupling as derived from the height of the histogram's peaks and the varying coupling modalities as shown by different preferred phases. Joint interval histograms have given stable relationships for at least one respiratory cycle. This should lead to integer ratios if the same phase reference is realized for longer periods of time. In this case a distinction between phase and frequency coordination is impossible, because constant phase reference implies whole number ratios in frequency.

On the other hand a different cardiorespiratory relationship was found in trained and untrained subjects. The ratio of 4:1 is normally observed in healthy untrained humans during sleep or several therapeutical processes /7/. The tendency to lowered ratios in the athletes therefore is interpreted in terms of altered dispositional autonomous functions. These are induced by morphological and functional improvement of cardiorespiratory efficiency. A basal preparatory disposition for a distinct ratio is supposed, which is superimposed by an intensification of temporal order under conditions of sleep. It is realized by subtle mechanisms of phase tuning. Thus, our results may hint at the functional significance of phase coordination in terms of a rather economic filling and outflow mechanics of the heart, supported by exact (optimal) respiratory timing. In the athlete, maximal coherence of the two systems seems to be realized, as manifested by a greater amplitude of respiratory heart rate modulation /18/ and a close synchrony of cardiovascular, inspiratory, and even expiratory timing, as previous investigations have shown /14/.

Decoupling with respect to respiratory heart rate modulation was found in numerous investigations under conditions of physical /19/

and mental /20/ strain. Even for different diseased states, such as arterial hypertension /21/, myocardial dysfunctions /18/, diabetes mellitus /22/, and increasing biological age of the myocard /23/. In our case, investigations on physical and psychovegetative strain /8/ have shown phase coordination to break down completely even for the slightest stressor. This gave evidence that phase reference is the most sensitive indicator, followed by magnitude of coupled oscillators, and finally by the mean frequency of cardiovascular and respiratory rhythms. Figure 5 gives an outline of the mechanisms involved for different functional states. Phase and frequency coordination is mainly found during the trophotropic state, including sleep, relaxation, repose, and recovery, whereas decoupling occurs under conditions of strain, including various diseases. With respect to decoupling of phase coordination we have recently observed a loss of coupling in patients who suffer from the sleep apnea syndrome /24/. We found, that during sleep with regular breathing, systolic inspiratory onsets occur which are comparable to the results of healthy young men as reported here. Frequency coordination took values of 5:1 and 6:1. But during hyperventilated breathing, intermitted to apneic phases, cardiorespiratory coherence was inhibited completely. These hyperventilation phases occur in the range of 20 to 80 times per hour of sleep, depending on the progression of the disease. We therefore conclude that an increase of temporal order is found during elevated functional efficiency, as seen in the athlete, and during progressive therapeutical processes /7/. This highly integrated activity of cardiovascular and respiratory systems is diminished under conditions of strain and disease, where elevated metabolic transport requires a larger nonphasic energy production. In this case a system-specific (proprioceptive) compensation of physiological dysfunction or deviation from the control values are balanced. The organisation of improved efficiency with respect to hemodynamics, gas exchange, meta-

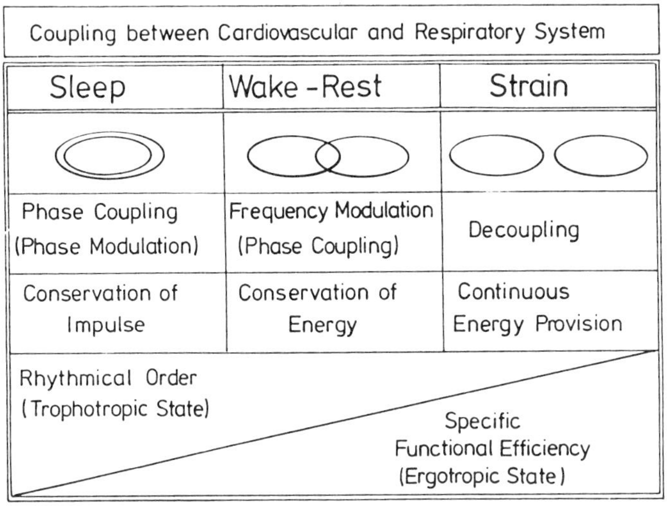

Fig.5 Outline of coupling mechanisms between cardiovascular and respiratory systems according to the functional state. During sleep the highest coherence is found (phase and frequency coordination most dominant, frequency modulation with largest magnitude). These are impaired in the waking state with an abrupt loss in phase reference and a gradual decrease in modulation amplitude. During strain, including the diseased state, decoupling occurs. In this state coherence is replaced by elevated tonic energy provision

bolic transport, and humoral economy are not yet understood, neither as a whole, nor in detail. But using the assessment of temporal coherence in the cardiovascular and respiratory systems, an easily measurable, undisturbing indicator of the functional state is available.

Literature

1. E. Gadermann, G. Hildebrandt, H. Jungmann: Z. Kreisl.-Forsch. 50, 805 (1961)
2. A. Bardou, B. Levy, P.J. Birkni, A. Tedgui, J.-M. Bazire, P. Saumont: Eur. J. Appl. Physiol. 46, 387 (1981)
3. G. Hildebrandt, H.R. Klein: Arch. Kreisl.-Forsch. 59, 235 (1969)
4. K. Golenhofen, G. Hildebrandt: Z. Kreisl.-Forsch. 46, 257 (1957)
5. F. Raschke, W. Bockelbrink, G. Hildebrandt: In Sleep 1976, Proc. 3rd Eur. Congr. Sleep Res., ed. by W.P. Koella, P. Levin (Karger, Basel, München 1977) p.298
6. G. Hildebrandt, H.R. Klein: Klin. Wschr. 57, 87 (1979)
7. G. Hildebrandt: J. Aut. Nerv. System, suppl., 253 (1986)
8. F. Raschke: In Cardiorespiratory and Cardiosomatic Psychophysiology, ed. by P. Grossman, K. Janssen, D. Vaitl (Plenum, New York 1986) p.207
9. H.P. Koepchen, K. Thurau: Pflügers Arch. 267, 10 (1958)
10. K. Bucher, H. Schwitter, B. Hool-Zulauf, E. Batschelet: Res. Exp. Med. 157, 281 (1972)
11. D.L. Eckberg, C.R. Orshan: J. Clin. Invest. 59, 780 (1977)
12. P. Langhorst, M. Stroh-Werz, K. Dittmar, H. Camerer: Brain Res. 87, 407 (1975)
13. K. Golenhofen, H. Lippross: Pflügers Arch. 309, 159 (1969)
14. F. Raschke: In ISAM-Gent-1981, 3rd International Symp. on Ambulatory Monitoring, ed. by F.D. Stott, E.B. Raftery, D.L. Clement, S. Wright (Academic Press, London, New York 1982) p.349
15. F. Raschke: Die Kopplung zwischen Herzschlag und Atmung (Ph. D. Diss., University of Marburg 1981)
16. H.-B. Klöppel: In Sleep 1978, Proc. 4th Eur. Congr. Sleep Res., ed. by L. Popoviciu, B. Asgian, G. Badiu (Karger, Basel, München 1980) p.397
17. A. Rechtschaffen, A. Kales: A Manual of Standardized Terminology, Techniques and Scoring System for Sleep Stages of Human Subjects (Public Health Service Publication 204, Washington D.C. 1968)
18. K. Eckoldt, B. Pfeifer, E. Schubert: In Central Interaction between Respiratory and Cardiovascular Control Systems, ed. by H.P. Koepchen, S.M. Hilton, A. Trzebski (Springer, Berlin, Heidelberg 1980) p.216
19. W. Rohmert, W. Laurig, U. Philipp, H. Luczak: Ergonomics 16, 33 (1973)
20. G. Mulder, W.R.E.H. Mulder-Hajonides van der Meulen: Ergonomics, 16, 69 (1973)
21. D. Gross: Z. Kreisl.-Forsch. 58, 699 (1969)
22. W. Wieling, C. Borst, M.A. von Dongen-Torman, J.W. van der Hofstede, J.F.M. Brederode, E. Endert, A.J. Dunning: Diabetologia 24, 422 (1983)
23. W.J.M. Hrushesky, D. Fader, O. Schmitt, V. Gilbertsen: Science 244, 1001 (1984)
24. F. Raschke: In Sleep Related Disorders and Internal Diseases, ed. by J.H. Peter, T. Podszus, P. von Wichert (Springer, Heidelberg 1987)

Part IV

Circadian Clocks

The Autonomous Time Structure and Its Reactive Modifications in the Human Organism

G. Hildebrandt

Institut für Arbeitsphysiologie und Rehabilitationsforschung,
Phillips-Universität Marburg, Robert-Koch-Straße 7a,
D-3550 Marburg/Lahn, Fed. Rep. of Germany

In the course of the last decades more and more indications have been accumulated showing that the entire spectrum of biological rhythms in man exhibits characteristic principles of biological time structures which also rule the functional behaviour of the rhythms in the different parts of the spectrum.

Looking at the functions listed in Fig. 1, one can derive that the rhythms are hierarchically ordered: With increasing period duration the rhythms become likewise increasingly complex. The processes in question begin with cellular high fre-

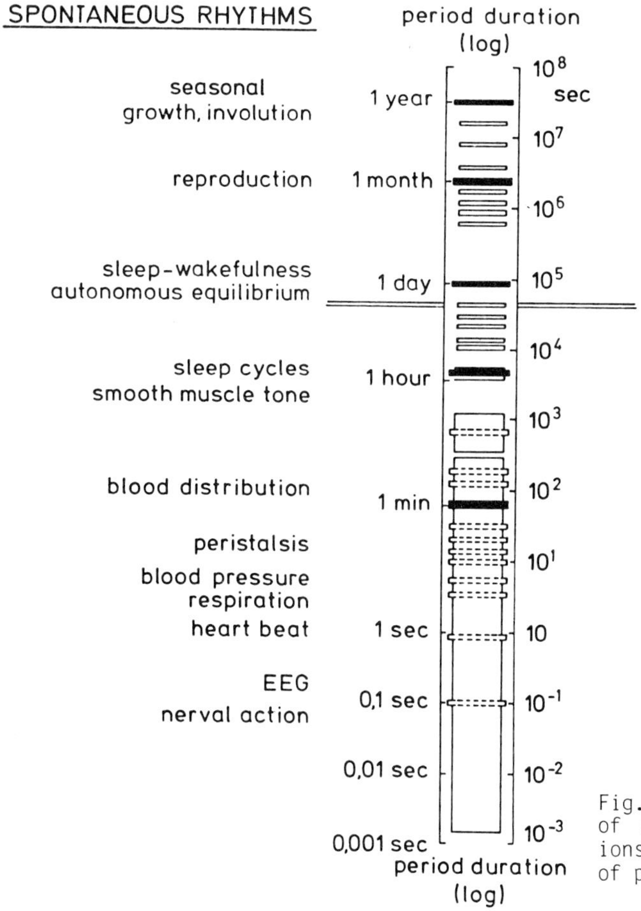

Fig. 1.: Spectrum of main types of spontaneous rhythmical functions in man. Logarithmic scale of period durations. (From /1/)

quency rhythms then go on to organ and systemic rhythms up to the circadian variations which already involve the entire organism, and finally to the reproductive functions and rhythms of whole populations. More and more single functions are comprised by the rhythms in the long wave section of the spectrum. At the same time, rhythms are increasingly controlled by hormonal mechanisms, whereas in the high-frequency section nervous control is dominating.

Furthermore, the spectrum can be divided into two parts: In the long wave section which is containing the circadian rhythm and the so-called infradian rhythms, the rhythmic functions are synchronized by external zeitgebers, or else find their corresponding cycles in the environment, whereas in the entire ultradian section we find only endogenous autonomous rhythms which maintain a more or less strong internal time order by means of frequency- and phase-coordination.

Figure 2 shows a compilation of all period lengths of rhythmic functions as observed in the different parts of the spectrum. Under strict resting conditions and in a state of complete adaptation only a few spontaneous rhythms dominate in the spectrum and can easily be detected by so-called macroscopic observation. However, in particular under loading conditions like stress or strain, as well as in pathological situations, quite a lot of further periodicities come up.

As demonstrated by the figure, the whole spectrum of rhythms can be divided into certain blocks, with the period lengths - as a rule - predominantly exhibiting

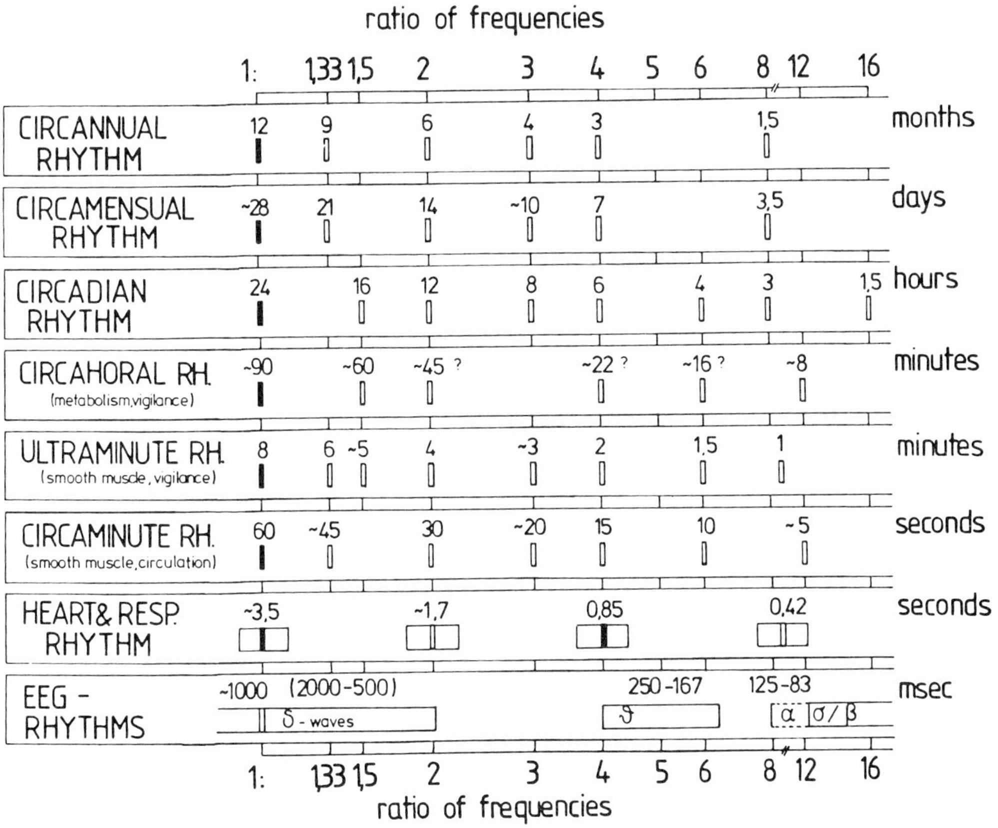

Fig. 2: Ratios of frequencies within the different "blocks" of spontaneous rhythmical functions as indicated by the preferred period lengths

in each of these simple whole number frequency ratios which form a harmonic system. The most common ratio is 2:1 or 4:1, forming a temporal equivalent to bifurcation or dichotomy and indicating frequency multiplication or demultiplication of periods as an important mechanism of temporal order in the organism. However, ratios of 3:1 and others also occur in the blocks of the spectrum, forming trifurcation or trichotomy, respectively.

The connections between the various blocks seem to be different. In some cases there is no gap between the harmonic intervals, in other cases the transition is more or less complicated.

During the last decades several authors have contributed to a better understanding of the harmonic structure of the rhythm spectrum in man. For instance, recently HEJL/2/ has presented a so-called "periodic system" of biological rhythms.

For some parts of the spectrum there exist already very clear indications for the strict harmonic structure of the temporal order. As shown in Fig.3, BROUGHTON /3/ has pointed out that the basic rest-activity REM-NREM cycle of about 90 min period length is part of a harmonic chain of submultiple periods of the 24-hour rhythm.

Period length 24 h	Circadian period
12 h	Sleep deprivation
6 h 3 h	Frequent ultradian superimposition
90 min	REM-NREM-sleep cycle

Fig. 3: Submultiple period lengths of the 24-hour period. (According to /3/)

By long-term observations GOLENHOFEN & VON LOH /4/ have been able to show that even small pieces of smooth muscle tissue (Taenia coli of the guinea pig) exhibit a spontaneous activity of rhythmic contractions with the preferred period durations of 1,2,3 etc. up to 8 minutes (Fig.4).

In the 1-min range, SINZ /5/ has detected a harmonic spectrum of rhythms(Fig.5) by using computer analysis of various bodily functions as e.g. heart rate, respiratory rate, peripheral blood flow, and reaction time.

Finally, our own group has stated over and over (Fig.6) that heart beat, respiration, blood pressure rhythm, and the 1-min rhythm of peripheral blood flow under resting conditions alike form a complex harmonically ordered system.

The mechanism of this harmonic coordination is not yet understood in every instance. Yet there exist several findings that internal phase coupling as a special mode of synchronization is mainly involved /6/,/7/,/8/. However, harmonic ratios of functional capacities and time constants respectively seem to play a role also /9/.

Concerning the functional significance of the harmonic temporal order of biological systems, there is already an overwhelming amount of evidence that frequency and phase coordination establish a system of economical co-action and hence - in general - can favour the functional economy of the organism.

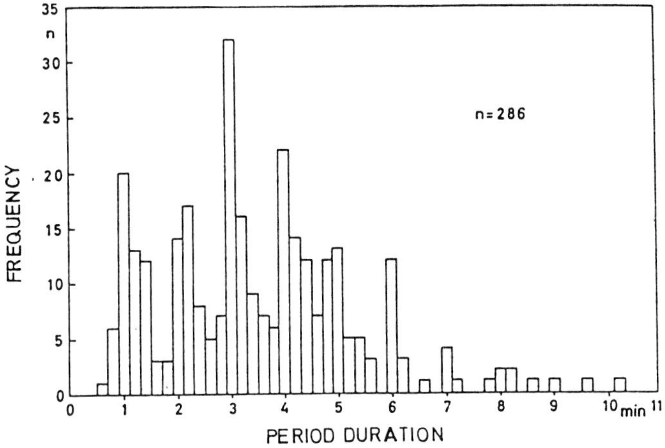

Fig. 4: Histogram of period lengths of spontaneous smooth muscle contractions (Taenia coli of the guinea pig). (After /4/)

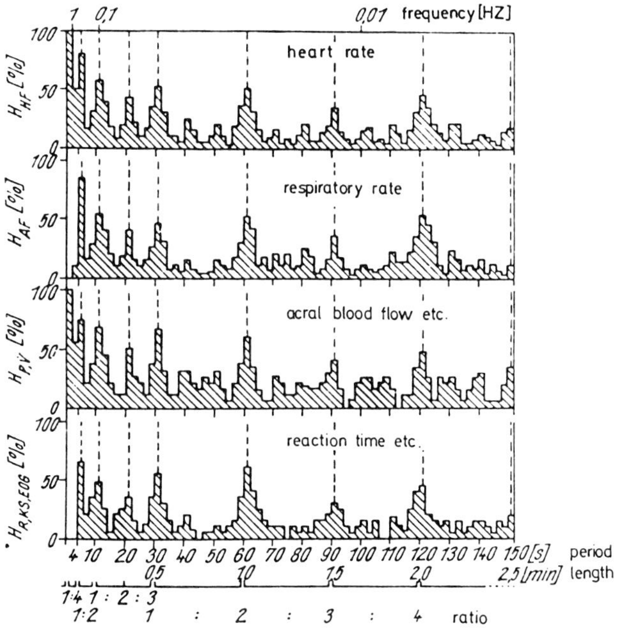

Fig. 5: Histograms of period lengths of a total of 7890 periods of circa-minute rhythms (heart rate H HF, respiration rate H AF, blood pressure waves H PV sensomotor reaction time R, short-term memory KS, saccadic eye movements' EOG). (After /5/)

Looking again at the general overview of periods (Fig.2), it is symbolized in the lower part by the broader ranges of period lengths that in the high-frequency range of the spectrum the strength of the harmonic time order decreases due to an increasing variability of the frequencies. For instance, in the EEG frequency spectrum we have not been able to establish empirically even during night sleep a strict temporal order of the different wave types. Even within the block of heart and respiratory rhythms, the preference of integer frequency ratios, as we have demonstrated, exists only in terms of a statistical preference during day- time, while various disturbing influences may modulate the frequencies of the rhythmic functions /1o/.

Frequency modulation as a response of rhythmic functions to stimulation or strain is, of course, the most disturbing effect on the strict harmonic temporal order of the biological rhythms. However, it is not the only mode of response. Checking again the whole spectrum of autonomous rhythms in man, another principle of functional organization becomes evident (Fig.7).

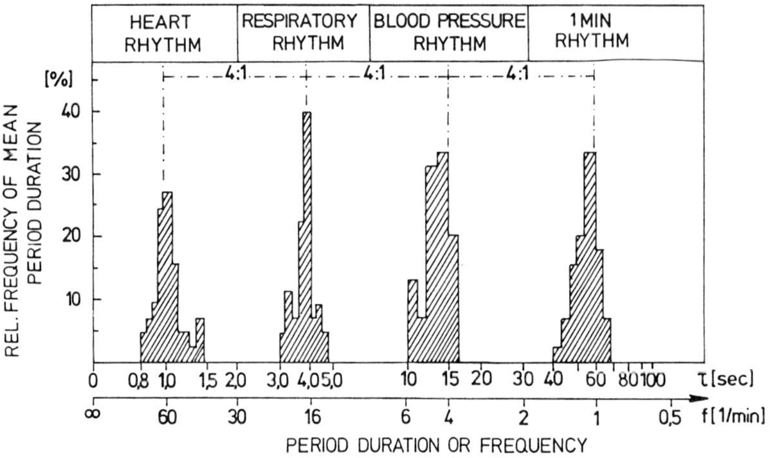

Fig. 6: Frequency histogram of the mean heart rate, respiratory rate, blood pressure waves, and minute rhythms during night sleep, from 18 healthy subjects totalling 53 nights. (From /11/)

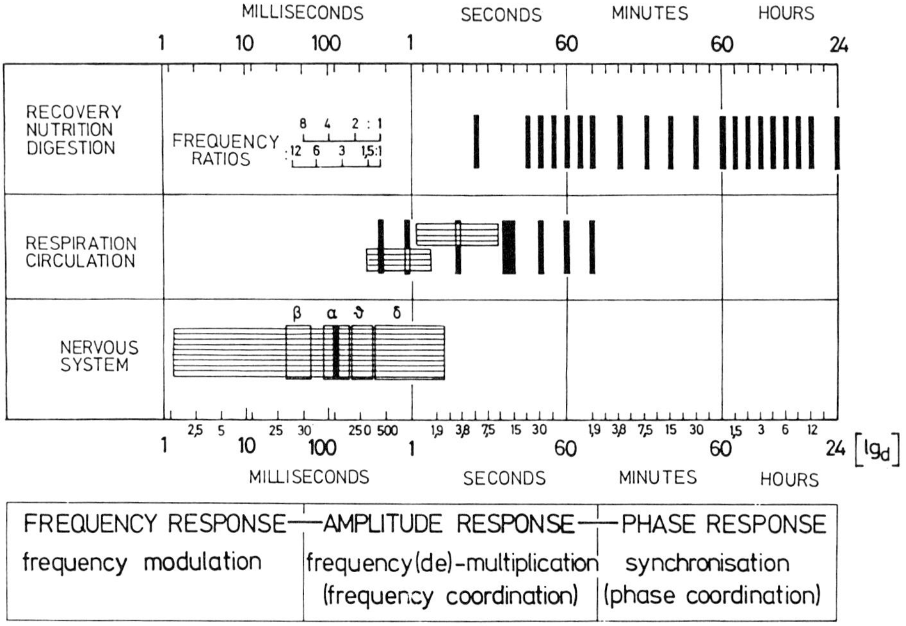

Fig. 7: Frequency behaviour and modes of interaction of the endogenous rhythmic functions in different parts of the spectrum. Black vertical bars indicate the preferred frequency bands, horizontal hatching indicates the range of frequency modulation. For further explanation, see the text. (After /12/)

Looking at their functional significance, we may discover in the longer wave section mainly rhythms of the metabolic system. e.g. nutritional, digestive, and recovery functions. By contrast, the short-wave section contains the rhythmic actions of the nervous system, forming an information system. In the intermediate range we find a predominance of rhythms serving the transportation and distribution functions, mainly of the circulatory, respiratory, and intestinal system.

This tripartite organization of the autonomous spectrum also involves different functional behaviours with regard to frequency, amplitude, and phase: As symbolized by the horizontal hatching, the rhythms of nerval action exhibit the greatest variability of frequencies. These rhythms are responsible for all the transmission and communication in the information system by portraying the momentary degree of excitation by means of frequency modulation. It is only during night sleep that the rhythmicity of the central nervous system becomes partially synchronized into certain frequency bands of the EEG. Thus we may speak of a frequency-responding system.

By contrast, the rhythms of the metabolic system in the longer wave section prefer distinct frequency bands, which are ordered into integer ratios. In the figure, the black bars mark the preferred frequency bands or frequency norms, respectively. Some of them have proved to dispose of stabilizing mechanisms, as for instance with regard to temperature. The abscissa represents a logarithmic scale, hence the frequency ratios as indicated apply to all parts of the spectrum. In order to maintain this temporal order, the rhythmic functions tend to respond to interferences by changing their amplitude or phase, whereby changes in frequency only occur by "jumping" into other preferred bands of the harmonic system. Therefore, these rhythms of the metabolic system are characterized by amplitude- and phase responses, leading to frequency multiplication, demultiplication and/or synchronization.

In the middle wave length section the rhythmical functions of the transportation- and distribution system exhibit both: frequency modulation response to functional load as well as changes in amplitude and setting of frequency norms by coordinating the rhythmical actions to a larger harmonic time structure of integer frequency ratios, based on the preference to phase response.

Concerning the interactions of the various rhythmic functions, as from the point of view of these structural principles, we must expect slower rhythms to be capable to act upon the faster rhythms preferably by modulating the frequencies, while on the other hand changes of the faster rhythms, as mostly evoked by external loads, may influence the slower ones preferably by enhancing their amplitudes, multiplying their period lengths and/or shifting their phases.

This can be verified, for example, by the frequency modulation of faster rhythms as induced by the circadian rhythm under resting conditions. As shown in Fig.8, circadian changes in frequency not only occur in pulse- and respiratory rates, but also in the alpha-frequency, in the arterial dicrotic wave length, in the blood pressure rhythm and circa-minute rhythm as well as in the rhythmic change of the laterality of the nasal respiration. The circadian amplitude of frequency modulation is similar in all these functions, amounting to about 10-12%. However, the slower rhythms like circa-minute rhythm and laterality rhythm exhibit multimodal frequency distributions of their period lengths. Therefore the question remains open whether or not the circadian changes of the mean frequencies are produced by frequency modulation or by frequency jumps within the spectrum of preferred frequency bands.

On the other hand, the circadian rhythm originates characteristic changes in the strength of the harmonic time order, as measured by the rates of phase coupling between the different rhythmical functions. Fig.9 shows, for example, daily courses of the coupling rates, leading to integer frequency ratios between various minute rhythms, between blood pressure rhythm and respiration, blinking rhythm and respiration, heart beat and respiration, as well as heart beat and dicrotic arterial oscillation. In all parameters, the coupling rates increase during the increasing trophotropic state of the autonomous system in the afternoon and night, whereas during the ergotropic phase of the circadian variation the coupling rates decline to a minimum.

It is important to point out that the increase of functional economy which is brought about by strengthening the harmonical time order represents an important

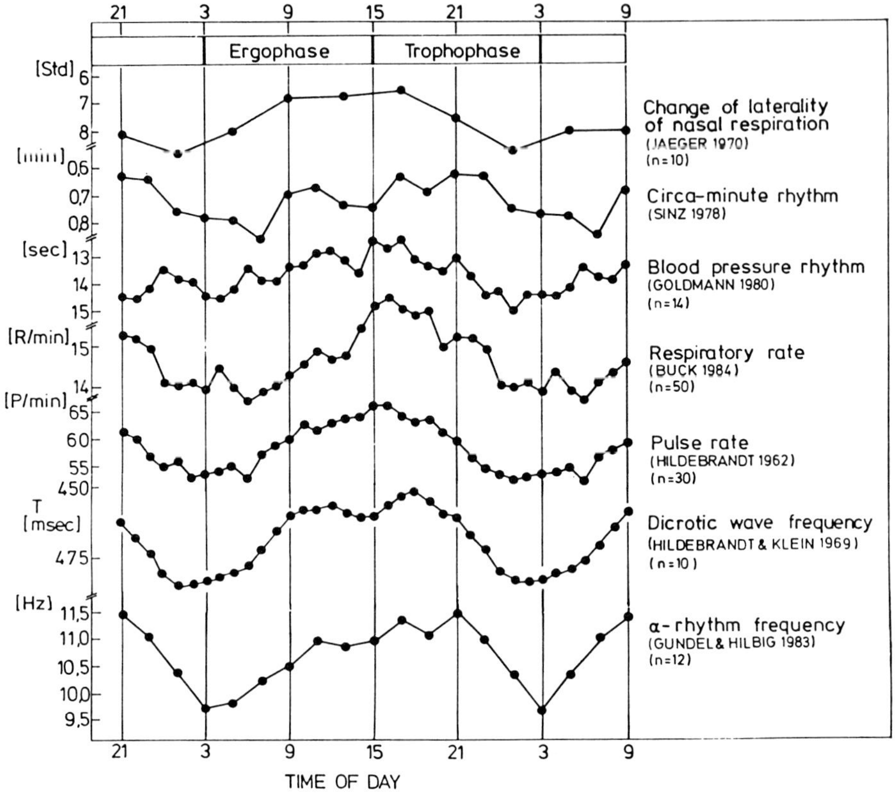

Fig. 8: Daily courses of the mean frequencies of various ultradian rhythms. A compilation of data from the literature.

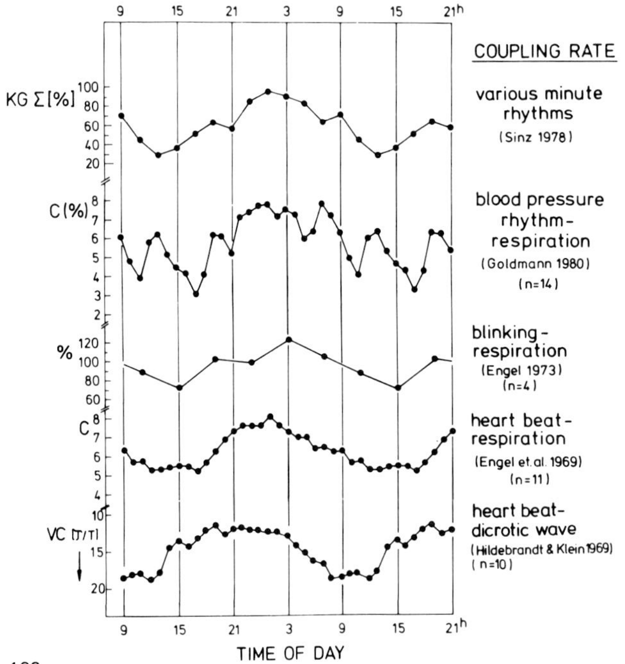

Fig. 9: Mean daily courses of the coupling rates between various ultradian rhtyhmic functions in man. Compilation of results from the literature.

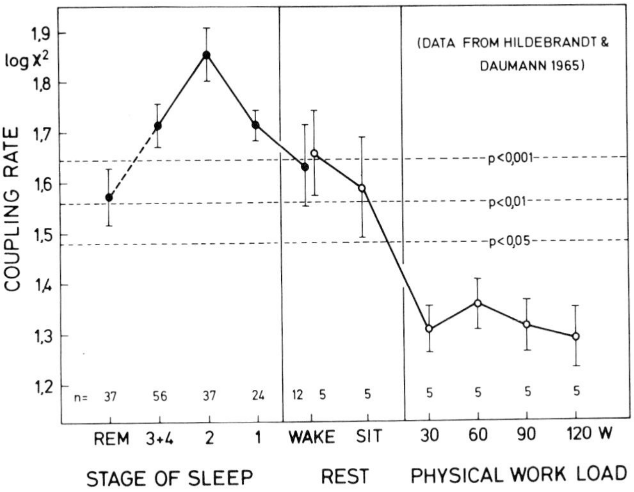

Fig.10: Mean coupling rates between onset of inspiration and heart beat in healthy subjects during different sleep stages, waking, and sitting, as compared to different amounts of physical work load (Data from /9/). (After /13/)

precondition for the recuperation and regeneration during night sleep. Several findings could prove that functional economy is, in general, favoured by an enhancement of the harmonic time structure. This will be demonstrated in more detail by RASCHKE in this volume.

By contrast, the destructive effects of physiological and pathological strain or stress on the harmonic temporal order have been demonstrated in the different parts of the rhythm spectrum. With respect to this I will not touch the well-known desynchronizing effects on the EEG. Fig.1o shows by a compilation from RASCHKE et al./19/ the rate of phase coupling between heart and respiratory rhythm at different sleep stages and at different amounts of work load. Whereas during sleep the coordination between both the rhythmic functions is strengthened with increasing depth of sleep, even small amounts of work load are able to abolish completely the rhythmic interaction.

Figure 11 shows histograms of the ratio between heart period and arterial dicrotic wave length in groups of subjects under resting conditions. In healthy individuals (center) the whole number ratio of 2:1 is markedly preferred. ECKERMANN /14/ has calculated that the economical effect of this coordination amounts to about 3o %. In trained subjects with increased trophotropy of the autonomous system the preference of the integer ratio is much more pronounced and (due to the bradycardia) the ratio of 3:1 is also preferred. In a group of patients, however, suffering from functional disorders of the circulatory system, we could observe a drastic deviation from the normal phase- or frequency coordination. Possibly, the preference of the ratio of 1.5:1 might indicate only a reduction of the coordinative effects.

A further example concerns the coordination between respiration and blood pressure rhythm in man. As shown in Fig.12, in a lying position the coupling rate is markedly increased, demonstrating again that ergotropic frequency modulation tends to weaken the autonomous temporal order /15/.

Most extensive studies on the effect of strain on the time structure of rhythmic functions have been performed in the range of circadian rhythms, and this preferably with respect to the response to the load of night and shift work. In prin-

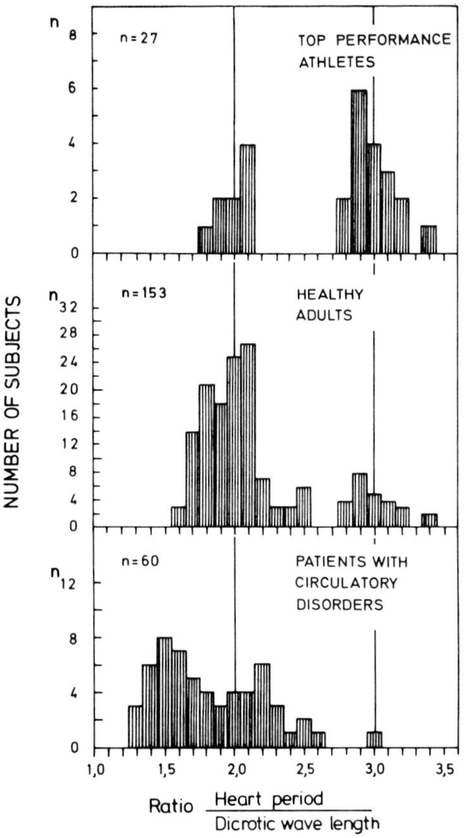

Fig.11: Histogram of the mean ratios between heart period and dicrotic wave length under resting conditions in top-performance athletes (top), healthy adults (center), and patients suffering from circulatory disorders (bottom). (From /16/)

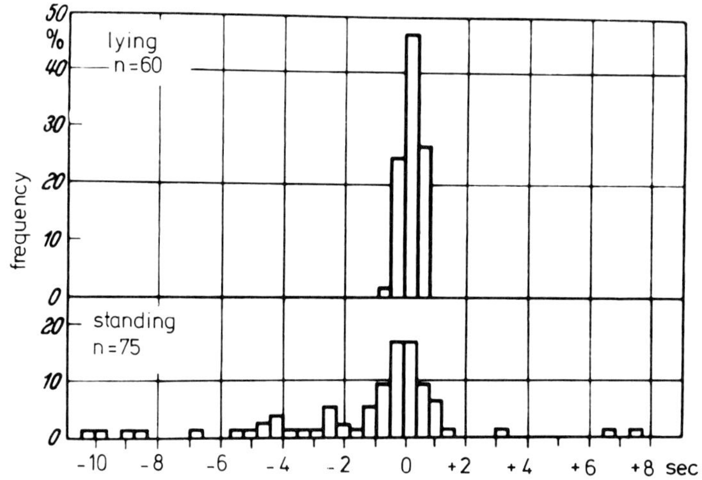

Fig.12: Frequency distributions of the deviations from the normal phase reference between respiration and blood pressure rhythm in a healthy adult in lying and standing position. (From /15/)

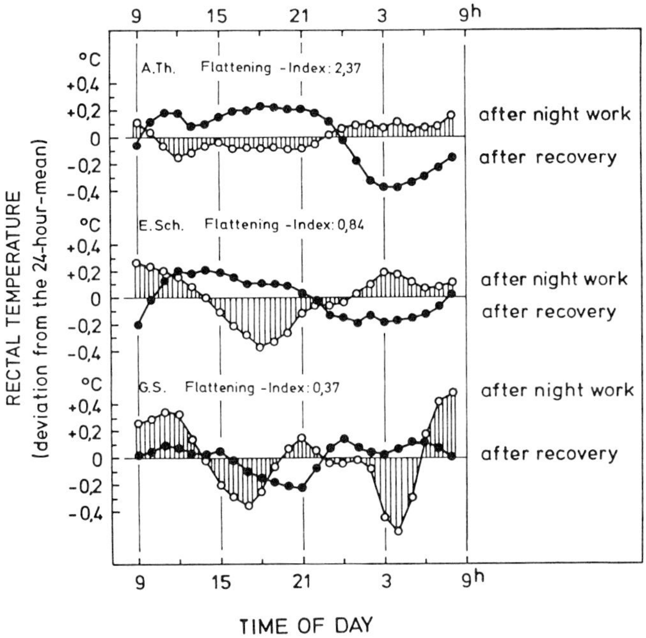

Fig.13: Three examples of the daily course of body temperature of night nurses after a period of night work and after a recovery period. Curves are plotted as deviations from the 24-hour average. For further explanations see text. (After /17/)

ciple, three different modes of response of the circadian system can be observed, as shown by the examples of three night nurses, whose circadian courses of rectal temperature were measured under strict resting conditions after normal daily routine (recovery) and after a period of three weeks of permanent night work (Fig.13).

In the upper example, the load of night work leads to a more or less complete flattening of the circadian amplitude. This mode of circadian response is also well known for pathological conditions. MENZEL /18/ was the first to point out that in patients the circadian amplitude decreases with increasing severeness of an illness.

In the second example, night work is responded to by a phase shift of the circadian rhythm of body temperature, corresponding to the shift of the daily routine.

In the lowest example, besides the increase in the circadian amplitude, after the night work period the subject exhibited a two-peaked 12-hour periodicity instead of the 24-hour rhythm. Such frequency multiplications mainly occur when the organism is loaded without having sufficient opportunity for recuperation. In studies on engine drivers we were able to show that the amplitude of the 12-hour period increases with increasing amount of tiredness. As demonstrated in Fig.14, the amplitude of the afternoon dip of performance,which is formed by the 12-hour periodicity, is a function of the foregoing clocking-on time.

MENZEL /18/ pointed out that patients suffering from sleep disorders exhibit a prominent 12-hour period of vegetative functions instead of the normal 24-hour rhythm. Furthermore, he observed in patients that with increasing loss of functioning the daily courses were superimposed by submultiple periods of the circadian rhythm.

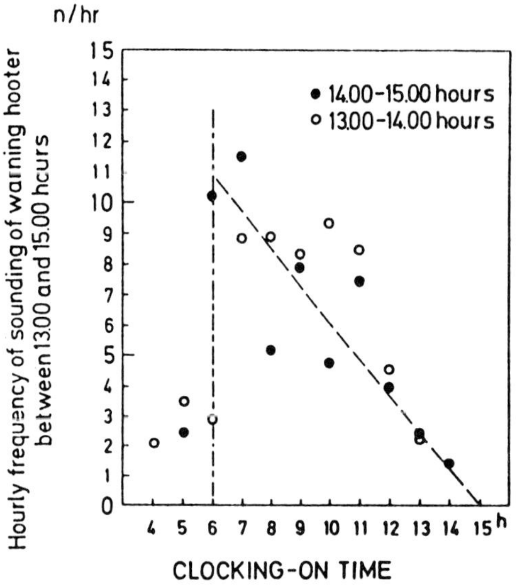

Fig.14: Mean hourly frequency of the warning hooter as caused by handling errors of the engine drivers between 13.oo and 15.oo h on the day related to the time of day when shift started. (After /19/)

In principle, it has been known for a long time that the reactions of living systems are periodically structured. However, up to now only few chronobiologists have tried to ascertain the particular properties of these reactive periodicities, and to examine their interrelations to the spontaneous rhythmic functions. The main interest has been focussed on the spontaneous rhythms. These, however, become overt only under undisturbed and unmasked conditions, when the organism is in a regulatory equilibrium with both the outer and the inner environment, that means in a state of complete adaptation.

Of course, reactions never represent a direct continuation of the stimulus, neither with regard to quality nor to quantity, but can be evoked by the stimulus. Hence, a periodicity, which is induced by a stimulus, brings to appearance an endogenous time structure, whether it be already active or in a latent state.

According to our results, reactive periodicity can be evoked by single, repeated, or continuous stimulation. As an important characteristic the phase position of reactive periods depends on the stimulus, the stressor acting as a synchronizer of the reacting functions.

The amplitudes of reactive periodicity dampen down with increasing compensation. Hence, reactive periods often appear to be transients during adaptive processes.

Concerning the time structure, the period lengths of reactive periodicities differ from those of the spontaneous rhythms, however, they prefer whole-number frequency relationships with the spontaneous ones. By this, they prove to be parts of the coordinated harmonic time structure of the organism. Under strain, rhythmic functions can transitorily undergo frequency multiplications or demultiplications, returning to the spontaneous rhythmicity after compensation is completed, or - as sometimes - reactive periodicity dampens down completely, indicating that the responding oscillator returns to latency.

These characteristic properties of reactive periodicity can be observed in all ranges of the spectrum: Fig.15 shows, as an example, two curves of human muscle blood flow, as observed by GOLENHOFEN /20/, representing an adaptive reaction of the blood vessels to the continuous infusion of adrenaline. In both cases the drug evokes a periodic response, the onset of which is strongly related to the begin of injection, and the amplitudes dampen down under the continuous action of the drug. The period duration amounts to 2 min, thus doubling the spontaneous 1-min rhythm of muscle blood flow in man

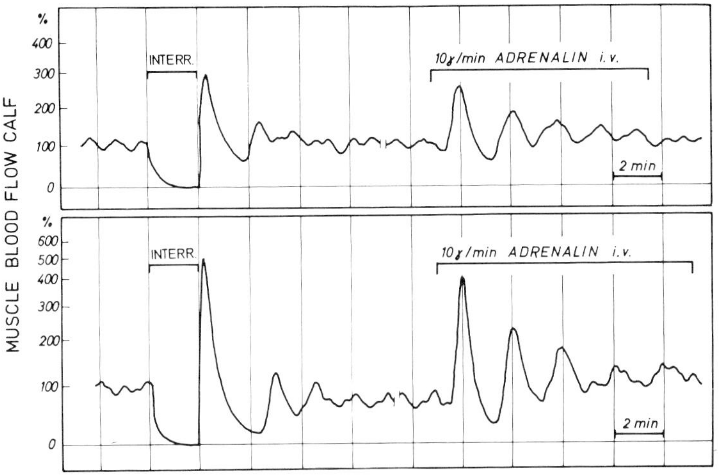

Fig.15: Two examples of reactive periodicity, evoked by a continuous infusion of adrenaline, in the course of muscle blood flow in man. Blood flow was measured by means of a heated thermocouple element. Interr.= interruption of the spontaneous blood flow by inflation of a cuff. Ordinates are calibrated in % of the average resting blood flow. (From /20/)

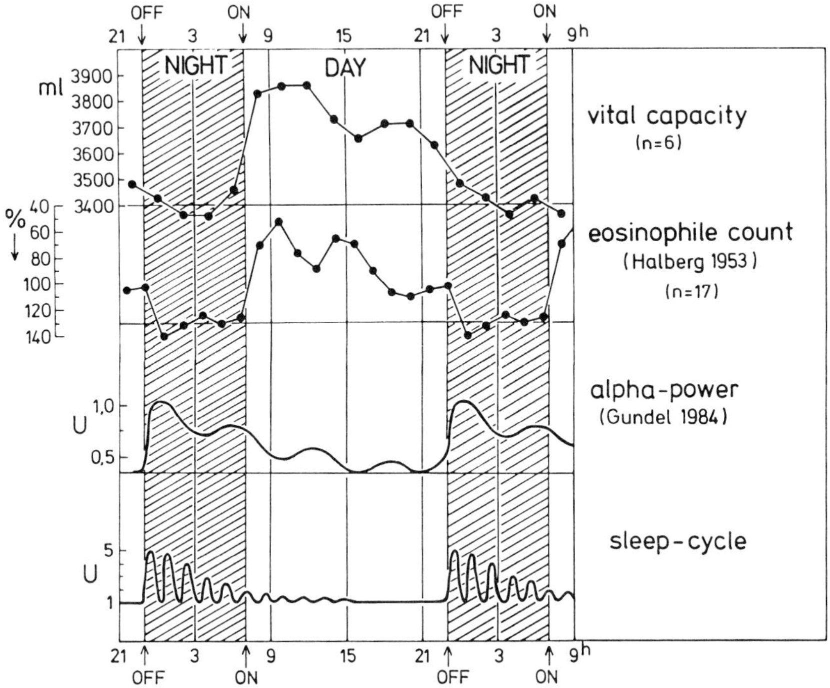

Fig.16: Two examples each of the ultradian periodic response to onset and offset of the day, respectively. For further explanation see text. (After /12/)

As shown in the next figure (Fig.16), in the ultradian range of the spectrum the more or less abrupt changes of the external milieu between day and night are responded to by periodic reactions. There are several functions, which respond to the morning onset of the day by a steep initial deviation continuing as a reactive periodicity, the amplitude of which is dampened down during the day. The period lengths mostly represent submultiples of the 24-hour period.

There are, however, other rhythmical functions, which respond to the offset of day or sleep begin by forming periodically structured reactions, the amplitudes of which dampen down during the night and the following day. There are, for instance, some indications that the sleep cycle as a basic rest-activity cycle continues only during the first half of the day /21/. The period lengths of the off-responses also represent submultiples of the circadian period.

From the medical point of view, periodic reactions, which are structured by multiple frequencies of the circamensual cycle, are of predominant interest. Here the preferred period length amounts to about 7 days. According to several authors, this so-called circaseptan periodicity can be seen in numerous adaptive and compensating processes, for instance in wound healing, in immunological adaptation like infectious diseases or in rejection of organ transplants. Furthermore, the circaseptan periodicity synchronizes the cycles of cell division of erythropoietic reactions to high altitude as well as of compensatory growth of organs.

Therapeutical induction of circaseptan periodicity during cure treatment could prove the decisive fact that this reactive periodicity is not simply a consequence of the social week cycle, but is evoked by the synchronizing onset of physical treatment. As shown in Fig.17, the circaseptan periodicity of reaction time and flicker fusion threshold in groups of patients is strictly synchronized over the days of treatment and does not show any phase difference according to the day of the week, when treatment was started. By the way, comparison with non-treated inhabitants of the same spa station did not show a significant periodicity.

Looking again at the whole spectrum of rhythmic functions, the complexity of the periodic reactions increases also with increasing period length, gaining more and more adaptive significance (Fig.18). In any part of the spectrum, the period durations of the reactive periods are ranged between the respective spontaneous rhythms, which dominate the time structure of the organism under resting conditions and in complete adaptation.

From the standpoint of a faster spontaneous rhythm, the appearance of a slower reactive periodicity involves a period multiplication, which at the same time increases the autonomous amplitudes, leading to longer lasting and more intensive recovery processes, thus preparing for increases in functional capacity.

From the standpoint of a slower spontaneous rhythm, however, the induction of a reactive periodicity of higher frequency represents a frequency multiplication, which is able to make use more economically of the actual capacity, according to the well-known principle of interval training. - Both mechanisms are decisive preconditions for proper compensation or adaptation.

Considering all the findings as exemplified by the figures demonstrated, one can summarize that there exist at least five different modes of rhythm response (Fig.19), each of them leading to different consequences with respect to the temporal order in the organism:

1. Rhythmic functions can react by frequency modulation. This mainly occurs in the high frequency section of the spectrum, and must originate a more or less complete loss of the harmonic time structure.

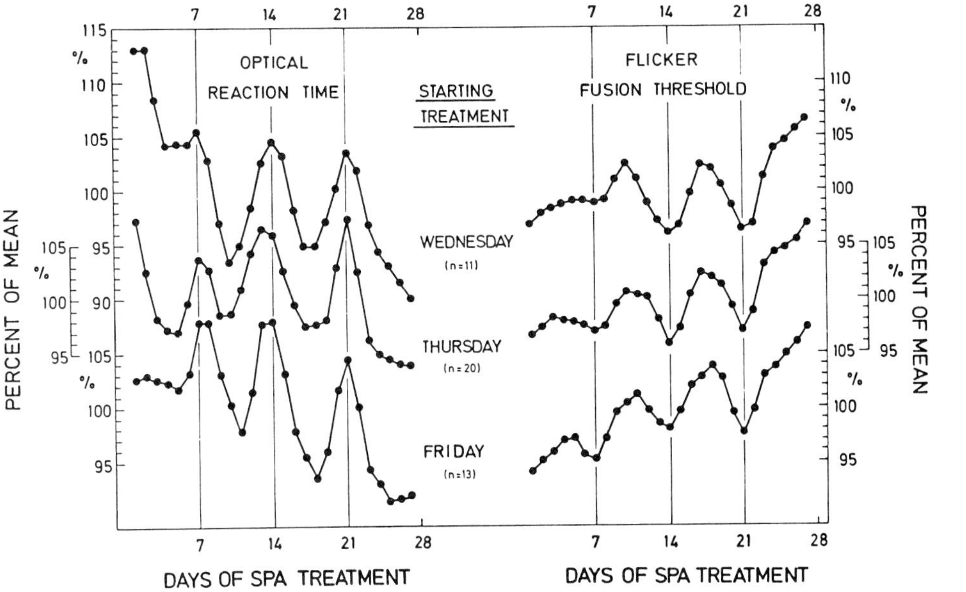

Fig.17: Mean courses of optical reaction time and flicker fusion threshold in 3 subgroups of patients starting spa treatment on different days of the week. (From /22/)

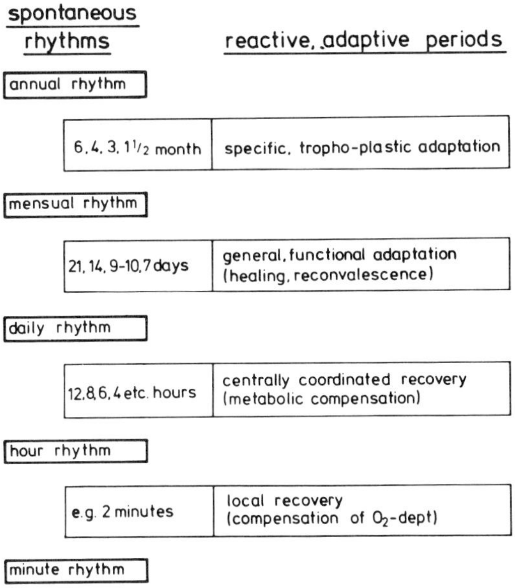

Fig.18: The positions of reactive periods between the spontaneous biological rhythms and their adaptive significance in the different parts of the rhythm spectrum. For further explanation see text. (From /1/)

2. Under strain, rhythmic functions can develop frequency jumps by frequency multiplication or demultiplication. The resulting reactive periods modify the harmonic time structure of the organism, using an "emergency time order" to improve compensatory or adaptive efficiency. This mode of rhythm response can be observed in all slower functions, which are not able to respond by frequency modulations.

MODE OF RHYTHM RESPONSE →	TEMPORAL DISORDER
1. Frequency Modulation	Loss of Time Structure
2. Frequency (De)-Multiplication Frequency "Jumps" Reactive Periodicity	Modification of the Harmonic Time Structure ("Emergency Order")
3. Phase Shifting through Zeitgeber Response	Internal Desynchronization (Preservation of External Order)
4. Phase Shifting through Transitory Uncoupling	External Desynchronization (Preservation of Internal Order)
5. Amplitude Response	No Change in Temporal Order

Fig.19: Modes of rhythm response leading to different types of temporal disorder. For further explanation see text

3. The - so to speak - classical mode of rhythm response by phase shift mainly occurs in the longer wave section of the spectrum. It has to be differentiated: There is phase shifting, which is induced by zeitgeber action. This may lead to internal desynchronization because of the different responsiveness of the compartments of the long wave system concerned.

4. Recent findings in night and shift work /23/ , which showed that the speed of phase shift of the circadian system does not depend on the rotation speed of the shift schedule, lead to the assumption that delaying phase shifts can be caused by a transitory uncoupling from the environmental zeitgeber regimen. In this case, the internal time order can be preserved at the cost of an external desynchronization.

5. Finally, rhythmic functions can respond by mere changes in amplitude. This mode of response will not change the temporal order of the organism, however, amplitude response implies high functional capacities. It is interesting to remember that well trained subjects prefer amplitude response, for instance in the stroke volume of the heart and, at the same time, they are able to strengthen the coordination of rhythmical functions, leading to higher economy.

To come to an end, I want to emphasize again that chronobiology up to now was mainly concerned with the spontaneous rhythmic functions and their harmonic temporal order. The reactive behaviour and the modifications of this time structure have not been taken sufficiently into consideration.

Besides of the resulting theoretical deficit, from the practical point of view, it is important to discriminate between the spontaneous rhythmicity under completely adapted resting conditions and the various modes of reactive modifications of the time structure as caused by rhythm response. This might contribute to a better understanding of the temporal order in the organism and help to avoid misjudgements of temporal disorders, as caused by physiological strain or pathological impacts, respectively.

References

1. G.Hildebrandt: The time structure of adaptive processes. In Biological Adaptation, ed. by G.Hildebrandt & H.Hensel (Georg Thieme-Verlag, Stuttgart, New York 1982) pp. 24-39
2. Z.Hejl: Periodisches System biologischer Rhythmen. In 3. DDR-UdSSR Symposium Chronobiologie und Chronomedizin, 1.-6.Juli 1986 in Halle(Saale)DDR, Ref. P 51

3. R.J.Broughton: Three Central Issues Concerning Ultradian Rhythms. In Ultradian Rhythms in Physiology and Behaviour, ed. by H.Schulz & P.Lavie (Springer-Verlag,Berlin,Heidelberg,New York,Tokyo 1985) pp. 217-233
4. K.Golenhofen & D.von Loh: Elektrophysiologische Untersuchungen zur normalen Spontanaktivität der isolierten Taenia coli des Meerschweinchens. Pflügers Arch ges.Physiol. 314: 312-328 (1970)
5. R.Sinz: Zeitstrukturen und organismische Regulation.(Akademie-Verlag, Berlin 1978)
6. K.Bucher, H.Schwitter, B.Hool-Zulauf & E.Batschelet: Links between cardiac and respiratory rhythmicity. Res.Exp.Med.157: 281-288 (1972)
7. E.von Holst: Die relative Koordination als Phänomen und als Methode zentralnervöser Funktionsanalyse. Ergebn.Physiol. 42: 228-3o6 (1939)
8. G.Hildebrandt: Die Koordination rhythmischer Funktionen beim Menschen. Verh.Dtsch.Ges.Inn.Med. 73: 922-941 (1967)
9. G.Hildebrandt & F.J.Daumann: Die Koordination von Puls- und Atemrhythmus bei Arbeit. Internat.Z.angew.Physiol. 21: 27-48 (1965)
1o. G.Hildebrandt: Coordination of cardiac and respiratory rhythms and effects thereon of therapeutic procedures. Journ.Auton.Nerv.Syst.Suppl: 253-263 (1986)
11. F.Raschke: Analysis of the Frequency and Phase Relationships of Circulatory and Respiratory Rhythms During Adaptive Processes. In Biological Adaptation, ed. by G.Hildebrandt & H.Hensel (Georg Thieme-Verlag, Stuttgart,New York 1982) pp. 52-63
12. G.Hildebrandt: Functional significance of ultradian rhythms and reactive periodicity. J.interdiscipl.Cycle Res. 1986 (In press)
13. F.Raschke & G.Hildebrandt: Coupling of the cardio-respiratory control system by modulation and triggering. In Cardiovascular System Dynamics - Models and Measurements, ed. by Th.Kenner, R.Busse & H.Hinghofer-Szalkay (Plenum Press, New York, London 1982) pp. 533-542
14. P.Eckermann: Untersuchungen an einem Kreislaufmodell mittels Analogrechner. Inaug.-Diss. Rostock (1969)
15. K.Golenhofen & G.Hildebrandt: Die Beziehungen des Blutdruckrhythmus zu Atmung und peripherer Durchblutung. Pflügers Arch.ges.Physiol.267: 27-45 (1958)
16. E.Gadermann, G.Hildebrandt & H.Jungmann: Über harmonische Beziehungen zwischen Pulsrhythmus und arterieller Grundschwingung. Z.Kreislaufforsch. 5o: 8o5-814 (1961)
17. G.Hildebrandt: Survey of current concepts relative to rhythms and shift work. In Chronobiology: Principles and Applications to Shifts in Schedules, ed. by L.E.Scheving & F.Halberg (Sijthoff & Noordhoff, Alphen aan den Rijn, Rockville,Md.USA 1980) pp. 261-292
18. W.Menzel: Therapie unter dem Gesichtspunkt biologischer Rhythmen. In Ergebnisse der Physikalisch-diätetischen Therapie, ed.by H.Lampert (Steinkopff, Dresden, Leipzig 1955) Band 5: pp.1-38
19. G.Hildebrandt, W.Rohmert & J.Rutenfranz: 12&24 H Rhythms of Error Frequency of Locomotive Drivers and the Influence of Tiredness on it. Int.J.Chronobiol. 2: 175-180
2o. K.Golenhofen: Zur Reaktionsperiodik der menschlichen Muskelstrombahn. Arch.Kreislaufforsch. 38: 2o2-223 (1962)
21. P.Lavie: Ultradian Rhythms: Gates of Sleep and Wakefulness. In Experimental Brain Research, Suppl.12 (Springer-Verlag, Berlin, Heidelberg, New York, Tokyo 1985) pp. 148-164
22. G.Hildebrandt, F.Geyer & W.Brüning: Circaseptan adaptive periodicity and weekly rhythm. In Biological Adaptation, ed. by G.Hildebrandt & H.Hensel (Georg Thieme-Verlag, Stuttgart, New York 1982) pp. 113-116
23. G.Hildebrandt: Individual differences in susceptibility to night- and shift work (Introductory remarks). In Night and Shiftwork: Longterm Effects and their Prevention, ed. by M.Haider, M.Koller & R.Cervinka (Verlag Peter Lang, Frankfurt am Main, Bern, New York 1986) pp. 1o9-122

Bright Light in Work-Sleep Schedules for Shift Workers: Application of Circadian Rhythm Principles

C.I. Eastman

Sleep Disorder Service and Research Center,
Rush-Presbyterian-St. Luke's Medical Center, 1753 West Congress Parkway,
Chicago, IL 60612, USA

1. Shift Work Problems Explained by Circadian Rhythms

Basic research on human circadian rhythms has revealed principles that could be applied to many practical problems such as shift work. Although the problems associated with shift work have been extensively documented and also studied in laboratory simulations [1, 15, 16, 18, 28, 31], there have been few major work-site interventions based on circadian principles [6, 29]. About 20% of the people in industrialized countries are engaged in shift work. Their major complaint is of sleep disturbances, especially in connection with the night shift, but also to some extent with morning work. Sleep after the night shift is short (4-6 hrs) and of poor quality. Other common complaints are persisting fatigue, impaired performance at work, and gastrointestinal difficulties.

Many of the physiologically based problems of shift work can be attributed to conflicts with the body's circadian rhythms [5, 28]. Although most workers believe that noise is the main factor that disturbs their sleep after the night shift, studies show that the shortened sleep results from the improper placement of sleep within the circadian cycle of body temperature [1, 2, 3]. It is difficult to sleep while body temperature is high, and especially when it is rising [9, 45]. Whether there is any causal link between temperature and sleep is not known. The important point is that body temperature is used as a convenient marker for the phase of the internal circadian oscillator. Some models of human circadian rhythms include a second "activity" or sleep-wake oscillator [21, 39], but this is not necessary [13], especially since sleep naturally occurs almost entirely in phase with the temperature rhythm [44]. Alertness and most measures of performance efficiency also have circadian rhythms that parallel the temperature rhythm. Fatigue and impaired performance during night work result when work is placed at an inappropriate phase of the temperature cycle (around the minimum instead of the maximum). The cumulative sleep loss associated with night shifts also contributes to fatigue and poor performance at work.

A typical shift work schedule for intensive care unit nurses at our hospital is shown in Fig. 1. The shift changes between days and nights every two weeks. Other nurses in the units work fixed evening or fixed night shifts. Nurse shift schedules that rotate between the day and night shifts are common [34]. This figure illustrates that sleep after the night shift is usually shorter than sleep before the day shift, although a few sleep episodes before the day shift are also fairly short. Sleep on days off is usually longer. There are some "replacement" naps around 18:00, especially during the night shift. The investigations of others [18, 28, 31] demonstrate that with a work-sleep schedule like this, there can be little adaptation

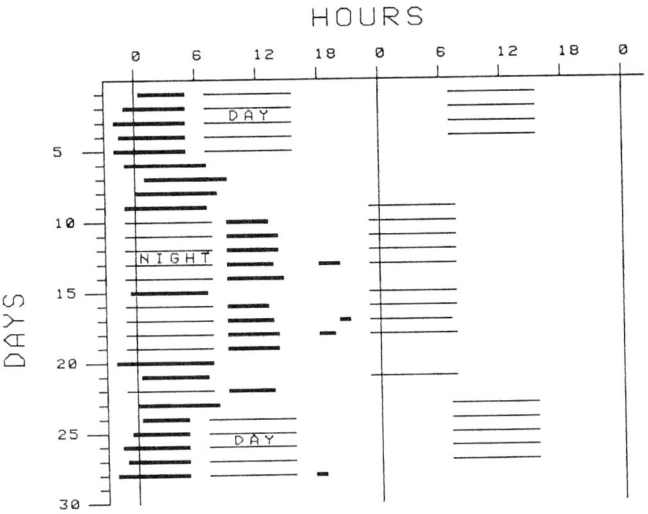

Fig 1. Typical work and sleep schedule for a nurse in an intensive care unit. Thin horizontal lines: work times. Thick horizontal lines: sleep times. The day shift is from 7:00 to 15:30. The night shift is from 23:00 to 7:30. The shift changes every two weeks. The work times are double-plotted. There are four days off in each two week period. The sleep times are chosen to represent those of the typical shift worker based on the survey data of Tepas et al. [35]. To allow for travel time, etc., there are two hrs between waking up in the morning and the beginning of work.

of the circadian rhythm of body temperature to the night shift. Although the temperature rhythm might shift during the five consecutive days of night work, the night sleep on the subsequent day off would reverse most of the change in phase. Thus for most of the days on the night shift, this nurse would be working and sleeping at inappropriate phases of his or her circadian cycle.

There is some controversy about whether a rapidly rotating or slowly rotating shift schedule is best [15, 28]. One advantage of a rapidly rotating system (2-3 days on a particular shift before changing to the next) is that the total number of consecutive days on the night shift are few, minimizing the cumulative sleep loss. A disadvantage is that the circadian rhythms have no time to adjust, and the worker is always forced to sleep and work out of phase with his or her circadian cycle. On the other hand, a slowly rotating system provides more opportunity for adaptation of circadian rhythms. In practice, however, adaptation to the night shift is rarely complete because either the shift changes as soon as adaptation is approached (typically after a week) or there are days off in which the worker reverts to a day-active, night-sleeping schedule. Even "permanent" night shift schedules do not produce complete adaptation because the worker typically reverts to sleeping at night on days off. Thus, the terms "fixed" and "permanent" are misleading because although the work schedule is fixed, the sleep schedule frequently shifts abruptly. Another reason cited for the incomplete adaptation of circadian rhythms even with permanent night work is that although the sleep and work schedule may be shifted, other potential zeitgebers (time givers) such as the natural light-dark (LD) cycle and some social cues do not shift. These stable 24-hr zeitgebers may actually oppose the shifting of the internal circadian rhythms.

2. A Work-Sleep Schedule for Shift Workers

Intensive care nurses must handle complicated equipment and manage critically ill patients at all hours. This is only one situation in which optimal performance is as important at night as during the day. Other pertinent examples with life and death consequences include nuclear power plant operators, air traffic controllers and pilots. Since the typical shift work systems are unsatisfactory for reasons discussed above, a radically different approach is needed. I designed sleep schedules to fit certain intensive care unit work schedules with the goal of producing better adaptation of circadian rhythms to the night shift. One version of this type of work-sleep schedule is shown in Fig. 2. The work times are identical to those in Fig. 1, but the sleep schedule is gradually delayed to facilitate the transition between shifts. If the temperature rhythm delays along with the sleep schedule (i.e., if the temperature rhythm entrains to the sleep schedule), then sleep and work will always fall closer to the appropriate phase of the circadian cycle. In other words, sleep will occur when temperature is low, and work will occur when temperature is high, even during the night shift. Thus, sleep after the night shift should be longer and "deeper" and there should be less fatigue and inefficiency at work. The sleep schedule shifts in a delaying (rather than advancing) direction because the range of entrainment of the temperature rhythm in most experiments is from about 23 to 27 hrs, symmetrical around the average free-running period of about 25 hrs [39, 42]. In other words, the temperature rhythm can be shifted faster in the delaying direction. The Ls and Ds in Fig. 2 will be explained later.

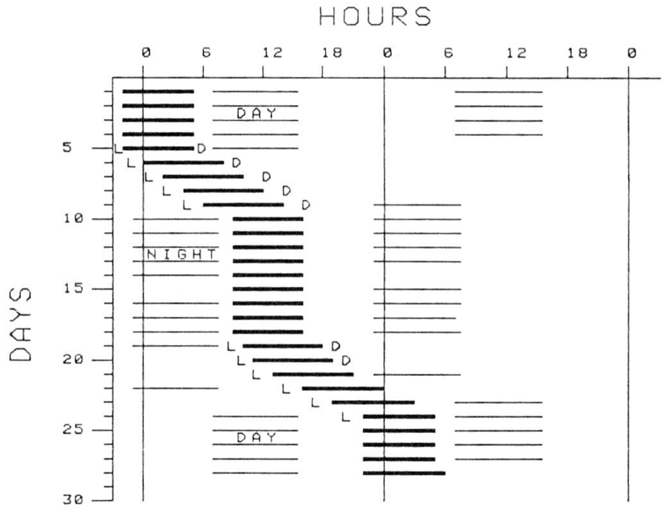

Fig. 2. Identical work schedule as in Fig. 1, but with a sleep schedule based on circadian principles designed to improve sleep and performance. Sleep is delayed by 1-3 hrs per day during certain portions of the schedule. For most days of the night shift sleep is taken in the beginning of the day to conform with the habits of the typical shift worker. However, sleep could be gradually delayed to later in the day starting before day 19 to give the nurse some days with free time in the morning. The Ls show when the worker should be exposed to sunlight (or very bright artificial light). The Ds show when the worker should not be exposed to sunlight.

The success of this plan depends on whether the circadian rhythm of temperature can be entrained to the sleep schedule. The temperature rhythm can be entrained to 26-27 hr sleep-wake schedules (acoustical signals for "get up" and "go to bed") in temporal isolation units where all other time cues are eliminated [40, 41]. However, there have been no studies to determine whether entrainment to such schedules is possible when people live in the real world exposed to the competing 24-hr zeitgebers.

3. Testing a 26-hr Sleep-Wake Schedule

To determine whether sleep and the temperature rhythm of shift workers could follow sleep schedules like that shown in Fig. 2, a 26-hr sleep-wake schedule was tested on four normal subjects (not shift workers) [14]. After a baseline period on a 24-hr sleep-wake schedule, the subjects followed a 26-hr schedule until sleep once again occurred at the baseline time (Fig. 3). Body temperature was continuously measured with a rectal probe and the Vitalog portable monitor. Daily sleep logs provided an estimate of sleep and wake times. Black vinyl was used to cover the bedroom windows to facilitate day sleeping. For further details see EASTMAN [14].

Two subjects followed the sleep schedule with little difficulty, and the temperature rhythm appeared to be entrained to the 26-hr schedule. The data from one of these subjects are shown in Fig. 3. Sleep occurred later in the temperature cycle during the 26-hr schedule compared to the 24-hr schedule. A similar delay in the phase of sleep relative to temperature was seen in subjects entrained to longer zeitgeber periods in the temporal isolation units [39]. Periodograms (not shown) were computed to determine the periodicity of the temperature rhythm [11]. The periodograms from the days of the 26-hr schedule had one significant peak near 26 hrs for both subjects, confirming that the temperature rhythm was synchronized to the 26-hr schedule.

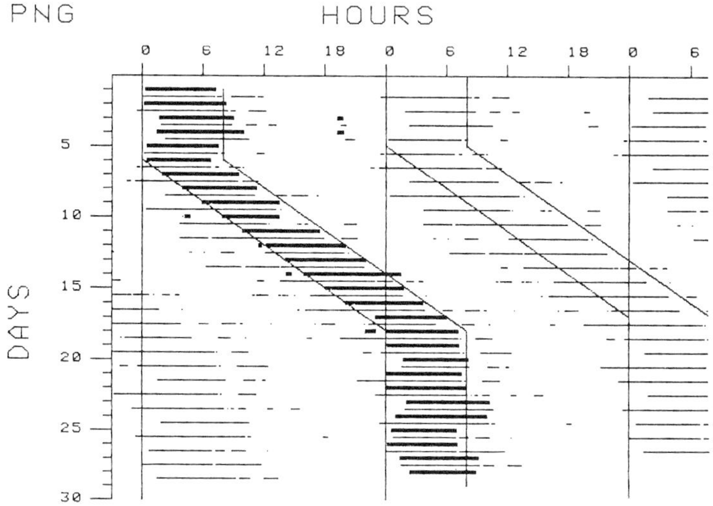

Fig. 3. Subject PNG, sleep and temperature chart. Thick horizontal lines: sleep time. Double lines bounding the sleep times: planned sleep schedule. Thin horizontal lines: temperature below the daily mean. Six days on a 24-hr schedule were followed by 13 days on a 26-hr schedule and 10 days back on the same 24-hr schedule. Sleep times are only plotted once to permit better viewing of the temperature rhythm in the second plot.

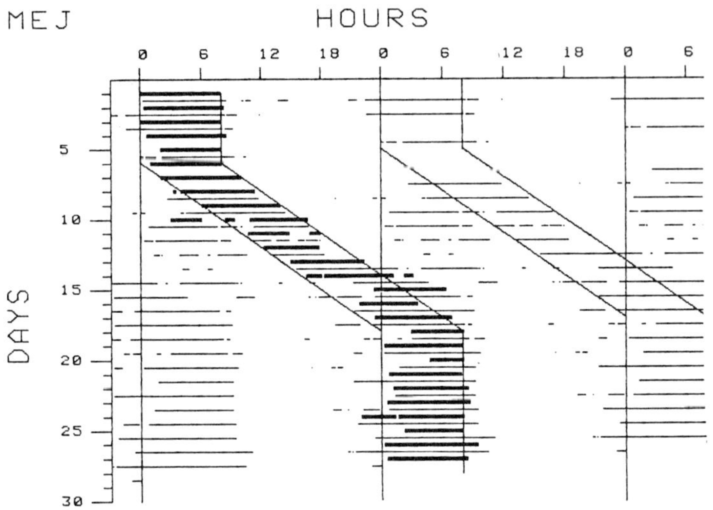

Fig. 4. Subject MEJ, sleep and temperature chart. Due to technical failures, temperature data were lost for days 4, 6 and 7.

On the other hand, two other subjects had considerable difficulty following the 26-hr schedule. The periodograms for temperature for these two subjects had two peaks, one near 24 hrs and one near 26 hrs. The sleep and temperature chart for one of these subjects is shown in Fig. 4. An unintentional nap occurred before the planned bedtime on day 10, and sleep onset was delayed for several hours on day 15 although the subject was in bed trying to sleep. One component of the temperature rhythm remained in phase with the 24-hr day (note the lines between hours 0-8 on days 9-13), and one component followed the 26-hr schedule. Clearly the temperature rhythm of this subject was not entrained to the 26-hr schedule.

4. Adding Bright Light to the 26-hr Sleep-Wake Schedule

At this point it appeared that a work-sleep schedule that incorporated a 26-hr sleep-wake schedule might produce the desired effect for some, but not all shift workers. Meanwhile, the importance of the natural LD cycle as a zeitgeber for man was being stressed by LEWY et al. [22, 23, 25, 26]. After discovering that sunlight or very bright artificial light, but not ordinary indoor light, could suppress nocturnal melatonin secretion, they suggested that human circadian rhythms might be entrained by the natural LD cycle, unperturbed by the use of indoor light. They further suggested that circadian rhythms might be phase-shifted by very bright light applied at the appropriate time as determined by the phase-response curve (PRC).

The PRC is typically generated by testing the effect of a short pulse of light (e.g., 15 min) on the circadian rhythms of animals that are free-running in constant dark or dim light. The PRC is a graph of the magnitude (hrs) and direction (advance or delay) of the phase shift vs. the time at which the light was applied [30]. Although a PRC has not been generated for humans, the PRCs for other animal species (nocturnal and diurnal) have similar shapes [17]. Thus we can assume that light would shift human circadian rhythms in the same way. The PRC predicts that light at the end of the day (light phase) and in the first half of the night (dark phase) should delay circadian rhythms, light in the second half of the night and in the beginning of the day should advance circadian rhythms, and light during the rest of the day should have little effect.

An experiment was designed to test whether bright light could facilitate entrainment to the 26-hr sleep-wake schedule. Since the 26-hr schedule requires a delay in circadian rhythms (2 hrs/day), bright light was applied before bed, a time predicted by the PRC to delay circadian rhythms. Sunlight was avoided after waking, a time predicted to advance circadian rhythms. The bright light was applied for two hrs with a bank of eight four-foot fluorescent Vita-lite bulbs (producing about 2000 lux at three feet). Similar banks of light have been used to treat winter depression [33]. Ordinary indoor light rarely exceeds 500 lux, and bright sunlight produces about 100,000 lux. The subjects wore dark welder's goggles if they went outdoors in the 6 hrs after waking, but they were encouraged to stay indoors at these times. The black vinyl over the bedroom windows prevented sunlight from reaching the subjects near the end of their sleep episodes and in the hours soon after waking.

To date four subjects have been studied. They followed the 26-hr sleep-wake schedule twice, separated by at least 12 days on a 24-hr schedule. The conditions during one of the 26-hr schedules were the same as for the four subjects discussed previously (the natural light condition). During the other 26-hr schedule exposure to bright light was manipulated as described above (the evening light condition). The results from one subject are shown in Fig. 5. She was able to sleep within the planned times throughout the entire experiment, but had more difficulty sleeping during the 26-hr schedules than during the 24-hr schedules. There was not a large difference in sleep times between the two 26-hr schedules. The pattern of sleep throughout the experiment was similar for two other subjects. The fourth subject had considerably more difficulty sleeping on the 26-hr schedule during the natural light condition than during the evening light condition.

Figure 5 shows that the temperature rhythm of subject EMP appeared entrained to the 26-hr sleep-wake schedule during the evening light condition, but not during the natural light condition. Notice that the temperature lines followed the 26-hr schedule during the evening light condition, but that there was a strong 24-hr component during the natural light condition (see hrs 2-10 on days 31-39). The temperature periodogram for the evening light condition had one peak at 26 hrs, but for the natural light condition there were two peaks, one near 24 hrs and one near 26 hrs.

An important consideration is the issue of masking, in which the alternation of sleep and wake produces a direct effect on temperature which can obscure (mask) the temperature variation generated by the endogenous oscillator [4, 27, 28]. In this case, the difference in the temperature rhythm between the evening and natural light conditions cannot be due to masking by sleep because sleep occurs at approximately the same times in both conditions.

The results from two other subjects were similar to those shown in Fig. 5. The periodograms from the natural light condition had two peaks, whereas those from the evening light condition had one peak at 26 hrs. These periodograms can be seen in EASTMAN [12]. In other words, the temperature rhythm of three subjects was entrained to the 26-hr sleep-wake schedule when bright light was used to delay

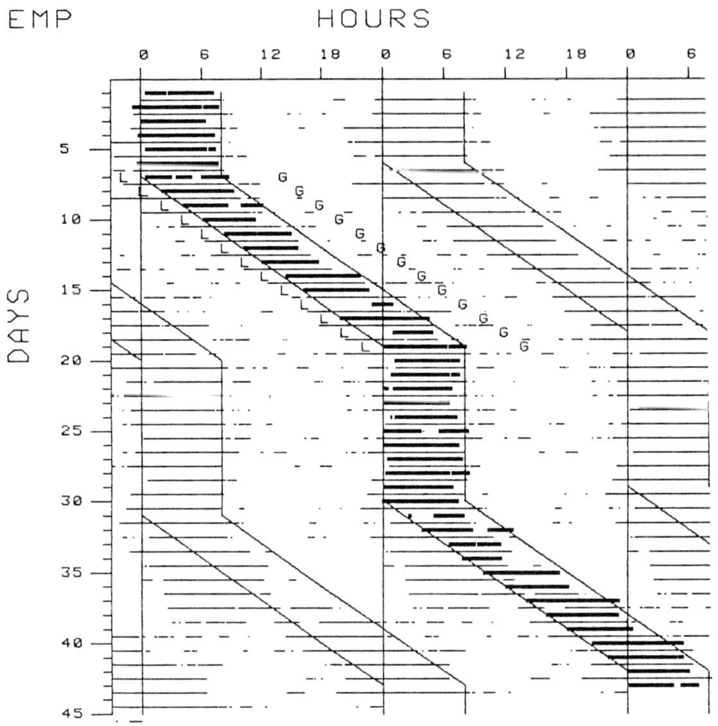

Fig. 5. Subject EMP, sleep and temperature chart. Ls and Gs mark the days when the subject sat in front of the bright lights for 2 hrs before bed, and wore the dark goggles if outside in the 6 hrs after waking.

circadian rhythms and sunlight was avoided at times that could advance circadian rhythms. The fourth subject was not entrained to either 26-hr schedule. The periodograms from the evening and natural light conditions both had two peaks [see EASTMAN, 12]. However, the strength of the 24-hr component was reduced and the 26-hr component was enhanced during the evening light condition for this subject. Thus, for all subjects studied so far, the manipulation of bright light exposure improved the entrainment of the temperature rhythm to a 26-hr sleep-wake schedule.

Another way to conceptualize the design is in terms of the periodicities of the zeitgebers. In the evening light condition there were two 26-hr zeitgebers, the sleep-wake schedule and the bright lights (2 hrs every 26 hrs). One of the 24-hr zeitgebers (the natural LD cycle) was partially blocked out. In the natural light condition the only 26-hr zeitgeber was the sleep-wake schedule. Bright light (sunlight) occurred with a 24-hr period. Changing the periodicity of bright light exposure was enough to produce entrainment to the 26-hr sleep-wake schedule in most cases despite the competing influence of all the other 24-hr zeitgebers, such as social cues.

Recently other investigators have also shown that bright light can shift human circadian rhythms. WEVER [38, 43] had special bright lights built into the temporal isolation unit. With these lights the lower and upper limits of the range of entrainment for temperature were extended beyond 18 and 29 hrs. No combination of zeitgebers had ever pushed the temperature rhythm to these limits. Bright lights also produced faster adjustment to a simulated westward flight across six time zones. LEWY et al. [25] applied morning or evening light and shifted the phase of the melatonin and temperature rhythm of depressed patients in the direction predicted by the PRC. Their earlier studies on normal subjects [23, 24] had shown that the phase of the melatonin rhythm could be advanced by blocking out evening sunlight (advancing dusk) and delayed by blocking out morning sunlight (delaying dawn). In other words, the circadian rhythm was shifted in the direction predicted by the PRC by the removal, rather than by the addition, of bright light. CZEISLER et al. [8] produced a six hr phase delay in the temperature rhythm of one woman by exposing her to bright light for four hours before bed. The large phase shift may be due in part to the facts that the light was brighter than that used by other investigators and the subject was kept indoors and thus away from morning sunlight that might cause a phase advance.

Most of the studies mentioned above are preliminary and involve measurements on very few subjects. Obviously more work needs to be done to determine the parameters of light (and dark) necessary to produce a desired phase shift (e.g., intensity, duration and timing). In other words we need to know the shape of the PRC for various stimuli in humans and the variability to be expected among subjects. Some of this work might best be performed in temporal isolation units. However, knowing the shape of the PRC is not enough to predict what will happen to the circadian rhythms of people during light manipulations in the natural environment where there are competing zeitgebers. This must be determined in field studies.

5. Adding Bright Light to the Work-Sleep Schedule for Shift Workers

Given the mounting evidence that bright light can shift human circadian rhythms, it makes sense to add light manipulations to the work-sleep schedule in Fig. 2. Accordingly, during the delaying portions of the sleep schedule the worker should be exposed to sunlight, or very bright artificial lights, before sleep and should avoid sunlight after waking. The Ls and Ds in Fig. 2 show when light should be applied and avoided. Note that there are only two Ds on the second delaying schedule (days 19 and 20) because after that the worker will be waking up after sunset. The delay shift from days 18 to 24 should be easier than the shift from days 5 to 10 for several reasons. First, natural sunlight will be available before bed and this might be more convenient and would be more effective (brighter) than artificial lights. Also, it should be easier to avoid sunlight in the morning because on most days the worker will wake up after sunset. Finally, the sleep-wake schedule will be moving toward, rather than away from, being in phase with the natural 24-hr zeitgebers. For these reasons this delaying schedule was designed with larger phase shifts, mostly three hrs/day, as compared to the first delaying schedule (days 5-10) in which the shift is usually only 2 hrs/day. Sleep schedules like that shown in Fig. 2 can be made to fit many different work schedules, and they are especially easy to design when evening work shifts are included, as long as the work shifts rotate in the delaying direction (from days to evenings to nights).

Of course more research is needed to determine whether the temperature rhythm of most shift workers can be entrained to schedules like these, and whether the expected benefits (e.g., improved sleep and performance) will be obtained. Even if sleep and performance are improved by these schedules, they may not be practical for all shift workers because of social constraints. The schedule requires sleeping at unusual hours during some days off. Many workers might refuse to adhere to this plan. However, there are large individual differences in tolerance to shift work [28, 32]. Those workers who suffer the most discomfort might be motivated to arrange their social lives to take advantage of these work-sleep schedules. Another possibility is that a nurse might follow the schedule only occasionally, two or three times a year or as needed, to permit a period of recovery and prevent "burn-out." Finally, schedules that are more socially convenient might be possible if future research yields practical methods to produce faster phase shifts of circadian rhythms with bright light. An advancing sleep schedule from the night shift to the day shift might even be feasible.

Other practical problems besides shift work can benefit from the application of bright light to shift or to stabilize circadian rhythms. Examples include jet-lag [10], circadian rhythm disorders such as poor entrainment or free-running in the natural environment [19, 20, 36], and the delayed sleep phase syndrome [7, 37].

Acknowledgements. I am grateful to my subjects for their diligent efforts and careful record keeping. Supported by NIH BRSG S07RR0547 and NIH NIRA 1 R23 NS23421.

References

1. T. Akerstedt: Experientia. 40, 417-422 (1984)
2. T. Akerstedt, M. Gilberg: Sleep. 4, 159-169 (1981)
3. T. Akerstedt, M. Gilberg: In Night and Shift Work: Biological and Social Aspects. ed. by Reinberg et.al. (Pergamon, Oxford 1981) p.127-138
4. J. Aschoff: In The 24-Hour Workday. A Symposium on Variations in Work-Sleep Schedules, ed. by L.C. Johnson, et.al., Washington, D.C., National Institute for Occupational Safety and Health, (1981) p. 13-50.
5. J. Aschoff, K. Hoffmann, H. Pohl, R. Wever: Chronobiologia. 2, 23-78 (1975)
6. C.A. Czeisler, M.C. Moore--Ede, R.M. Coleman: Science. 217, 460-463 (1982)
7. C.A. Czeisler, G.S.Richardson, R.M. Coleman, J.C. Zimmerman, M.C. Moore--Ede, W.C. Dement, E.D. Weitzman: Sleep. 4, 1-21 (1981)
8. C.A. Czeisler, J.S. Allan, S.H. Strogatz, J.M. Ronda, R. Sanchez, C. D. Rios, W.O. Freitag, G.S. Richardson, R.E. Kronauer: Science. 233, 667-671 (1986)
9. C.A. Czeisler, E.D. Weitzman, M.C. Moore--Ede, J.C. Zimmerman, R.S. Knauer: Science. 210, 1264-1267 (1980)
10. S. Daan, A.J. Lewy: Psychopharmacol. Bull. 20, 566-568 (1984)
11. J.G. Dorrscheidt, & L. Beck: J. Math. Biol. 2, 107-121 (1975)
12. C.I. Eastman: Sleep Res. 15, 271 (1986)
13. C.I. Eastman: In Mathematical Models of the Circadian Sleep-Wake Cycle, ed. by M.C. Moore--Ede, & C.A. Czeisler, (Raven Press, New York 1983) p.81-101
14. C.I. Eastman: IEEE/Seventh Annual Conference of the Engineering in Medicine & Biology Society, 1067-1072 (1985)
15. S. Folkard, D.S. Minors, J.M. Waterhouse: Chronobiologia. 12, 31-54 (1985)

16. S. Folkard, T.H. Monk, (eds): Hours of Work. (John Wiley & Sons, New York 1985)
17. T.M. Hoban, F.M. Sulzman: Amer. J. Physiol. 249, R274-R280 (1985)
18. L.C. Johnson, D.Tepas, W. Colquhoun, M. Colligan, (eds): The Twenty-Four Hour Workday: Proceedings of a Symposium on Variations in Work-Sleep Schedules. DHHS Publication No.81-127. U.S. Department of Health and Human Services, Cincinnati, OH, (1981)
19. B. Kamgar-Parsi, T.A. Wehr, G.J. Christian: Sleep. 6, 257-264 (1983)
20. C.P. Kokkoris, E. Weitzman, C. Pollack, A. Spielman, C. Czeisler, H. Bradlow: Sleep. 1, 177-190 (1978)
21. R.E. Kronauer, C. Czeisler, S. Pilato, M. Moore--Ede, E. Weitzman: Amer. J. Physiol. 242, R3-R17 (1982)
22. A.J. Lewy, A.J. Sack, R.L. Fredrickson, R.H. Reaves, M. Denny, D. Zielske: Psychopharmacol. Bull. 19, 523-525 (1983)
23. A.J. Lewy, R.A. Sack, C.L. Singer: Psychopharmacol. Bull. 20, 561-565 (1984)
24. A.J. Lewy, R. L.Sack, C. Singer: Annals N.Y. Academy of Sciences. 453, 253-259 (1985)
25. A.J. Lewy, R.L. Sack, C.M. Singer: Psychopharmacol. Bull. 21, 368-372 (1985)
26. A.J. Lewy, T.A. Wehr, F.K. Goodwin, D.A. Newsome, S.P. Markey: Science. 210, 1267-1268 (1980)
27. D.S. Minors, J.M. Waterhouse: Experientia. 42, 1-13 (1986)
28. D.S. Minors, J.M. Waterhouse: Circadian Rhythms and the Human (Wright P.S.G., Bristol, 1981)
29. K. Orth-Gomer: Psychosom. Med. 45, 407-415 (1983)
30. C.S. Pittendrigh: In Handbook of Behavioral Neurobiology Vol. 4: Biological Rhythms. ed. by J. Aschoff, (Plenum Press, New York 1981) p.95-124
31. A. Reinberg, N. Vieux, P. Andlauer (eds): Night and Shift Work: Biological and Social Aspects (Pergamon Press, Oxford 1981)
32. A. Reinberg, N. Vieux, P. Andlauer, M. Smolensky: Adv. Biol. Psychiat. 11, 35-47 (1983)
33. N.E. Rosenthal, D.A. Sack, C. Gillin, A.J. Lewy, F.K. Goodwin, Y. Davenport, P.S. Mueller, D.A. Newsome, T.A. Wehr: Arch. Gen. Psychiat. 41, 72-80 (1984)
34. D.L. Tasto, M.J. Colligan, E.W. Skjei, S.J. Polly, (eds): Health Consequences of Shift Work DHEW Publication No. 78-154, Cincinnati, Ohio, U.S. Department of Health, Education, and Welfare, (1978)
35. D.I. Tepas: J. Human Ergology. 11, 325-336 (1982)
36. A.L. Weber, M.S. Cary, N. Connor, P. Keyes: Sleep. 2, 347-354 (1980)
37. E.D. Weitzman, C.A. Czeisler, R.M. Coleman, A.J. Spielman, J.C. Zimmerman, W. Dement: Arch. Gen. Psychiat. 38, 737-746 (1981)
38. R.A. Wever: Annals N.Y. Academy Sciences. 453, 282-304 (1985)
39. R.A. Wever: The Circadian System of Man (Springer-Verlag, New York 1979)
40. R.A. Wever: In Rhythmic Aspects of Behavior ed. by F.M. Brown, R.C. Graeber (Lawrence Erlbaum Associates, Hillsdale, N.J. 1982) pp.105-171
41. R.A. Wever: In Circadian Rhythms in Psychiatry, ed. by T.A. Wehr, F.K. Goodwin, (Boxwood Press, Pacific Grove, CA. 1983) pp.17-31
42. R.A. Wever: Pflugers Arch. 396, 128-137 (1983)
43. R.A. Wever, J. Polasek, C.M. Wildgruber: Pflugers Arch. 396, 85-87 (1983)
44. J. Zulley, S.S. Campbell: Human Neurobiology. 4, 123-126 (1985)
45. J. Zulley, R. Wever, J. Aschoff: Pflugers Arch. 391, 314-318 (1981)

Disturbances of the Circadian System Due to Masking Effects

R. Moog

Institut für Arbeitsphysiologie und Rehabilitationsforschung, Phillips-Universität Marburg, Robert-Koch-Straße 7a, D-3550 Marburg/Lahn, Fed. Rep. of Germany

As e.g. MINORS & WATERHOUSE /1/ presumed, masking agents may act as zeitgebers also, because they may influence the circadian oscillator in the same ways as zeitgebers are believed to do.

Furthermore, as it was shown by HILDEBRANDT /2/ various masking agents cause the organism to respond with maximum amplitudes always at the same circadian phase, namely in the ascending circadian phase. He presumes that these amplitude responses are closely related to the phase response curves already found in animal studies.

If a masking agent acts as a zeitgeber, it should be able to evoke effects lastinq some hours, not only a stimulus response, as is already known for the specific dynamic action, rectal temperature, heart rate and other variables evoked by nutrition (e.g. FOERTSCH /3/).

The aim of the following two experiments is to proove whether the potent masking agent - activity - is able to produce similar long-lasting effects on rectal temperature.

In order to obtain a reference with minimal masking effects ten healthy male students were first observed on a control day during which subjects were kept in a sound proofed climatic chamber for 24 hours at the lowest possible activity level, while on a low and equally distributed protein diet and sleeping at their convenience. On this initial control day the courses of rectal temperature were continuously recorded. The same conditions were applied 24 hours later on a following strain day. On strain days, activities were interpolated in the routine.

In the first experiment subjects were sleep deprived from 2.30 p.m. to 9.00 a.m.. During sleep deprivation subjects were kept awake by physical activities (HR 100 P/min.). The interindividual phase differences were standardized by phase-shifts of the individual rhythms to the pooled phase of the group (arithmetic mean; s.fig.:1).

On strain days rectal temperature decreased during the ascending circadian phase of rectal temperature for several hours as compared to the control days. An indication for a phase shift of the circadian rhythm could not be detected.

Differences between morning- and evening-types in respect to the rectal temperature reactions were not found, as it may be presumed from the differences between morning- and evening-types while adapting to incoherent zeitgeber-regimen (e.g. HILDEBRANDT

/2/; MOOG /4/). Moreover the above masking effect could be phase dependent.

Therefore, low physical activities (30 min. of pedal work; max 100 beats/min;) were inserted four times in the strain day with respect to the phases of rectal temperature on the foregoing undisturbed control day. The 12 subjects did not know at which times they would be exposed to this strain, so, from the subjects point of view, these sessions were randomly distributed over the day. Short-term masking effects were omitted by linear interpolations. Interindividual phase differences within the groups of morning/indifferent- and evening-types were standardized by phase shifts to the means of the respective groups. Short-term effects were omitted by linear interpolation. Start of strain days were balanced for the groups.

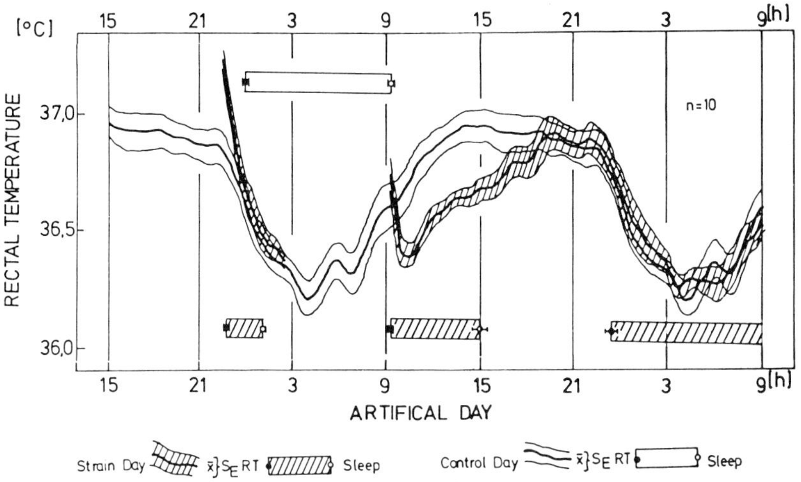

Fig.:1 Mean courses of rectal temperature on the first controlday and after sleep deprivation on the following strain day (n=10).

Evidently, morning types did raise their average temperature at the minimum and in the ascending phase of their circadian rhythms, while evening types lowered their temperature during the respective phases. Again, there was no hint for a phase shift of the circadian system, but the effect was phase-dependent.

Consequently, foregoing physical activity may alter rectal temperature for several hours, and this differently in subjects with different circadian phase positions.

Our present results give no evidence for phase shifts of the circadian system and therefore no direct evidence for a zeitgeber effect of our masking agents. But such a response can only be expected if the stimulus is given repetitively and cyclically. Furthermore, in the second experiment the effects may be related to the different circadian responses of the morning- and evening-types, as caused by incoherent phase-shifts of zeitgebers.

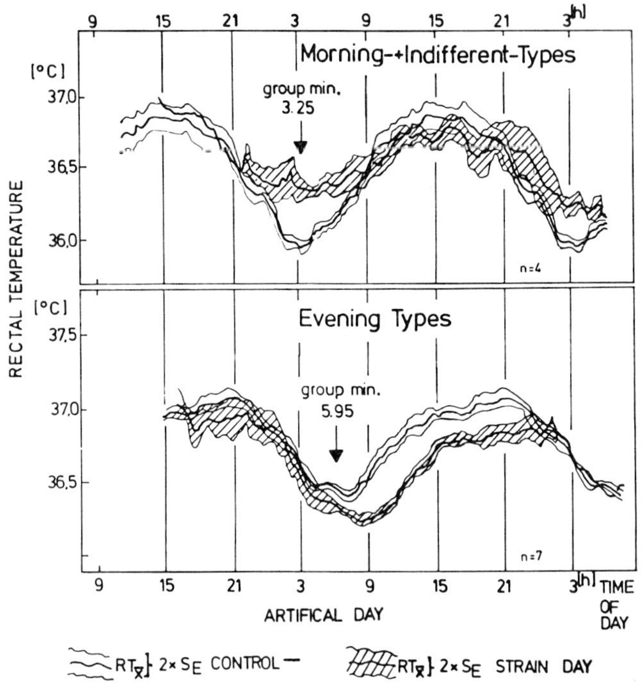

Fig.:2 Different long-lasting masking effects on circadian rhythms of rectal temperature in groups of subjects of different circadian phase positions

However, experiments of our design which expose subjects to agents of masking while other masking agents are minimized, should allow us to learn more about the ways zeitgebers act, if the agents are given repetitively and/or cyclic, coherent or incoherent to each other and/or to the nycthemeral zeitgebers.

REFERENCES

1. D.S. Minors and J.M. Waterhouse: Proceedings of the 2nd Meeting of the European Society of Chronobiology, Marburg 1986, in press
2. G. Hildebrandt, In Night- and Shiftwork: Longterm Effects and their Prevention, M. Haider, M. Koller and R. Cervinka, Edts. P. Lang Frankfurt, 1986 pp 109-116
3. H.U. Foertsch. Dissertation Universität Münster, 1968
4. R. Moog, in Intern. Symposium on Sleep-Related Disorders and Internal Diseases, Marburg 1986, in press

Simulation of the Circadian Response to Time Zone Transitions by a Van der Pol Oscillator

A. Gundel

DFVLR-Institute for Aerospace Medicine, P.O. Box 906058,
D-5000 Köln 90, Fed. Rep. of Germany

1. Introduction

When a zeitgeber advance shift is increased from about 6 to 12 hours, the response of the entrained circadian body temperature rhythm changes from a phase advance to a phase delay. The shift at which this transition occurs is called "critical shift" in this context. In general, it is not an integer number of hours. The term critical is to describe an unstable equilibrium. That is the state of a pendulum which stands upright and will swing by more than 180° in either direction towards its stable equilibrium due to any infinitesimal force.

Phenomena related to critical shifts are investigated by simulations with a Van der Pol oscillator. The aim is to derive predictions about jet lag.

2. Van der Pol Oscillator

The Van der Pol equation describes a second order system in which a non-linear damping term is added to the differential equation for damped linear oscillations:

$$\frac{d^2x(t)}{dt^2} - \mu(1-x^2(t))\frac{dx(t)}{dt} + \omega^2 x(t) = z(t) \ , \quad \mu > 0 \ .$$

The parameter μ determines the degree of non-linearity or the stiffness of the oscillator which is introduced by the term $\mu x^2 dx/dt$ into the equation. For small μ, the free-running period T_f of a Van der Pol oscillator with period $T=2\pi/\omega$ is approximately given by $T_f \approx T/(1-\mu^2/16)$, i.e. the period T_f is always greater than T and increases quadratically with increasing stiffness.

The oscillator is subjected to an external force z(t), i.e. the zeitgeber. We have solved the equation with z(t) being zero for 12 hours and taking a positive constant (symbol Z) for the other 12 hours of a 24-h zeitgeber period. The selection of a zeitgeber with a different shape would have only minor influences on qualitative results.

The external force is conceived as a composition of different internal and external zeitgebers like rest-activity cycle, light-dark cycle, and others. Our model seems to be suitable to describe experiments in which zeitgebers are abruptly shifted, including the rest-activity cycle. By considering the rest-activity cycle a zeitgeber, our model concept differs from others given in the literature for simulations of the circadian response to zeitgeber shifts. Wever

/1/ proposed a one-oscillator model which consists of the Van der Pol oscillator with additional terms. The model does not incorporate the rest-activity cycle as a potential zeitgeber, but properties of this cycle are derived from the oscillator solutions using thresholds. Gander et al. /2/ emphasized the multi-oscillatory nature of the circadian system. In their simulations endogenous body temperature rhythm and sleep-wake cycle were represented by two coupled oscillators. A simple zeitgeber effect of the rest-activity cycle was not taken into account by this two-oscillator model.

3. Simulations

Figure 1 shows the desynchronization between oscillator and zeitgeber, i.e. the deviation from their phase relationship in the entrained state, following different shifts. Parameter values T=24.5 hours, Z=0.5, and μ=0.4 have been used for these simulations, and result in an approximate free-running period of T_f=24.75 hours. This lies between the average period of 24.86 hours (N=33) observed in free-running experiments after spontaneous internal desynchronization /3/ and the period of T=24.57 hours (N=7) derived from fractional desynchronization experiments /4/. The external force intensity Z is close to an average value obtained from quantitative interpretations of temperature data from a transmeridian flight experiment /5/. The shift has been modelled by shortening (advance) and lengthening (delay) of an interval in which the rectangular external force is constant. Phases have been simply determined by evaluating the zero crossings of the oscillations transformed to zero mean. With the specified parameter values, the critical shift is found between +7 and +8 hours. Resynchronization to zeitgebers shifted nearly critically takes the longest time with only little phase adaptation during the first few days. Resynchronization times become shorter at both sides of the critical shift. Especially, reentrainment times following the 12-hour shifts are shorter than those after nearly critical shifts.

In model simulations, the size of the critical shift depends on the parameter values. Regarding the parameter space with the coordinates μ, Z, and T, we find for each specified shift, in our simulations +9 hours, a plane in the space which separates oscillators showing advance and delay responses to this shift. According to the term critical shift, the parameter values on the plane will also be called "critical" values with regard to the defined shift. Figure 2

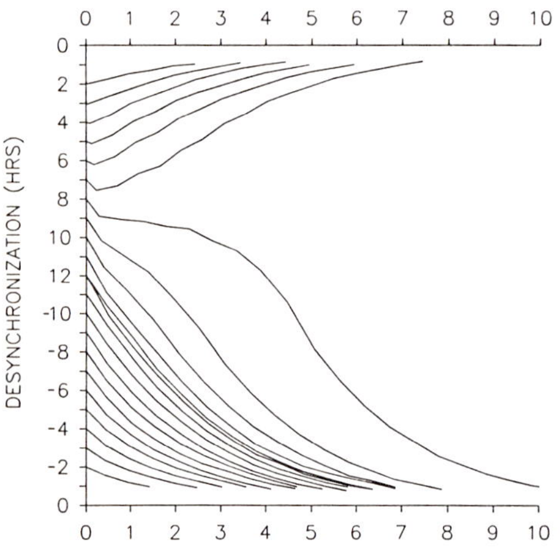

Fig. 1
Desynchronization between oscillator and zeitgeber following shifts between +12 and -12 hours. Positive shifts (advance) correspond to eastbound, negative shifts (delay) to westbound flights. Desynchronizations of less than one hour are not displayed

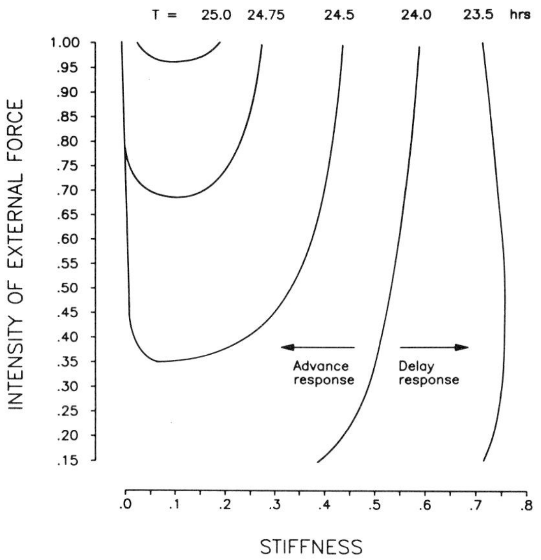

Fig. 2
The lines of parameter values (5 different periods T in a μ-Z plane) for which a +9h shift is critical

shows cuts through the critical plane for five oscillator periods between 23.5 and 25.0 hours represented by lines in the μ-Z plane. On the right-hand side of each line, where the stiffer oscillators with longer free-running periods are found, the solutions respond with a delay, and on the left-hand side with an advance. If the stiffness is very low, i.e. the oscillator is almost linear, again a delay can be observed with oscillator periods greater than 24 hours.

The evaluation of critical lines (for $T \geqq 24$ hrs) revealed that by increasing T (keeping μ and Z constant) and/or increasing μ (keeping T and Z constant) both leading to a longer free-running period, the size of the critical shift becomes smaller. The critical lines also show that a weak zeitgeber strength facilitates a delay response to an advance zeitgeber shift.

Figure 3 shows resynchronization times in a μ-Z plane (T=24.0 hrs) after a 9-hour advance shift. The times are given by the integer number of days on which the phase difference to the adapted state is more than one hour. Around the line of critical parameters (compare with Fig. 2) the times are longer than they are for parameter values in the neighbourhood forming a ridge in the map of resynchronization times. This ridge appears more pronounced when the "critical" stiffness is relatively high. Therefore, resynchronization times are shorter at the critical line for the oscillator period T=24.5 hours compared with T=24.0 hours.

Not only phase and period adaptation but also circadian amplitudes exhibit characteristic alterations after nearly critical shifts. The simulations in Fig. 4 are to exemplify this. Solutions of the Van der Pol equation with T=24.5 hours and Z=0.5 are shown for increasing stiffness. On the third day, a 9-hour advance shift is modelled. Subsequently the solutions undergo transient changes with patterns being dependent on stiffness. The critical shift is found between μ=0.20 and μ=0.30 .

Oscillation amplitudes are reduced for up to 5 days. The reduction can be observed with stiffnesses on both sides of the critical shift, but it is more pronounced when the oscillators adapt by an

INTENSITY OF EXTERNAL FORCE		.1		.2		.3		.4		.5		.6		.7		.8
1.00	4	3	3	2	2	2	2	3	3	3	3	3	3	3	3	3
.95	4	4	3	3	2	2	2	3	3	4	4	4	4	3	3	3
.90	5	4	3	3	3	2	2	3	3	4	4	4	4	4	4	4
.85	5	4	4	3	3	3	2	3	3	4	4	4	4	4	4	4
.80	5	4	4	4	4	3	3	3	4	5	5	5	5	4	4	4
.75	5	4	4	4	4	4	3	4	3	5	5	5	5	5	5	5
.70	6	5	5	5	4	4	4	4	3	6	6	6	5	5	5	5
.65	7	5	5	5	5	5	5	5	5	7	7	6	6	6	6	6
.60	7	6	5	5	5	5	6	6	7	8	7	7	6	6	6	6
.55	8	6	6	6	6	6	7	7	7	9	8	8	7	7	7	6
.50	8	7	7	7	7	7	7	8	9	12	9	8	8	8	7	7
.45	8	8	7	7	7	8	8	9	10	16	11	9	9	8	8	8
.40	9	9	8	8	8	9	9	10	12	15	12	10	10	9	9	9
.35	11	10	10	10	10	10	11	12	14	19	13	11	11	10	10	10
.30	12	11	11	11	12	13	13	14	18	17	14	13	12	12	11	11
.25	14	13	14	14	14	15	16	19	4W	19	16	15	14	13	13	13
.20	17	17	17	17	18	19	21	27	25	20	18	17	16	15	X	X
.15	25	24	23	25	27	4W	4W	4W	4W	23	20	X	X	X	X	X

STIFFNESS

Fig. 3
Resynchronization times in a μ-Z plane for an oscillator period of T=24.0 hours (zeitgeber shift +9h)
X: oscillator is not entrained
4W: resynchronization time is longer than 4 weeks

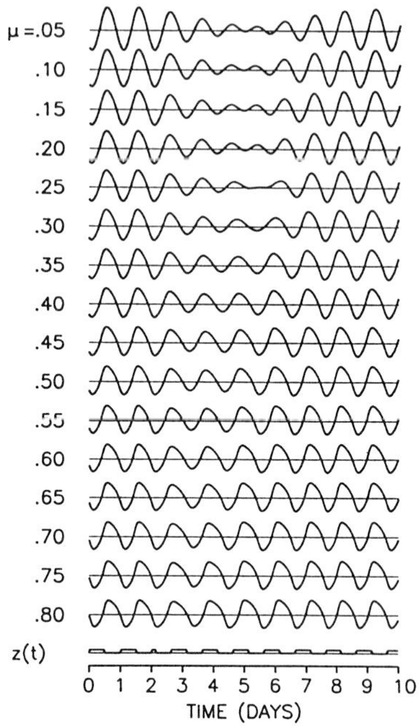

Fig. 4
Simulations of the response to a +9h shift (on the third day) for increasing stiffness (T=24.5 hrs and Z=0.5). Following the shift, amplitude reduction systematically changes depending on stiffness

advance. Amplitudes turned out to be especially diminished after nearly critical shifts if the "critical" stiffness is relatively low.

Furthermore, detailed simulations show that the time for which amplitudes are reduced shortens if the zeitgeber intensity Z is increased.

4. Discussion and Predictions about Jet Lag

Experiments and general ideas about jet lag have been reviewed by Klein and Wegmann /6/ and by Graeber /7/. One of the most discussed issues is the question whether people suffer more from jet lag after east- or after westbound flights. From the simulations, predictions about the severity of jet lag symptoms after nearly critical shifts are inferred. The experimental validation of the results will be discussed elsewhere.

Jet lag can be considered to depend on four discernible phenomena:

1.) Circadian amplitudes are reduced without an important change of daily means. The reduction is strongest in somebody for whom the shift is nearly critical. For performance measures which often parallel the body temperature rhythm, the reduction implies that pre-shift peak performance is not reached during any time of the day.

2.) During the adaptation to the abruptly shifted ensemble of external and internal zeitgebers, the circadian acrophase, e.g. of body temperature, occurs at unusual local times and is desynchronized from the sleep-wake cycle. With nearly critical shifts phase differences may even be 12 hours.

3.) Following a zeitgeber shift, circadian components may lose their internal synchronization and dissociate transiently (a multioscillatory phenomenon). Most likely, this affects the regulation of various body functions. The dissociation reaches a phase difference of 12 hours following nearly critical shifts if there are delay as well as advance responses.

4.) Resynchronization times are longest for critical shifts. Therefore, amplitude reduction and internal dissociation may not only be strongest after a critical shift but can also affect the circadian system for the longest time.

In summary: the most severe consequences of jet lag are predicted to occur with nearly critical shifts. This means in particular, eastbound flights which lead to a nearly critical zeitgeber shift are followed by jet lag with stronger impairments of e.g. performance as compared with westbound flights crossing the same number of time zones.

References

1. R. Wever: J. Theoret. Biol. 13, 187 (1966)
2. P.H. Gander, R.E. Kronauer, R.C. Graeber: Am. J. Physiol. 249, R704 (1985)
3. R.A. Wever: Experientia 40, 1226 (1984)
4. R.A. Wever: Pflügers Arch. ges. Physiol. 396, 128 (1983)
5. A. Gundel, H.M. Wegmann: In Proc. XVII International Conference of the International Society for Chronobiology (Little Rock, in press)
6. K.E. Klein, H.M. Wegmann: Significance of Circadian Rhythm in Aerospace Operations, AGARDograph No. 247 (AGARD, Neuilly-Sur-Seine 1980)
7. R.C. Graeber: In Rhythmic Aspects of Behavior, ed. by F.M. Brown, R.C. Graeber (Lawrence Erlbaum Associates, Hillsdale 1982)

ːcadian Rhythms and Depression

ˀflug

Department of Psychiatry, Johann Wolfgang Goethe-Universität, D-6000 Frankfurt, Fed. Rep. of Germany

I. Depression as illness

1. Depression is a common illness; it is estimated that about 3 or 4 percent of the population suffer from a depression requiring treatment. It is characterized by a syndrome of varying intensity with a varying combination of psychological, psychomotor and somatic symptoms. The patients are downcast and sad, incapable of being glad. Thought is experienced as inhibited and turns on guilt and hopelessness. Fear is important, and is almost always present. Patients complain of a feeling of emptiness, that they have no ideas, and cannot concentrate. A marked disturbance of mood is characterized by indecisiveness, apathy, a sensation of loss of feeling, a loss of selfesteem and thoughts of suicide. A withdrawal from social contact takes place, the patients isolate themselves. The psychomotor symptoms may consist of great restlessness, agitation and nervousness or loss of drive, inhibition, even stupor. The patients appear rigid and tormented; everything is felt to proceed slowly.

The somatic symptoms consist of insomnia, loss of appetite, constipation, a tendency to perspire, vague feelings in the head, chest or abdomen and the extremities (usually described as feeling of pressure or heaviness). Dryness of the mouth, tachycardia and libido disturbances are common.

2. Many of us are familiar with similar but transitory depressive complaints - perhaps following a setback, or accompanying a situation of exhaustion. Such disturbances are part of the spectrum of human affective reactions and do not have the character of morbidity. Depression is to be regarded as illness when the depressive mood reaches a certain intensity and dictates behaviour, that is to say, everything that is experienced, thought, planned or felt has mainly a depressive aspect. "Depression" as an illness can have widely differing backgrounds and courses of development. Together with certain symptoms these lead to different nosological groups. Some depressions arise as a reaction to a psychological trauma or as an expression of an abnormal personality development (neurotic depression) or as a result of chronic conflict situations (depressive development). The endogenous depression proceeds in phases, with or without mania. Finally, depressions may result from organic lesions, which are either directly cerebral or due to extracerebral causes.

Why have I given this survey of types of depression? Because there is no one "depression" as such, and nearly all investigations into the connection between depression and circadian system relate only to the endogenous depression, and do not permit generalization. The reasons for this lie in the phenomenology and the courses of the illness, both of which suggest such a connection. The following remarks therefore refer to the endogenous depression and findings relating to this form of depression which indicate relevant changes in the circadian system.

3. The endogenous depression occurs in phases, frequently with no perceptible external causes. During a phase there is often a very deep depressive mood, which can go as far as a delusion. The duration of a phase is very variable. In the case of untreated depressions phases last about six months on average. The end of a phase is followed by an interval free of complaints. Where manic phases occur in the course of a depression, one speaks of a bipolar depression or cyclothymia; when only depressive phases occur, one speaks of monopolar depression. Bipolar and monopolar depressions and manias are subsumed under the term "affective psychoses or disorders". The following phenomena suggest a disturbance in the circadian rhythm: diurnal variations, sleep disturbances, seasonal dependencies and a cyclic course.

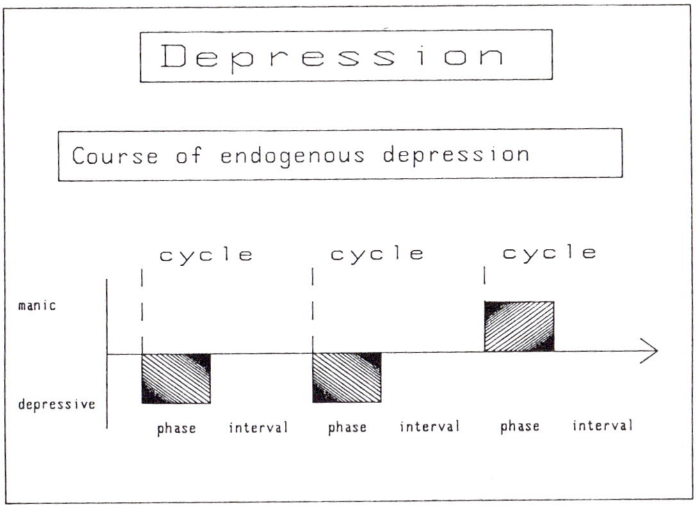

Fig.1

3.1. Diurnal variations of mood and drive

HAMPP (1) found 18 percent of a healthy population to be definite morning types (or "larks"), and 34 percent definite evening types (or "owls"), while the remaining percent stated no clear regular diurnal variation. According to MIDDELHOFF (2), by contrast, the following picture resulted in a group of 81 patients with endogenous depression during symptom-free intervals: 49 percent were morning types, 35 percent evening types and only 16 percent unclassified. This means that there was among the depressive patients a significant accumulation of morning types, and overall a clear preponderance of rhythmics in comparison with the healthy population. Approximately half of the patients investigated by MIDDELHOFF reported a complete reversal of their diurnal rhythm during depression, which disappeared after the depressive phase. During depression about eighty percent of patients wake deeply depressed, after a fragmented, frequently interrupted and superficial sleep (3). In the course of the day, especially in the afternoon and evening, an improvement in mood and drive takes place. At the climax of a depressive phase the diurnal variation described may be absent; the improvement has successively moved later and later in the day. The reoccurrence of diurnal variations is a prognostically favourable sign for the course of the phase. According to PAPOUSEK (4), early waking in the morning and the diurnal variation can be interpreted as an internal dissociation of circadian rhythms, by which the readiness for achievement while awake is delayed relative to the advanced sleeping-waking periodicity. This may be connected with an oscillator which has recently been described for mental performance (5).

3.2. Sleep disturbances

Depressive phases begin in 50 percent of cases with a sleep disturbance (2). Sleep is described as superficial and interrupted by frequent waking. Waking early in the morning is felt as very painful, the patient does not feel rested. Neurophysiological investigations have been able to objectivize depressive sleep disturbances: delay in going to sleep, frequent waking, reduction or even absence of synchronized sleep (stage III and stage IV in EEG); compared with healthy persons, the REM-sleep variables together with the other sleep parameters show increased inter- and intraindividual variability. According to PAPOUSEK (4), sleep disturbance in the case of cyclothymia can be described as a disturbance of the time structure caused by a change in circadian rhythms. The signs of this are above all more frequent and unusual changes in the sleep stages with fragmentation of sleep continuity (7), a greater variability in the duration of the REM-cycle and chronological displacement of the maxima and minima of REM-sleep and synchronized sleep in the course of the night (6, 7, 8, 9).
The shortening of the REM-latency (6) and the waking periods occurring in the last third of sleep with early waking (10) led, together with other parameters (especially body temperature, biochemical variables), to the formulation of the "phase-advance"-hypothesis of depression (11).

3.3. Seasonal dependence

Annual rhythms have a circadian basis, which is connected with photoperiodic mechanisms, corresponding to the changes in the amount of light during the day (12). Affective disorders commonly show seasonal variation in their occurrence. This has been described for depression with a peak in spring and one in the autumn (13, 14, 15) - the times of noticeable alteration in the length of the day. ROSENTHAL et al. (16) described a particular group of affective disorders (seasonal affective disorder, SAD, winter depression), which are mostly of bipolar type II and start in autumn and winter, particularly between October and December, with a depressive mood which lasts about four months, and remits in the spring. The depression of these patients differs from the majority of endogenous depressions in that they eat more, with a particular tendency to carbohydrates, put on weight and sleep longer. Many of these patients felt an improvement of their depression on travelling south from northerly latitudes. This led to the question of the effect of light on depression. LEWY et al. (16) has reported on this.

3.4. Cyclic course

A phase of illness and an interval are designated as a cycle. According to E. KRETSCHMER (18) the manic-depressive or circular phases are the pathogenic model case of oscillations which return to a starting-point. This periodicity differs only in degree from the periodic phenomena in the life course of healthy persons. The dependence of the beginning of a phase on sleeping-waking rhythm is known (19, 20, 21); the times of change into or out of depression are above all in the early hours of the morning. Social influences are of significance in provoking a depressive phase, especially when they involve a change in accustomed situations requiring adaptation. Particular times at which the risk of a phase provocation is increased, so-called "tempora minoris resistantiae" (4), are the early morning hours within the twenty-four hour rhythm, spring and autumn within the annual rhythm, the premenstruum within the menstruation cycle, and the beginning of pregnancy and puerperium within the cycle of pregnancy; furthermore, certain phases of development and involution, certain meteorological and atmospheric influences, as well as phases of social changes.

II. The circadian system in depression

There are several models based on the concept of hereditary insuffiency of circadian synchronisation mechanisms in endogenous depression (4) and which are the starting-point of new therapeutic approaches.

Fig. 2 is a schematic representation of the disturbances in phase position and period length observed under natural conditions in manic-depressive patients.

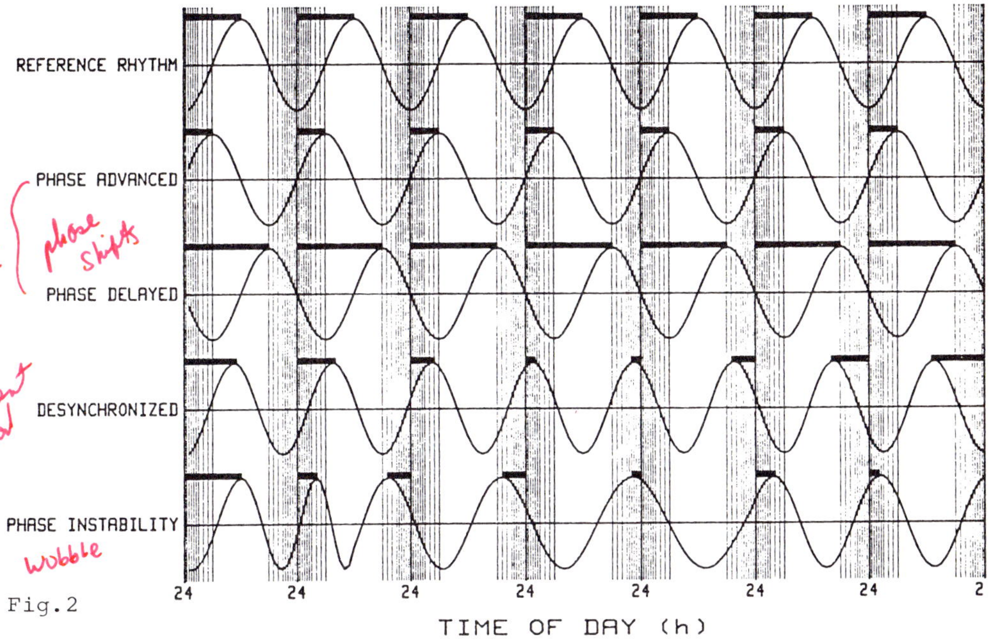

Fig.2

1. Phase advance

In this model the phase position of one or more oscillators is advanced in relation to the 24-hour rhythm of the environment. In an analysis of 19 studies of circadian variations of various physiological and biochemical functions, WEHR and GOODWIN (11) were able to observe an advancing of the phase positions in depression of from one to several hours. These findings correspond to a changed chronological distribution of the occurrence of REM-phases, which frequently occur with shortened latency in the first third of the night (6, 8), the first REM-phase being abnormally long (22). The effects of partial sleep deprivation (23), after staying awake in the second half of the night (from 1.30 h) lead to an improvement of the depression, can be cited in support of the phase advance hypothesis. The results of various experiments imply, according to WEHR and WIRZ-JUSTICE (24), that the depressive process is sleep-dependent and that the sleeping-waking rhythm governed by the weak oscillator coincides with advanced circadian rhythm (which governs for example body temperature and REM-phases) in a sleep-sensitive phase. This is supported by the times of change into and out of depression, which are in the early hours of the morning, and also the diurnal variation, with the strongest depression in the early hours of the morning. The postulated internal coincidence between different oscillators which affect sleep and temperature rhythm was modified by KRIPKE (12) by the assumption of an external coincidence dependent on a photosensitive period during the critical interval in the morning. Experiments with bright light with depressives have shown that the time for an optimum therapeutic effect is dependent on the phase disposition. According to LEWY et al. (17) this time is in the evening for patients with "phase advance".

2. Phase delay

The description of winter depression and the findings of studies on circadian secretion of melatonin and body temperature have indicated a further change in phase relations, the circadian rhythms being delayed. Most winter depressions appear to be characterized by this (LEWY et al. (17)). Experiments with exposure to bright light at different times of day seem to confirm this hypothesis.

3. Phase instability

In several longitudinal studies on circadian temperature rhythm in monopolar and bipolar depressions, no systematic changes in phase position or frequency were found; instead the circadian phase relation was highly variable during depression, while being stable in the symptom-free interval (25, 26). A high correlation between phase lability and subjective self-rating could be observed; the more marked the depressive symptoms were, the greater were the phase deviations (27).

4. Desynchronisation

In long-term studies it was observed in a subgroup of manic-depressive patients that the circadian rhythms of temperature and other psychological and behavioral variables during depression were free-running with a somewhat shorter period (12, 28). These findings supported the thesis put forward by HALBERG (29) according to which manic-depressive episodes may represent beat phenomena between a free-running physiological clock and the 24-hour periodicity of the environment. In the case of the patients concerned, the free-running period was up to 21.8 hours, while the sleeping-waking rhythms remained synchronized with the environment. For MHPG excretion too a free-running rhythm of 20.5 hours could be measured in a manic-depressive patient during depression; in the symptom-free interval the period length was again 24.0 hours (30). This finding is interesting inasmuch as MHPH largely originates from the norepinephrin metabolism in the brain. The VMA, which is an exclusively peripheral norepinephrin metabolite, shows no change in its secretion rhythm, nor does body temperature. KRIPKE et al. (12) pointed out that there are also patients with prolongation of circadian periodicity.

III. Therapeutic aspects

The findings of studies of the circadian system in manic depressive patients have raised completely new questions as to the mode of action of certain forms of therapy.

1. Antidepressants

The tricyclic antidepressant imipramine and the monoaminooxydase-inhibitor clorgyline prolong the circadian periodicity of the rest-activity rhythm in animal experiments under free-running conditions; under normal conditions they lead to a delaying of the phase position (31, 32). The phase positions of various rhythms of the neurotransmitter receptors in the brain are also delayed (31, 33). The antidepressant effect of imipramine and clorgyline and their chronobiological activity are in agreement with the "phase advance" model. However, both these medicaments also induced a dissociation from components of the circadian activity rhythm. Switches to manic or hypomanic moods are connected with this tendency to dissociation of oscillatory components.

2. Lithium

Lithiumsalts are chronobiologically active. In most studies they show prolongations of the circadian periodicity, as ENGELMANN has reported. About 20 % of patients with affective psychoses show no prophylactic effect under treatment with lithiumsalts (34). Possibly these are patients whose circadian system does not tend to shortening of autonomous periodicity or to advancing the phase position (12).

3. Sleep deprivation

If monopolar and bipolar depressive patients are deprived of sleep for a night, in about 60 - 80 % mood and drive are significantly better the following day (35). As a rule the improvement takes place during the sleepless night, and an abrupt dramatic change can often be overserved in the early hours of the morning (between about 2.00 and 6.00 o'clock, the so-called "critical time"). When sleep deprivation is carried out partially in the second part of the night (staying awake from 1.30), the result, in contrast to partial sleep deprivation during the first half of the night, therapeutic effects comparable to those of total sleep deprivation (23). Selective sleep deprivation consists in the patient being prevented from sleeping in particular stages of sleep. This has been demonstrated by an improvement on deprivation of REM-stages over a certain period (3 weeks) (22). All forms of sleep deprivation can be seen as an intervention in the 24-hour rhythm upon which the therapeutic effect rests. As yet, however, there are no definite findings to support or refute these assumptions in relation to human beings.

4. Modification of the course of the day

Proceeding from the "phase-advance" model, WEHR et al. (36) advanced the sleeping-waking periodicity corresponding to the advanced oscillator of REM- and temperature rhythm. In one phase-changing experiment, a depressive patient was able to come out of her depression when sleeping time was advanced by six hours. The effect lasted for two weeks. After a relapse, the same experiment had the same effect; a third repetition produced no improvement. This therapeutic experiment is comparable with chronotherapeutic experiments in the case of certain sleep disorders (37, 38).

5. Light therapy

This has already been described by LEWY.

Conclusion

Studies carried out up to now indicate that the circadian system is of great importance in affective disorders. Various models and hypotheses which have emerged from the studies are calculated to explain certain pathogenetic mechanisms. It may be expected that therapeutic problems also can be brought closer to solution by the chronobiological approach.

REFERENCES

1. H. Hampp: Arch. Psychiat. u.Z. ges. Neurol. 201, p.355 (1961)
2. H.D. Middelhoff: Arch. Psychiat. u. Z. ges. Neurol. 209, p. 315 (1967)
3. H. Waldmann: Fortschr. Neurol. Psychiat. 40, p. 83 (1972)
4. M.Papousek: Fortschr.Neurol. Psychiat. 43, p. 381(1975)
5. S. Folkard, R. Wever, C.M. Wildgruber: Nature 305,p. 223-226 (1983)
6. D.J. Kupfer: Biol. Psychiat. 11, p. 159 (1977)
7. D.J. Kupfer, F.G. Foster: Lancet 2, p. 684 (1972)
8. S.C. Gresham, W.F. Agnew, R.L. Williams: Arch. Gen. Psychiat. 13, p. 503 (1965)
9. H. Schulz, R. Lund, C. Cording, G. Dirlich: Biol. Psychiat. 14, p. 595 (1979)
10. J.C. Gillin, W. Duncan, K.D. Pettigrew, B.L. Frankel, F. Snyder: Arch. Gen. Psychiat. 36, p. 85 (1979)
11. T.A. Wehr, F.K. Goodwin: Biological rhythms and psychiatry. In. American Handbook of Psychiatry, ed. by S. Arieti and H.K.H. Brodie, 7th. Vol. 2nd Ed., p. 46 (New York: Basic books 1981)
12. D.F. Kripke, D.J. Mullaney, M. Atkinson, S. Wolf: Biolog. Psychiat. 13, p. 335 (1978)
13. G.H. Leuthold: Arch. Psychiat. Nervenkr. 111, p. 55 (1940)
14. E. Slater: Z. ges. Neurol. Psychiat. 192, p. 794 (1938)
15. J. Angst, P. Grof, H. Hippius, W. Pöldinger, E.Varga, P. Weis, F. Wyss: In: Das depressive Syndrom, ed. by Hippius, H. und H. Selbach, p. 93 (Urban u. Schwarzenberg, München 1969)
16. N.E. Rosenthal, D.A. Sack, J.C. Gillin, A.J. Lewy, F.K. Goodwin, Y. Davenport, P.S. Mueller, D.A. Newsome, T.A. Wehr: Arch. Gen. Psychiat. 41, p. 72 (1984)
17. A.J. Lewy, R.L. Sack, C.M. Singer : Psychopharmacol. Bull. Vol. 21 N° 3, p. 368 - 372 (1985)
18. E. Kretschmer: Körperbau und Charakter. (Springer: Berlin (1940)

19. W.E. Bunney, D.L. Murphy, F.K. Goodwin, G.F. Borge: Arch. Gen. Psychiat. 27, p. 295 (1972)

20. W.E. Bunney, D.L. Murphy, F.K. Goodwin, K.M. House, E.K. Gordon: Arch. Gen. Psychiat. 27, p. 304 (1972)

21. W.E. Bunney, F.K. Goodwin, D.L. Murphy: Arch. Gen. Psychiat. 27, p. 312 (1972)

22. G.W. Vogel, F. Vogel, R.S. Mc. Abee, A.J. Thurmond: Arch. Gen. Psychiat. 37, p. 247 (1980)

23. B. Schilgen, R. Tölle: Arch. Gen. Psychiat. 37,p. 267 (1980)

24. T.A. Wehr, A. Wirz-Justice: Pharmacopsychiat. 15, p. 31 (1982)

25. B. Pflug, W. Martin: Arch. Psychiat. Nervenkr. 229, p. 127 (1980)

26. B. Pflug, A. Johnsson, W. Martin: In: Circadian rhythms in psychiatry, ed. by T.A. Wehr and F.K. Goodwin, p. 71 (Boxwood Press 1983, Pacific Grove)

27. B. Pflug, A. Johnsson, A. Tveito Ekse: Acta psychiat. scand. 63, p. 227 (1981)

28. M. Atkinson, D.F. Kripke, S.R. Wolf: Chronobiologia 2, p. 325 (1975)

29. F. Halberg: In: Cycles biologiques et psychiatrie, ed. by J. de Ajuriaguerra, p. 73 (Masson et Cie. Paris: 1968)

30. B. Pflug, W. Engelmann, J.J. Gaertner: J. Neutral. Transm. 53, p. 213 (1982)

31. A. Wirz-Justice, M.S. Kafka, D. Naber, I.C. Campell, P.J. Marangos, L. Tamarkin, R.A. Wehr: Brain Res. 241, p. 115 (1982)

32. A. Wirz-Justice, T.A. Wehr: Uncoupling of circadian rhythms in hamsters and man. In: Sleep 1980, ed. by W.P. Koella, p. 64 (Basel: Karger 1981)

33. A. Wirz-Justice, M.S. Kafka, D. Naber, T.A. Wehr: Life sciences 27, p. 341 (1980)

34. W. Greil, M. Schölderle: In: Die Lithiumtherapie,ed. by B. Müller-Oerlinghausen u. W. Greil, p. 138 (Springer: Berlin-Heidelberg-New York - Tokyo, 1986)

35. B. Pflug: Depression und Schlafentzug. Neue therapeutische und theoretische Aspekte. Habil. Schrift Tübingen 1973

36. T.A. Wehr, A. Wirz-Justice, F.K. Goodwin, W. Duncan, J.C. Gillin: Science 206, p. 710 (1979)

37. E.D. Weitzman, C.A. Czeisler, R.M. Coleman, W.C. Dement, G.S. Richardson, C.P. Pollak: Sleep Res. 8, p. 221 (1979)

38. H. Moldofsky, S. Musisi, E.A. Phillipson: Sleep 9, p. 61-65 (1986).

Lithium Effects on Circadian Rhythms

W. Engelmann

Institut für Biologie I, Universität Tübingen,
Auf der Morgenstelle 1, D-7400 Tübinge, Fed. Rep. of Germany

1. Introduction

The circadian system of people suffering from endogenous depression differs from that of healthy subjects (different articles in [1], [2,3]). It has been speculated that the symptoms of this disorder are caused by an abnormality of the circadian system [1], as indicated in Fig. 1a. Alternatively, the circadian system could have been altered by the particular mental disorder (Fig. 1b), or both, mental disorder and change in the circadian system could result from a third factor F (Fig. 1c)

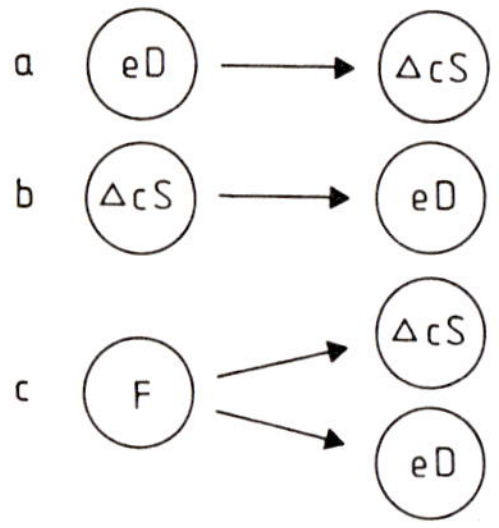

Fig. 1. Causal relationships between endogenous depression (eD) and changes in the circadian system ΔcS. See text.

Support for a causal relationship between endogenous depression and an altered circadian system (Fig.1a) comes from findings where methods or substances that are used to treat the disease are also known to influence the circadian system. Thus, light is a Zeitgeber for almost all circadian rhythms including those of man [4] and has recently been used for the treatment of mood disorders [5]. Li has definite therapeutic [6] and prophylatic effects [7] in endogenous depression and also interferes profoundly with circadian rhythms in plants, animals and man . However, the mechanism by which it exerts an effect on circadian rhythms is not known, since the basic mechanisms of circadian rhythms themselves are not yet understood in detail [8]. It is not even known, whether the same mechanism is utilized in the different rhythms of one organism or in those of different species. For the effect of Li on biochemical, cellular and physiological processes see [9].

2. Effects of Li on Circadian Rhythms in Unicellulars, Plants and Animals

In unicellulars Li was found to increase the period of circadian cell division in Skeletonema [10]. In *Euglena* the period length of the circadian rhythm of mobility is lengthened [11], but no effect was found in the phototactic response rhythm in *Chlamydomonas* [12] and the bioluminescence rhythm of *Gonyaulax* [13].

In fungi the rhythmic formation of conidia in the bd strain of *Neurospora* is slowed by Li [14].

In higher plants photoperiodic responses are changed by Li [15,16]. Since photoperiodic timing uses the circadian clock [17], Li might have affected the period of the circadian system. The petal movement of *Kalanchoe* is lengthened by Li in a dose dependent way [18], as is the leaf movement rhythm in *Oxalis* [19], *Trifolium* [20], and *Phaseolus* [21], and the K uptake rhythm in *Lemna* [22].

In lower animals Li produces dose dependent increases in the period of the compound action potential rhythm of nerves of isolated eyes of *Aplysia* [23]. The locomotor activity rhythm of *Drosophila* [24], *Musca* [25] and *Leucophaea* [26] is increased by Li, and the range of entrainment broadened in the latter [27].

In vertebrates Li increases the period of the circadian swimming activity in isolated goldfish [28], shortens the roosting activity cycle in self-selected light/dark cycles in canaries [29], and shortens the locomotor activity rhythm in the bat *Taphozous* [30]. The diurnal pattern of neurotic behaviour, emotional reactivity, and central nervous activation is phase displaced under Li in mice [31], suggesting a change in period length of the underlying oscillator. Diurnal rhythms of food and water intake and urine flow [32], of different hormones and electrolytes [33], and of the locomotor activity rhythm [34] are shifted by Li in rats. The circadian food intake rhythm is slowed by Li in blinded rats [35]. Li increases the period of the running wheel activity rhythm in rats [3], Syrian hamsters [18,36,37] and *Meriones* [26]. A different strain of hamsters showed lengthening of period by Li in the animals with a shorter rhythm and shortening in those with a longer rhythm [38]. The range of entrainment is shifted to longer periods in rats [39] and hamsters [38,40].

In man Li changes the diurnal sleep cycle, sleep latency and REM latency [41], the time of the temperature minimum [2] and temperature maximum [42]. The circadian rhythm of core temperature, urinary electrolytes and urine volume was slightly longer under therapeutic doses of Li [43], and the rhythms of temperature, activity and sleep/wake-cycle were lengthened in four of 8 volunteers in an experiment performed under arctic conditions [44,45,46].

There is thus ample evidence for an effect of Li on circadian rhythms, which consists in most cases of a period lengthening, but in some cases of a period shortening. Other alkali ions such as Rb and Cs change also the period of circadian rhythms [47,48,25].

ıɾcadian system of man has a multi-oscillatory structure [49,50]. Most of the rhythmic properties are due to a hierarchical control by pacemakers. Details are under debate. According to one view [51], a Y oscillator in the SCN of the hypothalamus drives locomotor activity, the sleep-wake cycle and a variety of behavioural, psychological, physiological, and biochemical processes. A X oscillator, the localization of which in the CNS is not yet established, drives core temperature, REM sleep and other processes. The X oscillator has a period of about 25 h, the Y oscillator a longer period of about 36 hours, as deduced from the occurrence of internal desynchronization. X and Y oscillators are normally coupled with each other, and the X oscillator is the stronger one. Zeitgeber were proposed to influence the Y oscillator directly and the X oscillator indirectly via coupling. However, this view has been abandoned due to new experimental findings [52]. Under normal conditions the circadian system is synchronized internally and with the 24 h time structure of the environment. The intra- and interindividual variability of physiological functions seems to be rather small [53], although differences in period length and amplitude might lead to different chronobiological phase types (morning- and evening types, [54]).

A number of chronobiological alterations have been reported to occur in endogenous depression of humans [1, but see also 55]

- a changed phase relationship between the X- and Y-oscillator as shown by phase advanced REM, a phase-advanced core temperature rhythm and a higher number of morning types [2]
- aberrant frequencies in the core temperature rhythm and the methoxyhydroxyphenylglycol (a metabolite of brain noradrenaline rhythm)
- lower amplitudes of rhythms [9]
- larger variabilities of the circadian system [2]
- hypersensitivity to light [56]
- the occurrence of internal desynchronization in an environment without Zeitgeber is more often found in elderly people [43], and this part of the population also more frequently shows affective symptoms [57].

These results could result from an abnormally short period length of the X oscillator leading to phase-advanced rhythms of the processes driven by this oscillator, or in extreme cases to relative coordination or even internal desynchronization.

However, other explanations are possible such as

- a Y oscillator which is even slower than normal (i.e. beyond 36 h),
- a difference in the coupling properties of the pacemakers
- an altered entrainment by environmental Zeitgeber.

It is, for instance, claimed that supersensitivity to light is a trait shown by certain types of endogenous depression [56].

Since the human PRC to light has very likely stronger advance than delay phase shifts, to allow for the correction of the longer than 24 h free run period in synchronizing it to the 24 h environment, this hypersensitivity would lead to a phase advance of the pacemaker.

A completely different understanding of endogenous depression has been reviewed recently [58]. Annual rhythms that drive in vertebrates phenomena such as hibernation, torpor, migration and molting in birds have been proposed to be responsible for this mental disease (which would then be rather an atavism than a disease). In support of this hypothesis Li has been found to suppress hibernation in the Turkish hamster [59].

4. Li Effects on the Circadian System in Endogenous Depression

According to the phase advance hypothesis of endogenous depression, the X oscillator of the human circadian system is faster than normal in people suffering from this disorder. This would lead to an advanced phase relationship or, in extreme cases, to a situation where the oscillator cannot be synchronized by the 24 h Zeitgeber anymore and will therefore free run with its innate short period, whereas the slower Y oscillator will continue to be entrained by the environment. Li would slow the fast X oscillator and thus allow synchronization with the Y oscillator and/or the 24 h environmental time structure. Alternatively, Li could slow both the X and the Y oscillators thus and bring the fast X oscillator within the range of entrainment by the environmental Zeitgeber.

In a LD cycle of a 24 h day, Li delays in rats the phase of the rhythm of plasma prolactin, corticosterone, parathyroid hormone, Ca and Mg [33], whereas the rhythms of serotonin and melatonin are not affected. Since the former rhythms are driven by the X oscillator and the latter by the Y oscillator, only the X oscillator seems to be affected by Li [60]. Patients suffering from endogenous depression should therefore show a normal melatonin rhythm. This was reported to be the case [61]. Furthermore, although Li selectively affects suppression of melatonin by light, it has no influence on the entraining of the melatonin rhythm by light [62].

A parallel case illustrating this situation of two oscillators reacting differently to Li is the petal movement rhythm of *Kalanchoe*. It seems to be composed of two different oscillations, one initiated by light-on, the other by light off [63]. Li affects only the light-off-rhythm, whereas in continous weak light Li does not change the period. The dark oscillator is perhaps identical with the one described by Wilkins [64] controlling the pumping of malate into the vacuole of the plant cell, whereas the oscillation in LL is perhaps identical with the one controlling malate metabolism via photosynthetic pathways [65].

5. Models

Circadian oscillations have been simulated in the form of mathematical or control system models. The feedback model of Johnsson and Karlsson [66] has been particularly successful in simulating the circadian petal movement rhythm of Kalanchoe and its responses to light and temperature [67,68]. This model was modified to simulate the locomotor activity rhythm of nocturnal insects and effects of light and temperature [69]. We have used it also to simulate experimental phase response curves to light with and without Li treatment in hamsters [36,70]. The effects, which consist of smaller advances by light pulses and a small displacement of 0.5 h of the phase response curve, can be simulated if it is assumed that Li increases the time delay in the model and decreases the sensitivity of the oscillator to light pulses. An increase in time delay leads to longer periods. Period lengthening is a known property of Li and is probably connected with changes in membrane properties or transport on a cellular level. It is unknown whether decreased sensitivity to light takes place at the retinal, SCN or neurotransmission levels. Hypersensitivity to light in endogenous depression might be corrected by Li acting as a kind of pharmacological sun glass.

Models might help in sorting the different possibilities in which Li, light and other Zeitgeber influence the circadian system in healthy man and in those with affective disorders. It might also shed light on the ways in which pacemakers are coupled. It has, for instance been found that period change by Li or Rb depends on the period length before treatment, in that there was a shortening of the period in animals which had a long rhythm prior to treatment and a lengthening in animals which had a short rhythm (e.g. the effect on locomotor activity rhythm in *Musca* of both Li and Rb [25] and of Li on *Taphozous* [30], Syrian hamsters [38]) locomotor rhythms, and the estradiol rhythm in rats [7]).

These findings can be explained by a model of coupled oscillators [38], but the kind of coupling and the identification of the pacemakers is still uncertain.

Acknowledgements I am thankful to Dr. Silyn Roberts and Dr. Lewis for reading the manuscript.

References

1. T.A. Wehr and F.K. Goodwin: Circadian Rhythms in Psychiatry, (Boxwood Press, 1983)
2. B. Pflug: In Temporal Disorder in Human Oscillatory Systems, ed. L.Rensing, U.an der Heiden and M.C.Mackey (Springer, Berlin, Heidelberg, New York, Tokyo 1986)
3. B. Pflug: In Die Lithium-Therapie, ed. B.Müller-Oerlinghausen (Springer, Berlin, Heidelberg, New York, Tokyo, 1986) p. 46-50
4. C.I. Eastman: In Temporal Disorder in Human Oscillatory Systems, ed. L.Rensing, U.an der Heiden and M.C.Mackey (Springer, Berlin, Heidelberg, New York, Tokyo 1986)
5. A. Lewy: In Temporal Disorder in Human Oscillatory Systems, ed. L.Rensing, U.an der Heiden and M.C.Mackey (Springer, Berlin, Heidelberg, New York, Tokyo 1986)

6. M. Schölderle and W. Greil: In Die Lithium Therapie, ed. B. Müller-Oerlinghausen (Springer, Berlin, Heidelberg, New York, Tokyo, 1986) p. 130-137
7. A. Kukopulos and A. Tondo: In Die Lithium-Therapie, ed. B. Müller-Oerlinghausen (Springer, Berlin, Heidelberg, New York, Tokyo, 1986) p. 173-182
8. W. Engelmann and M. Schrempf: In Photochemical and Photobiological Reviews, ed. K.C. Smith, Vol. 5 (Plenum Press, New York, London, 1980) p. 49-86
9. W. Engelmann: In Neuropsychiatric Disorders and Disturbances in the Circadian System of Man, ed. A. Halaris, in preparation
10. K. Östgaard, A. Jensen and A. Johnsson: Physiol. Plant 55, 285-288 (1982)
11. O. Kreuels, unpublished
12. J.E. Goodenough, V.G. Bruce and A. Carter: Biol. Bull. 161, 371-381 (1981)
13. D. Lloyd: personal communication
14: W. Engelmann: unpublished
15. R. Kandeler: Planta 90, 203-207 (1970)
16. W. Engelmann, I. Bollig and R. Hartmann: Arzneimittelforsch.26, 1085-1086 (1976)
17. E. Bünning: Ber. Deutsch. Bot. Ges. 54, 590-607 (1936)
18. W. Engelmann: Z. Naturforsch. 28c, 733-736 (1973)
19. A. Johnsson, P.I. Johnsson, T. Rinnan and D. Skrove: Physiol. Plant. 53, 361-367 (1981)
20. W. Engelmann: unpublished
21. W.-E. Mayer: unpublished
22. T. Kondo: Plant Physiol. 75, 1071-1074 (1984)
23. J.C. Woolum and F. Strumwasser: J. Comp. Physiol. A151, 253-269 (1983)
24. J. Mack: Thesis Tübingen (1980)
25. H.P. Schmid and W. Engelmann: J. Interdisc. Cycle Res, in press (1986)
26. K. Hofmann, M. Günderoth-Palmowski, G. Wiedenmann and W. Engelmann: Z. Naturforsch. 33c, 231-234 (1978)
27. J. Rauch, P. Reinhard and W. Engelmann: J. Interdisc. Cycle Res. 17, 51-68 (1986)
28. M. Kawaliers: Physiol. and Behav. 27, 625-628 (1981)
29. G. Wahlström: In Bell Air Symposium Vol.3, (G. George et Cie., Geneve, Masson et Cie., Paris 1968)
30. R. Subbaraj: Z. Naturforsch. 36c, 1068-1071 (1981)
31. C. Poirel, M. Briand and O. Hengartner: In Chronopharmacology and Chronotherapeutics, ed. C.A. Walker (1981) p. 103-108
32. S. Christensen and T. Agner: Physiol. and Beh. 28, 635-640 (1982)
33. D.I. McEachron, D.F. Kripke, M. Eaves, L. Lenhard, D. Pavlinac and L. Deftos: Psych. Res. 7, 121-131 (1980)

34. A. Wirz-Justice: In Basic Mechanisms in the Action of Lithium ed. by H.M. Emrich, J.B. Aldenhoff and H.D. Lux (Excerpt. Med., Amsterdam, Oxford, Princeton, 1982) p. 249-258
35. A. Wirz-Justice, G.A. Gross and T.A. Wehr: In Vertebrate circadian Systems: Structure and Physiology, ed. by J. Aschoff, S. Daan and G. Gross (Springer Berlin, Heidelberg 1982) p. 187-193
36. S.Z. Han: J. Interdisc. Cycle Res. 15, 139-145 (1984)
37. P. Reinhard: Thesis Tübingen (1983)
38. K. Delius, M. Günderoth-Palmowski, I. Krause and W. Engelmann: J. Interdisc. Cycle Res. 15, 289-299 (1984)
39. D.L. McEachron, D.F. Kripke and V.G. Wyborney: Psych. Res. 5, 1-9 (1981)
40. P. Reinhard: J. Interdisc. Cycle Res. 16, 227-237 (1985)
41. L. Judd and D. Janowsky: In Biological Psychiatry, ed. by C. Perris, G. Struwe and B. Janssen (Elsevier, Amsterdam, New York, Oxford, 1981) p. 657-660
42. Sasaki, M. Suzuki, M. Onda, H. Itoh, T. Kitahara, T. Takahashi, H. Kasahara and A. Mori: Adv. Biosc. 40, 303-308 (1982)
43. P. Wever: The Circadian System of Man (Springer New York, Heidelberg, Berlin, 1979)
44. A. Johnsson, B. Pflug, W. Engelmann and W. Klemke: Pharmacopsych. 12, 423-425 (1979)
45. A. Johnsson, W. Engelmann, B. Pflug and W. Klemke: Z. Naturforsch. 35c, 503-507 (1980)
46. A. Johnsson, W. Engelmann, B. Pflug and W. Klemke: Int. J. Chronobiol. 8, 129-147 (1983)
47. W. Engelmann and H. Casper: J. Interdisc. Cycle Res. 15, 17-22 (1984)
48. T. Rinnan and A.Johnsson: Physiol.Plant. 66, 139-143 (1986)
49. R. Wever: In Temporal Disorder in Human Oscillatory systems, ed. L.Rensing, U.an der Heiden and M.C.Mackey (Springer, Berlin, Heidelberg, New York, Tokyo, 1986)
50. P.E.M. Rietveld: In Temporal Disorder in Human Oscillatory systems, ed. L.Rensing, U.an der Heiden and M.C.Mackey (Springer, Berlin, Heidelberg, New York, Tokyo, 1986)
51. R.E. Kronauer, C.A. Cseisler, S.F. Pilato, M.C. Moore-Ede and E.D. Weitzman: Am.J. Physiol. 242, R3-R17 (1982)
52. C.A. Czeisler, J.A. Allan, S.H. Strogatz, J.M. Ronda, R. Sanchez, C.D. Rios, W.O. Freitag, G.S. Richardson, and R.E. Kronauer, Science 233, 667-671 (1986)
53. J.Aschoff and R. Wever: Klin. Wochenschr. 58, 323-335 (1980)
54. G.A. Kerkhoff: Biol. Psych. 20, 83-112 (1985)
55. D.v. Zersen, H. Barthelmes, G. Dirlich, P. Doerr, H.M. Emrich, L. v. Lindern, R. Lund and K.M. Pirke: Psych.Res. 16, 51-63 (1985)
56. A.J. Lewy, J.I. Nurnberger, T.A. Wehr, D. Pack, L.E. Becker, R.-L. Powell and D.A. Newsome: Am.J.Psychiatr. 142, 725-727
57. J. Angst: In: Zur Ätiologie und Nosologie endogen depressiver Psychosen. (Springer, Berlin, Heidelberg, New York, 1966).

58. H. Giedke: Pharmacopsychiatry 19, 192-193 (1986)
59. H. Giedke and H. Pohl: Exp. 41, 1391-1392 (1985)
60. D.L. McEachron, D.F. Kripke, F.R. Sharp, A.J. Lewy and D.E. McClellan: Abstr. Soc. Neurosc., 13th Ann. Meet. Boston (1983)
61. J.C. Jimerson: Life Sc. 20, 1501-1508 (1977)
62. N.V.P. Nair and N. Hariharasubramanian: Brit. J. Psych. 145, 557-558 (1984)
63. W. Engelmann: Nachr. Akad. Wissensch. Göttingen II, Math. Phys. Kl. 10, 141 (1967)
64. M.B. Wilkins: Planta 157, 471-480 (1983)
65. M.B. Wilkins: Planta 161, 381-384 (1984)
66. A. Johnsson, H.G. Karlsson: J. Theor. Biol. 36, 153-174
67. W. Engelmann, H.G. Karlsson and A. Johnsson: Int. J. Chronobiol. 1, 147-156
68. W. Engelmann, I. Eger, A. Johnsson and H.G. Karlsson: Int. J. Chronobiol. 2, 347-358 (1974)
69. P.H. Gander, R.D. Lewis: Int. J. Chronobiol. 6, 263-280 (1979)
70. W. Engelmann and R.D. Lewis: unpublished
71. H.E. Albers: Am. J. Physiol. 241, R62-R66 (1981)

Treatment of Chronobiologic Sleep and Mood Disorders with Light: Theory and Practice

A.J. Lewy and R.L. Sack

Departments of Psychiatry, Ophthalmology, and Pharmacology,
Oregon Health Sciences University, Portland, OR 97201, USA

1. Suppression of Human Nighttime Melatonin Production by Exposure to Bright Light

Melatonin is produced by the pineal gland only at night during the dark in both diurnal and nocturnal animals [1,2]. Exposure to light during the night acutely suppresses melatonin production [3,4]. Most animals are exquisitely sensitive to light and will completely suppress their melatonin production when exposed to 10 - 500 lux light.

Humans were thought not to be affected by light: in addition to negative results obtained in temporal isolation studies in which light appeared to be an ineffective zeitgeber [5], studies attempting to suppress human melatonin production with light failed to produce any effect [6-12]. Thus, both types of studies suggested that humans did not respond to light in ways that other animals did. In 1980, however, we showed that 2500 lux light and sunlight (which is generally brighter than 2500 lux) can suppress melatonin production in humans [13].

This finding had at least two important implications. One was that humans had circadian and seasonal rhythms that might be cued to sunlight unperturbed by ordinary-intensity indoor light. A second implication was that bright artificial light could be used experimentally, and perhaps therapeutically, to manipulate these rhythms.

2. Bright Light Treatment of Winter Depression

We first tested these ideas in 1980 when we treated a patient who generally became depressed as the days shortened and came out of his depressions as the days lengthened [14]. We exposed him to 2500 lux light between 6 and 9 a.m. and between 4 and 7 p.m. for several days to extend day length (animals tell day length by measuring the time interval between dawn and dusk; melatonin is thought to mediate this response in many animals through the change in duration in nighttime secretion throughout the year [15]). After four days, he came out of his depression.

Since then, over a hundred patients with winter depression (or seasonal affective disorder, as it is sometimes called) have been identified and treated with bright light. Investigators most experienced with this disorder generally agree that the intensity and duration of the light exposure are critical. However, there is disagreement as to whether or not the timing of the light is critical.

3. Phase Shifting Effects of Bright Light

We [16] have hypothesized a human phase response curve (PRC) that is similar to those described for other animals [17-19]. We originally hypothesized [16] and later demonstrated [20-24] that humans advance their circadian rhythms in response to bright light exposure in the morning and delay them in response to bright light exposure in the evening. The delay response has since been confirmed by EASTMAN [25] and by CZEISLER et al. [26]. In addition, WEVER et al. [27] were the first to show that bright light could increase the range of entrainment of the human temperature circadian rhythm.

4. One vs. Two Pacemakers for the Melatonin Production Circadian Rhythm

There remain some unresolved areas here. One area is whether there are one or two pacemakers that regulate the timing of the melatonin production circadian rhythm. One school of thought [28] maintains that there are two separate (but functionally coupled) pacemakers for melatonin production - one that regulates the onset and is cued to dusk and one that regulates the offset and is cued to dawn. These investigators also state that the suppressant effect of light rarely, if ever, occurs in nature and then only under extremely long photoperiods. On the other hand, we [29] have held that the suppressant effect of light in humans occurs when photoperiods are approximately 12 hours or longer. This would explain what we have the termed the seasonal onset-offset phase paradox without the need to postulate two pacemakers [30].

The seasonal onset-offset phase paradox refers to the shorter duration of melatonin production in the summer than in the winter that results in a later onset and an earlier offset in the summer. To explain this, some investigators have postulated two pacemakers, since it is difficult to imagine how one pacemaker could shift its phase earlier and later at the same time. However, we have explained this paradox without the need for more than one pacemaker and have proposed a "clock-gate" model [29] in which the pacemaker in humans is shifted earlier in the summer and later in the winter (this prediction has been borne out by two different groups of investigators [31,32]). The later onset that is observed in the summer may be due to a suppressant effect from late evening sunlight on the signal that initiates melatonin production. We have, therefore, used the two known effects of light - the suppressant effect and the synchronizing effect - to explain how the pattern of melatonin production changes during the year, without the need to postulate two pacemakers.

5. The Clock-Gate Model and the Dim Light Melatonin Onset

The clock-gate model has led us to hypothesize that the pacemaker for melatonin production is phase advanced in the summer compared to winter in animals whose intrinsic circadian periods are greater than 24 hours [29]. The model has also led us to recommend that bright light be avoided after 5 or 6 p.m. when using the onset of melatonin production to mark circadian phase position. We call this the dim light melatonin onset, or DLMO [21].

We think that the onset of melatonin production is the most accurate part of the melatonin curve for marking circadian phase position. This is because the pineal secretes only basal levels of melatonin during the day. Consequently, the onset is clearly demarcated. Furthermore, the onset is less affected by amplitude than the other portions of the melatonin curve. The peak, acrophase and offset are all potentially confounded by factors that might affect amplitude, such as substrate depletion and changes in beta-adrenergic sensitivity that occur during the night. If there is one pacemaker for melatonin production, then the DLMO represents it. If there are two pacemakers for melatonin production (which we do not think is the case), then the DLMO would primarily reflect the evening pacemaker.

6. One vs. Two Pacemakers for the Human Circadian System

The clock-gate model has also helped us to conceptualize the entire circadian system as one pacemaker [33,34], although there is no certain proof on this point either. Although many circadian oscillators may exist (perhaps one or more for each overt circadian rhythm), in our opinion there is only one pacemaker that is ordinarily cued to the environmental zeitgeber(s). We think that a PRC should be demonstrated in order for an oscillator to be called an endogenous pacemaker. Otherwise, it might be a slave oscillator that is driven by the pacemaker which in turn is entrained to the light-dark cycle. A PRC in humans has only been demonstrated (albeit preliminarily) for bright light [20-26], and - to our knowledge - a PRC has not yet been demonstrated for social cues.

Our preference for a one-pacemaker model differs from the other pioneering light therapy groups and may account in part for different theoretical ideas regarding light therapy. For example, the Bethesda group has relied on the two-pacemaker model [5,35] for describing two-to-one coupling between two putative pacemakers in bipolar (manic-depressive) patients. The sleepless night often accompanying the switch from depression into mania has also been interpreted as an advance in the strong (X) pacemaker relative to the weak (Y) pacemaker [36]. Although some studies support an advance in some circadian rhythms in these patients, this area is at present controversial.

KRIPKE has also relied on the two-pacemaker model. Furthermore, he [37] has referred to the model [35] in which the zeitgeber(s) act indirectly (through the Y pacemaker) on the X pacemaker (WEVER [5] has theorized that zeitgebers act equally on these putative pacemakers). Thus, the two-pacemaker model makes it very difficult to know when to schedule bright light exposure to change internal phase relationships between pacemakers. In other words, do you use light in the evening to delay the advanced pacemaker or do you use light in the morning to advance the delayed pacemaker?

If there are two pacemakers, our thinking has been that the Y pacemaker is more sensitive to social cues and the X pacemaker is more sensitive to bright light [38]. Furthermore, since we are more impressed with phasic responses to bright light than to social cues, we have been leaning towards a one-pacemaker model [33,34], conceptualizing the sleep-wake cycle as a slave oscillator, driven by the endogenous pacemaker which in turn is cued to the bright light cycle. One of the leading advocates [26] for the two-pacemaker model has recently abandoned it, because of phasic responses obtained after shifting the bright light cycle while holding the sleep-wake cycle constant [20-26]. In summary, we have for several years been leaning towards a one-pacemaker model, although conclusive proof is lacking for any model, either with regard to one or two pacemaker(s) for the onset and offset of melatonin production or with regard to a separate endogenous pacemaker for the activity-rest rhythm.

7. Chronobiologic abnormalities

The one-pacemaker model has helped us to conceptualize abnormalities in the circadian system. If any rhythms seem abnormally advanced or delayed with respect to real time, we phase type [23] the individual to select the best time for light therapy: bright light in the morning should help phase-delayed individuals, whereas bright light in the evening should help phase-advanced individuals. Endogenous circadian rhythms seem to be primarily synchronized only to the bright light cycle, whereas sleep can be manipulated both through social cues and through the action of bright light on the pacemaker, which in turn influences the timing of sleep. Thus, through the use of bright light we can reset the phases of all of the circadian rhythms with respect to real time and through social cues we can also change the phase of sleep relative to the other circadian rhythms. We have further conceptualized chronobiologic sleep disorders as being different from chronobiologic mood disorders, in that in the former all circadian rhythms - including the sleep-wake cycle - are phase-disturbed to the same extent.

Thus, similar to WEHR et al. [39] and KRIPKE [40], we think that there is an internal phase angle disturbance between sleep and the other circadian rhythms involved in chronobiologic mood disorders [23]. However, we differ from them in two ways. One, we do not think that an internal phase angle disturbance between sleep and the other circadian rhythms necessarily means that sleep is controlled by a separate endogenous pacemaker. Furthermore, we think that there may be a phase delay type [20,23] of disturbance as well as a phase advance type [36,37,39-41], and we [23] think that there is a second type of internal phase angle disturbance in which circadian rhythms are abnormally delayed with respect to sleep (this is opposite to, and is an extension of, what has previously been proposed by WEHR et al. [39] and KRIPKE [40], in which circadian rhythms in affective disorders were thought to be abnormally advanced with respect to sleep).

8. The Melatonin and Photon Counting Hypotheses for Light Therapy of Winter Depression

With regard to winter depression, the Bethesda group has proposed two hypotheses for light therapy of winter depression. Their first hypothesis was the melatonin hypothesis [43]. According to the melatonin hypothesis, patients become depressed in the winter because of an abnormally long duration of melatonin production. They first began testing this hypothesis when they administered melatonin in the morning and evening to patients who were concurrently responding to bright light exposure morning and evening. Replacement of melatonin brought back some, but not all, of the depressive symptoms [43]. These investigators concluded that melatonin may be mediating part of the syndrome but then the next year they [44] were unable to mimic the antidepressant effect of light with the administration of atenolol in the evening (a beta-adrenergic blocker that reduces melatonin production). Following this study they concluded that the melatonin hypothesis was not correct. We think that this area is still inconclusive, because the first study was not repeated with a prospective prediction that the same symptoms and only those symptoms would worsen again when melatonin levels were reinstated and because the second study administered atenolol in the evening (it should also have been tried in the morning).

These investigators then proposed the photon counting (incident photon) hypothesis [44-47]. According to this hypothesis, the brightness and duration of light exposure are critical, but not the timing. We [48] have discussed in detail the studies they cite in support of this hypothesis elsewhere: in most of these studies, sleep time or bright light exposure around twilight were not controlled [43,45,46].

9. The Phase Shift Hypothesis

In a study in which sleep and bright light exposure around twilight were controlled, we found that morning bright light exposure (6 - 8 a.m.) was more effective than bright light exposure in the evening (8 - 10 p.m.) and that the combination was intermediate in reducing depression ratings in a group of eight winter depressive patients [22,49,50]. In our study, in both patients and normal controls, morning light exposure advanced their DLMOs and evening light delayed them with the combination causing a shift to intermediate phase positions. Patients also seemed to advance more and delay less than normals suggesting a phase-delayed PRC in the patients. Whether or not the DLMOs of the winter depressive patients are phase delayed at baseline (our data also indicate that this is so), the most likely explanation for the antidepressant effect of light exposure in these patients is that the light is working through phase advancing their circadian rhythms.

A less likely explanation is that the light is having some sort of "energizing" effect. We think this second explanation is less likely for at least three reasons. One is that we and others have identified a typical two-to three-day time course for the initiation and disappearance of the antidepressant response after beginning and stopping light exposure, respectively; the energizing effect appears to be immediate. The other two reasons have to do with two studies done this past winter.

In one study we compared one-half hour (6 - 6:30 a.m.) to two hours (6 - 8 a.m.) of morning light. On average there was no difference between the two durations. However, there seemed to be a subgroup of patients who responded best to two hours of morning light and a subgroup of patients who responded best to one-half hour of morning light. The remainder of the patients didn't seem to show a preference. In this study, we also noted an order effect in that any light treatment that was begun the first week (and therefore simultaneously occurred with advancing the sleep-wake cycle) was not as effective as compared to the same light treatment administered towards the end of the study (when patients had adapted to the earlier sleep schedule). We hypothesized that light treatment did not work the first week because sleep had just been advanced.

The second study was on three in-patients. In this study, sleep was delayed four hours while bright light exposure occurred between 11 a.m. and 1 p.m. The depression ratings declined in response to delaying sleep relative to the other circadian rhythms. This result is consistent with our hypothesis that their depressive pathology is related to an internal phase angle disturbance in which sleep is not as delayed as the other circadian rhythms. These data also provide further evidence that the light is working through advancing circadian rhythms with respect to sleep and argue against an emergizing effect.

10. Phase Typing Chronobiologic Sleep and Mood Disorders

We have proposed phase typing and phase shifting other types of sleep and mood disorders that are suspected of having a chronobiologic component

[16,20-23,50]. In depressed patients who have early morning awakening, we agree with KRIPKE that this subgroup is probably phase advanced. KRIPKE [51,52] originally used bright light exposure in the morning for these patients. Apparently, KRIPKE [37] has suggested that bright light in the morning might preferentially shift the sleep-wake cycle earlier with respect to the other circadian rhythms; our data suggest the opposite - bright light in the morning shifts circadian rhythms earlier with respect to the sleep-wake cycle. Consequently, we [16,20,23] think that the evening is the best time to test bright light exposure: in our experience, evening light delays their circadian rhythms and corrects the sleep disturbance. The effect of evening light on the other symptoms of depression is less clear and requires further study.

In the treatment of advanced and delayed sleep phase syndrome, we [16,20,23,50] have also used bright light exposure in the evening and in the morning, respectively. The scheduling of bright light (including avoiding it at critical times) has also been applied to the treatment of jet lag [53].

11. Conclusion

The study of melatonin physiology in humans has helped us identify three critical parameters for light to be chronobiologically active in humans: intensity, wavelength [54] and timing. We have proposed that the mechanism of action of bright light's antidepressant effect in winter depression is related to phase-advancing circadian rhythms with respect to sleep. We have extended this thinking to other chronobiologic sleep and mood disorders: phase-delayed disorders should respond best to bright light in the morning which would provide a corrective phase advance, whereas phase-advanced disorders should respond best to bright light in the evening which would provide a corrective phase delay. Sleep time should be held constant as soon as it reaches a normal phase position, because the phase angle between sleep and the other circadian rhythms may be pathogenic for chronobiologic mood disturbances. Our data also seem to be consistent with a one-pacemaker model for the timing of the human circadian system.

12. References

1 W.B. Quay: Proc. Soc. Exp. Biol. Med. 115 710 (1964)
2 H.J. Lynch, C.L. Ralph: Am. Zool. 10, 300 (1970)
3 K.P. Minneman, H. Lynch, R.J. Wurtman: Life Sci. 15 1791 (1974)
4 S.M. Reppert, M.S. Perlow, L. Tamarkin, D. Orloff, D.C. Klein: Brain Res. 223 313 (1981)
5 R.A. Wever: The Circadian System of Man, (Springer-Verlag, New York 1979)
6 D.C. Jimerson, H.J. Lynch, R.M. Post, R.J. Wurtman, W.E. Bunney: Life Sci. 20 1501 (1977)

7 H.J. Lynch, D.C. Jimerson, Y. Ozaki, R.M. Post, W.E. Bunney, R.J. Wurtman: Life Sci. 23 1557 (1977)
8 J. Arendt: J. Neural. Transm. Suppl. 13 265 (1978)
9 E.D. Weitzman, U. Weinberg, R. D'Eletto, H.J. Lynch, R.J. Wurtman, C.A. Czeisler, S. Erlich: J. Neural. Transm. Suppl. 13 325 (1978)
10 L. Wetterberg: J. Neural. Transm. Suppl. 13 289 (1978)
11 T. Akerstedt, J.E. Froberg, Y. Friberg, L. Wetterberg: Psychoneuroendocrin. 4 219 (1979)
12 G.M. Vaughan, R. Bell, A. De La Pena: Neurosci. Lett. 14 81 (1979)
13 A.J. Lewy, T.A. Wehr, F.K. Goodwin, D.A. Newsome, S.P. Markey: Science 210 1267 (1980)
14 A.J. Lewy, H.E. Kern, N.E. Rosenthal, T.A. Wehr: Am. J. Psychiat. 139 1496 (1982)
15 B. Goldman, V. Hall, C. Hollister, S. Reppert, P. Roychoudhury, S. Yellon, L. Tamarkin: Biol. Reprod. 24 778 (1981)
16 A.J. Lewy, R.L. Sack, R.H. Fredrickson, M. Reaves, D.D. Denney, D.R. Zielske: Psychopharmacol. Bull. 19 523 (1983)
17 P.J. DeCoursey: J. Cell. Comp. Physiol. 63 189 (1964)
18 C.S. Pittendrigh, S. Daan: J. Comp. Physiol. 106 291 (1976)
19 S. Binkley, G. Muller, T. Hernandez: J. Neurochem. 37 798 (1981)
20 A.J. Lewy, R.L. Sack, C.M. Singer: Psychopharmacol. Bull. 20 561 (1984)
21 A.J. Lewy, R.L. Sack, C.M. Singer: Ann. N.Y. Acad. Sci. 453 253 (1985)
22 A.J. Lewy, R.L. Sack, L.S. Miller, T.M. Hoban, C.M. Singer: In Biological Psychiatry 1985, ed. by C. Shagass, R. Josiassen, W. Bridger, K. Weiss, D. Staff, and G. Simpson, (Elsevier, New York 1986) p. 984
23 A.J. Lewy, R.L. Sack, C.M. Singer: Psychopharmacol. Bull. 21 368 (1985)
24 R.L. Sack, A.J. Lewy, L.S. Miller, C.M. Singer: Biol. Psychiat. 21 410 (1986)
25 C.I. Eastman: Sleep Res. 15, 271 (1986)
26 C.A. Czeisler, J.S. Allan, S.H. Strogatz, J.M. Ronda, R. Sanchez, C.D. Rios, W.O. Freitag, G.S. Richardson, R.E. Kronauer: Science, 233 667 (1986)
27 R. Wever, J. Polasek, C. Wildgruber: Pfluger's Arch. 396 85 (1983)
28 H. Illnerova, J. Vanecek: J. Comp. Physiol. 145 539 (1982)
29 A.J. Lewy: In The Pineal Gland, ed. by R.M. Relkin, (Elsevier North-Holland, New York 1983) p. 77
30 A.J. Lewy: In The Pineal Gland: Endocrine Aspects, ed. by G.M. Brown, S.D. Wainwright, (Pergamon Press, New York 1985) p. 203
31 H. Illnerova, P. Zrolsky, J. Vanecek: Brain Res. 328 186 (1985)
32 J. Arendt, J. Broadway: J. Physiol. P77 (1986)
33 S. Daan, D.G.M. Beersma, A.A. Borbely: Am. J. Physiol. 246 R161 (1984)
34 C.I. Eastman: In Mathematical Models of the Circadian Sleep-Wake Cycle, ed. by M.C. Moore-Ede, C.A. Czeisler, (Raven Press, New York 1984) p. 81

35 R.E. Kronauer, C.A. Czeisler, S.F. Pilato, M.C. Moore-Ede, E.D. Weitzman: Am. J. Physiol. 242 R3 (1984)
36 T.A. Wehr, F.K. Goodwin: In Circadian Rhythms in Psychiatry, ed. by T.A. Wehr, F.K. Goodwin, (Boxwood Press, Pacific Grove 1983) p. 129
37 D.F. Kripke: Ann. N.Y. Acad. Sci. 453 270 (1985)
38 A. J. Lewy: In Circadian Rhythms in Psychiatry, ed. by T.A. Wehr, F.K. Goodwin, (Boxwood Press, Pacific Grove 1983) p. 203
39 T.A. Wehr, A. Wirz-Justice, F.K. Goodwin, W. Duncan, J.C. Gillin: Science 206 710 (1979)
40 D.F. Kripke: Chonobiol. Int. 1 73 (1984)
41 M. Papousek: Fortschr. Neurol. Psychiatr. 43 381 (1975)
42 D.F Kripke, D.J. Mullaney, M.L. Atkinson, S. Wolf: Biol. Psychiat. 13 335 (1978)
43 N.E. Rosenthal, D.A. Sack, S.P. James, B.L. Parry, W.B. Mendelson, L. Tamarkin, T.A. Wehr: Ann. N.Y. Acad. Sci. 453 260 (1985)
44 N.E. Rosenthal, D.A. Sack, S.P. James, B.L. Parry, F. Jacobsen, C. Carpenter, T.A. Wehr: IVth World Congress of Biological Psychiatry Abstracts, September 8-13 (1985) p. 327
45 S.P. James, T.A. Wehr, D.A. Sack, B.L. Parry, N.E. Rosenthal: Brit. J. Psychiat. 147 424 (1985)
46 C.J. Hellekson, J.A. Kline, N.E. Rosenthal: Am. J. Psychiat. 143 1035 (1986)
47 T.A. Wehr, F. M. Jacobsen, D.A. Sack, J. Arendt, L. Tamarkin, N.E. Rosenthal: Arch. Gen. Psychiat. 43 870 (1986)
48 A.J. Lewy, R.L. Sack: Proc. Soc. Exp. Biol. Med. 183 11 1986
49 A.J. Lewy, R.L. Sack, L.S. Miller, T.M. Hoban: Antidepressant and circadian phase-shifting effects of light. (Submitted)
50 A. J. Lewy, R.L. Sack, C.M. Singer: In Photoperiodism, Melatonin and the Pineal, ed. by D. Evered, S. Clark, (Pitman, London 1985) p. 231
51 D.F. Kripke: In Biological Psychiatry 1981, ed. by C. Perris, G. Struwe, B. Jansson (Elsevier, Amsterdam 1981) p. 1249
52 D.F. Kripke, S. Risch, D. Janowsky: Psychopharmacol. Bull. 19 524 (1983)
53 S. Daan, A.J. Lewy: Psychopharmacol. Bull. 20 566 (1984)
54 G.C. Brainard, A.J. Lewy, M. Menaker, R.H. Fredrickson, L.S. Miller, R.G. Weleber, V. Cassone, D. Hudson: Ann. N.Y. Acad. Sci. 453 376 (1985)

13. Acknowledgement

The authors wish to thank Rick Boney, Gregory B. Clarke, Susan Fogg and Carol Simonton for their assistance in the preparation of this paper.

Free-Running Melatonin Rhythms in Blind People: Phase Shifts with Melatonin and Triazolam Administration

R.L. Sack, A.J. Lewy, and T.M. Hoban

Sleep and Mood Disorders Laboratory, Oregon Health Sciences University, Portland, OR 97201, USA

1. Introduction

The study of circadian rhythms in totally blind individuals offers an obvious strategy for understanding the effects of light on the human biological timekeeping system. Early investigations of circadian rhythms in blind people commonly found diminished amplitude in the rhythms of sleep, temperature and cortisol production [1-5], which were probably the result of averaging rhythms that were out of phase with each other. Subsequently, two single-case longitudinal studies demonstrated free-running plasma cortisol in blind subjects [6,7]. In these two studies, many blood samples (and extraordinary subject commitment) were required to discriminate the underlying free-running cortisol rhythm from background noise produced by stress and other masking effects. Since the plasma melatonin rhythm is not influenced by stress [8] and is an excellent marker for the rhythm of the circadian pacemaker in the hypothalamus, it offers a valuable strategy for studying circadian rhythms in humans, including the blind.

SMITH et al. [9] first reported that melatonin rhythms might be abnormal in blind people. Using a highly sensitive and specific GC-MS assay [10], LEWY and NEWSOME [11] studied overnight plasma melatonin production for a single 24-hour period in 10 totally blind subjects and found that the timing of melatonin production was abnormal in 7 of the 10. They then studied two subjects longitudinally and found that one subject consistently produced melatonin at the same time each day but at an unusual time (about 180 degrees out of phase); the other subject had an apparent free-running melatonin rhythm with a period (tau) of 25.1 hours, very similar to the average tau for core body temperature observed in sighted human subjects living in temporal isolation. The free-running melatonin rhythm appeared to reflect the rhythm of the hypothalamic pacemaker, even though the subject was maintaining a conventional sleep-wake schedule. Based on this study, LEWY and NEWSOME [11] concluded that the circadian rhythms of totally blind people were heterogeneous and could be classified as: 1) normally entrained, 2) abnormally entrained or 3) free-running.

2. Recent Studies of Melatonin Rhythms in Blind People

Since 1984 we have studied five newly recruited totally blind subjects at the Sleep and Mood Disorders Laboratory in Portland using the GC-MS method of LEWY and MARKEY [10]. Of the five, two appeared to have normally entrained melatonin rhythms; one had an unstable rhythm; and two (described below) had free-running rhythms. Clinical features of age, sex, etiology, duration of blindness and age of onset did not seem to differentiate subjects with normally entrained from those with abnormally entrained rhythms.

The study of the two free-running subjects has generated some remarkable findings. First, we found the circadian rhythm for melatonin production to be quite stable. The stability of the rhythm was assessed by sampling plasma melatonin hourly for 24-hour periods (weekly or bi-weekly) for 4-8 weeks; the procedure was then repeated one year (subject 02) or two years (subject 01) later. During the study period, the subjects maintained a conventional sleep-wake cycle (although they both complained of periodic difficulty with insomnia and daytime sleepiness). Tau was remarkably consistent for these subjects (Table 1).

Table 1

Subject	Tau_{1984}	Tau_{1985}	Tau_{1986}
01	24.5	--	24.6
02	--	25.1	25.1

A second remarkable finding was the precision of the melatonin rhythm. When a linear regression was fitted to the onsets of melatonin secretion, the average standard error for the two subjects around the regression line was $\pm$ 0.6 hours. In other words one could predict the free-running onset of melatonin secretion to within $\pm$ 36 min. at the 68% confidence level. This standard error is about equal to the sampling interval (one hour) so might possibly be reduced in future studies by more frequent sampling. The precision of the melatonin rhythm allowed us to reasonably interpolate (and extrapolate) the timing of melatonin production for at least 14 days before and after the day of actual measurement. Greater variability resulted in predicting the timing of melatonin production if the period of the melatonin rhythm were estimated from peak secretion; thus an assay that is sufficiently sensitive to detect the onset of melatonin production is important.

3. Melatonin and Triazolam Administration

After defining the period (tau) of the melatonin rhythm under baseline conditions, we tested the effects of administering exogenous melatonin or triazolam on the circadian melatonin production rhythm. Melatonin has been shown to entrain the rhythms of free-running rodents [12] and to phase advance the endogenous melatonin rhythm in normal (sighted) human volunteers [13]. Melatonin has been shown in most studies to have sedative activity [14-18] or to induce fatigue [13,19,20]. Triazolam is an approved benzodiazepine sedative-hypnotic that has been shown to phase-shift activity rhythms of free-running hamsters kept in constant darkness.TUREK and LOSEE-OLSEN [21]. Either drug might be able to induce sleep at the appropriate time and thus "anchor" the melatonin rhythm to the sleep cycle MINORS and WATERHOUSE [22].

Using a single-blind placebo-controlled cross-over design, we administered melatonin orally (5 mg) or triazolam (0.25 or 0.5 mg) at bedtime. Treatment was begun on the day when the melatonin onset was approaching a normal phase relationship to clock time (i.e. 2000 h). Melatonin was given for 18 days and triazolam for 30 or 34 days.

Both melatonin and triazolam produced phase advances in the free-running melatonin rhythm. However, the effects were of different magnitude in the two subjects. In subject 02 exogenous melatonin administration produced an apparent 7.6 hour phase advance but triazolam had an equivocal effect. In subject 01 melatonin caused a smaller (1.6 hour) phase advance, whereas triazolam caused a 6.9 hour phase advance.

4. Melatonin Rhythms and Sleep

Subject 02 kept a daily dairy of sleep times and quality. These data were related to the interpolated melatonin onset. Sleep quality clearly varied with melatonin phase position, deteriorating as the rhythm was maximally out of phase (0800h) and improving when melatonin phase position normalized.

For subject 02, self-rated estimates of sleep time were also plotted against melatonin onsets. Although he was attempting to maintain a conventional sleep-wake schedule, sleep onsets and wake-up times varied considerably and showed an apparent relationship to melatonin onset. When melatonin onset was advanced with respect to sleep, sleep onset was typically several hours early. When melatonin onset was delayed with respect ot sleep, sleep onset was typically several hours late. As the melatonin rhythm went from being maximally delayed to being maximally advanced, sleep time reverted from a late to an early time. Thus sleep times appeared to be a compromise between clock time and body time.

Because of the relationship between the melatonin rhythm and sleep tendency in subject 02, we prescribed a sleep schedule based on the endogenous melatonin rhythm rather than clock time, i.e., three hours after melatonin onset. In other words, he was going to bed about an hour later each day,thus synchronizing his sleep rhythm to his melatonin rhythm. Using this schedule, he was able to maintain much improved sleep and better wake-time alertness.

5. Discussion

We have shown that measuring 24-hour melatonin production at 1-2 week intervals provides an efficient strategy for detecting and classifying circadian rhythm abnormalities in blind subjects. The presence of stable, free-running melatonin rhythms in some blind people argues against an entraining influence of social cues in these subjects. However, the fact that other totally blind subjects have normally entrained rhythms leaves open the possibility that nonphotic time cues may be sufficient to entrain some blind people.

While early temporal isolation studies in sighted individuals concluded that light was a relatively unimportant time cue for entraining human circadian rhythms [23], the existence of pronounced circadian rhythm abnormalities in blind people adds to the evidence from recent studies (in sighted subjects) that has prompted a reconsideration of the importance of light [24-29].

It is perplexing that melatonin produced a robust 7.6 hour phase advance in subject 02 but produced only a modest (1.6 hour) advance in subject 01. Conversely, triazolam produced a 6.9 hour phase advance in subject 01 and only on equivocal advance in subject 02. Clearly, more free-running blind subjects need to be studied to be sure that either drug produces a consistent effect. There is some evidence that melatonin and the benzodiazepines might share a common receptor site [30]; therefore, it is intriguing to think that both drugs might be capable of acting on some common target in the circadian timekeeping system.

It is not yet clear whether triazolam or melatonin altered the intrinsic period or caused phase shifts in the melatonin rhythm. Administration of these drugs at different times of the day may resolve this question. If the effect were mainly on period, then one would see a change in the same direction whatever time of day the drug was given. However, if the effects were opposite in the evening compared to the morning (advances vs. delays), this would constitute evidence for a phase response curve (PRC) DECOURSEY [31]. A PRC has been shown for melatonin administration on activity-rest cycles in lizards UNDERWOOD et al. [32] and similarly, for triazolam administration in hamsters TUREK and LOSEE-OLSEN [21]. It is of interest that melatonin was shown to increase prolactin in prepubertal human subjects when given in the afternoon but had no effect when given in the morning (MAURI et al. [33]).

The phase advances produced by evening administration of melatonin and triazolam are opposite to the phase delays produced by evening bright light exposure [28,29]. In animal studies, phase advances have been found to result from exposure to dark pulses in the early subjective night [34,35]. Perhaps the effect of these drugs is similar.

Symptoms suggesting circadian rhythm difficulties, such as insomnia and daytime sleepiness, have been anecdotally reported in blind people, but no systematic surveys have been done. Subject 02 in our study was particularly symptomatic when sleeping out of phase with his melatonin rhythm and enjoyed improved alertness when encouraged to sleep in phase. Interestingly, the patient described by MILES et al. [6] had intuitively adopted that strategy, i.e., his activity-rest cycle had a 24.9 hour period. Subject 01 was less affected by the phase angle variations between melatonin and sleep. These differences suggest that the coupling strength between sleep and melatonin rhythms may be quite variable in humans.

In summary, our pilot studies of blind subjects indicate: 1) circadian rhythm abnormalities in melatonin production are clearly present in some totally blind people, but that other totally blind individuals have normally entrained melatonin rhythms; 2) free-running melatonin rhythms can give rise to periodic bouts of insomnia and excessive daytime sleepiness; 3) the regularity of melatonin rhythm in free-running blind subjects provides a way to test the chronobiological effects of drugs; and 4) preliminary data suggest that bedtime administration of triazolam or exogenous melatonin may phase advance the endogenous melatonin rhythm. These drugs may be useful for the treatment of chronobiologic disorders in sighted people.

6. References

1 C.J. Migeon, F.H. Tyler, J.P. Mahoney, A.A. Florentin, H. Castle, E.I. Bliss, L.T. Samuels: J. Clin. Endocrin. Metab. 16 622 (1956)

2 D.T. Krieger, F. Rizzo: Neuroendocrinol. 32 165 (1971)

3 F. Hollwich, B. Dieckhues: In Contemporary Opthalmology, ed. by J.G. Gellows, (Williams and Wilkins, Baltimore 1972) p. 472

4 S. Bodenheimer, J.S.D. Winter, C. Faiman: J. Clin. Endocrin. Metab. 37 472 (1973)

5 B. D'Alessandro, A. Bellastella, V. Esposito, C.F. Colucci, N. Montalbetti: Brit. Med. J. 2 274 (1974)

6 L.E.M. Miles, D.M. Raynal, M.A. Wilson: Science 198 421 (1977)

7 D.N. Orth, G.M. Besser, P.H. King, W.E. Nicholson: Clin. Endocrinol. 10 603 (1979)

8 G.M. Vaughn, S.D. McDonald, R. Bell, E.A. Stevens: Psychoendocrinology 4 351 (1979)

9 J.A. Smith, J. O'Hara, A.A. Schiff: Lancet ii 933 (1981)

10 A.J. Lewy, S.P. Markey: Science 201 741 (1978)

11 A.J. Lewy, D.A. Newsome: J. Clin. Endocrinol. Metab. 56 1103 (1983).

12 J. Redman, S. Armstrong, KT Ng: Science 219 1089 (1983)

13 J. Arendt, C. Bojkowski, S. Folkard, C. Franey, V. Marks, D. Minors, J. Waterhouse, R. Wever, C. Wildgruber, J. Wright: In Photoperiodism, Melatonin and the Pineal, ed. by D. Evered and S. Clark, Ciba Foundation Symposium 117 (Pitman, London 1985) p. 266

14 F. Anton-Tay, J. Diaz, A. Fernandez-Guardiola: Life Sci. 10 841 (1971)
15 F. Anton-Tay: Adv. Biochem. Psychopharm. 11 315 (1974)
16 H. Cramer, J. Rudolph, U. Consbruch, K. Kendel: Adv. Biochem. Psychopharm. 11 187 (1974)
17 A. Lerner, J. Nordlund: J. Neural. Transm. (Suppl.) 13 339 (1978)
18 L. Vollrath, P. Semm, G. Gammel: In Melatonin: Current Status and Perspectives, ed. by N. Birau and N. Schloot, (Pergamon Press, New York 1981) p. 327
19 H. Lieberman, F. Waldhauser, G. Garfield, H. Lynch, R.J. Wurtman: Brain Res. 323 201 (1984)
20 M.A. Sherer, H. Weingartner, S.P. James, N.E. Rosenthal: Neurosci. Lett. 3 277 (1985)
21 F.W. Turek, S. Losee-Olsen: Nature 321 167 (1986)
22 D.S. Minors, J.M. Waterhouse: J. Physiol. 308 92P (1980)
23 R. Wever: The Circadian System of Man (Springer-Verlag, New York 1979) 171 213 (1970)
24 C.A. Czeisler, G.S. Richardson, J.C. Zimmerman, M.C. Moore-Ede, E.D. Weitzman: Photochem. Photobiol. 34 239 (1981)
25 A.J. Lewy: Psychopharm. Bull. 18 127 (1982)
26 A.J. Lewy, R.L. Sack, R.H. Fredrickson, M. Reaves, D.D. Denney, D.R. Zielske: Psychopharm. Bull. 19 523 (1983)
27 R.A. Wever, J. Polasek, C.M. Wildgruber: Pflugers Arch. 396 85 (1983)
28 A.J. Lewy, R.L. Sack, C.M. Singer: Ann. N.Y. Acad. Sci. 453 376 (1985)
29 C.A. Czeisler, J.S. Allan, S.H. Strogatz, J.M. Ronda, R. Sanchez, C.D. Rios, W.D. Freitag, G.S. Richardson, R.E. Kronauer: Science 233 667 (1986)
30 P.J. Marangos, J. Patel, F. Hirata, D. Sondein, S.M. Paul, P. Skolnick, F.K. Goodwin: Life Sci. 29 259 (1981)
31 P.J. DeCoursey: Science 131 33 (1960)
32 H. Underwood: J. Pineal Res. 3 187 (1986)
33 R. Mauri, P. Lissoni, M. Resentini, C. DeMedici, F. Morabito, S. Djemal, L. DiBella: J. Endocrinol. Invest. 8 337 (1985)
34 Z. Boulos, B. Rusak: J. Comp. Physiol. 146 411 (1982)
35 S. Binkley, K. Mosher, B. H. White: J. Neurochem. 45 875 (1985)

Effects of Pacemaker Lesions on the Temporal Organization in Mammals

W.J. Rietveld

Dept. of Physiology and Physiological Physics, Div. of Med. Chronobiology, University of Leiden, P.O. Box 9604, NL-2300 RC Leiden, The Netherlands

1. INTRODUCTION

Many physiological, biochemical and behavioural processes show functionally significant circadian rhythms. A host of recent experiments mainly in rats and hamsters have led to the recognition of the suprachiasmatic nuclei (SCN) of the hypothalamus as a major regulator of circadian rhythmicity (1). The natural starting point of the search for the central pacemaker has been to trace the pathway for entrainment, as in the hierarchical multi-oscillator model the pacemaker interacts with the entrainment mechanism. Since in mammals the light-dark cycle is the predominant synchronizing agent, the zeitgeber can be assumed to enter the organism via the retina. The possibility that extraretinal photoreception plays any significant role in the process of photic entrainment in adult mammals can at present be considered very unlikely.

2. THE SCN AS A MAJOR PACEMAKER

In the late sixties it was established that a retinal projection to the hypothalamus existed in lower vertebrates. Using the autoradiographic tracing method Moore (2) demonstrated this pathway in the rat forming a direct connection between the retina and the SCN, the retino-hypothalamic projection, (RHP).

In addition to this anatomical finding there is other empirical support for the assumption that the SCN are a major pacemaker. Many behavioural circadian rhythms are abolished by complete SCN lesions or surgical isolation, (3). Electrical stimulation of the SCN alters the phase of circadian rhythms in locomotor activity in rodents (4). With the aid of 2-DG method, Schwartz et al. (5) demonstrated a circadian rhythm in metabolic activity in the SCN, glucose utilisation being high during the light phase. No other brain area exhibits a similar rhythm. In accordance with this are electrophysiological studies (6) showing that in vivo and in vitro the multi-unit activity within the SCN is high during the light period, low during darkness.

From the anatomical point of view the SCN are two small nuclei lying immediately above the optic chiasm. Each nucleus contains about 10 000 neurones. Recent data indicate that the SCN in the rat has a number of subdivisions. The rostral part, about one-fourth of the total nucleus, contains small neurones with a scant cytoplasm and relatively few organelles. The, few, dendrites have a limited arborization. The caudal part consists of a dorsomedial part, quite similar to the rostral part. The neurones of the ventrolateral part are larger with more cytoplasm and a more extensive arborization. This latter region is characterized by the presence of terminals of the RHP. Each SCN is interconnected with the contralateral SCN by a highly topographically ordered fibre system.

Within the SCN several neuropeptides are found in neurones as well as in terminals (7). Vasopressin-containing neurones are located exclusively in the rostral and

dorsomedial part. Vasoactive intestinal peptide (VIP) is present in neurones of the ventrolateral part, whereas neurones containing GABA, somatostatin, substance P or avian pancreatic polypeptide (APP) are present throughout the whole SCN. Several other peptides are found in terminals (serotonin, moluscan cardio-excitatory peptide, leu-enkephalin, cholecystokinin).
The basic question to answer while studying the properties of these SCN is how a group of cells is able to generate a periodic 24 hour frequency signal.

3. CELL OR NETWORK FUNCTION

According to Moore (2) the SCN neurones are initially produced as a set of genetically determined, independent oscillators that become interconnected during development so that individual neuronal function now becomes a network function.

If all cells of the SCN had the same pacemaker properties and were able to generate the same circadian signal, then the amount of cells within the SCN would not be very critical.
Lesion experiments in blinded rats, described by Rietveld (8), while recording food intake and locomotor activity, show that after a lesion of the rostral part of the SCN the pattern of activity splits into several ultradian components. After a couple of days to weeks the circadian pattern returns, but in all cases with a period length shorter than before the lesion (figure 1).

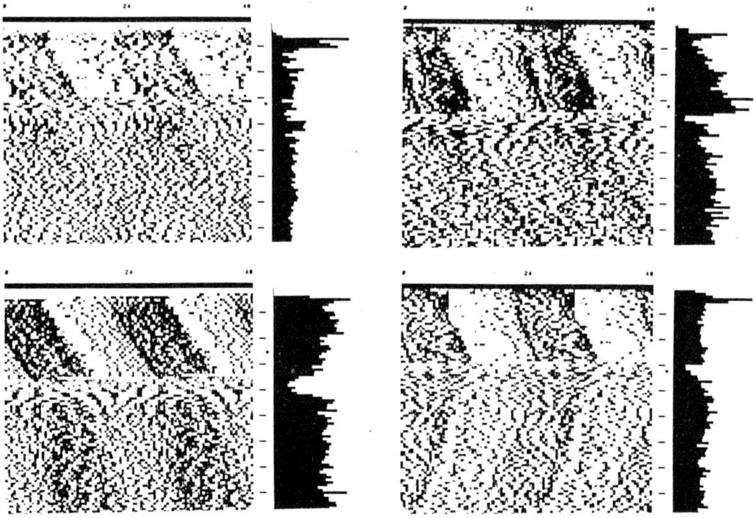

Figure 1. Effect of a lesion of the SCN on the circadian rhythm of food intake in 4 different rats. In the actograms the total amount of food per 30 minute period is given. The data are double plotted in the conventional manner. The total amount of activity per 24 hours is plotted at the right hand side of each actogram. Horizontal bars indicate 10 days period. After 30 days of free running (the animals have been blinded), they received a bilateral lesion of the SCN. Immediately after the lesion the pattern becomes irregular showing in some cases ultradian components. In the lower two animals a rhythm returns after about a month but now with a period shorter than before the lesion. In the upper left animal the lesion appeared to be localized in the caudal part of the SCN, in the three other animals the lesion was situated in the rostral areas. In all cases the amount of SCN that had been destructed was about 60 percent.

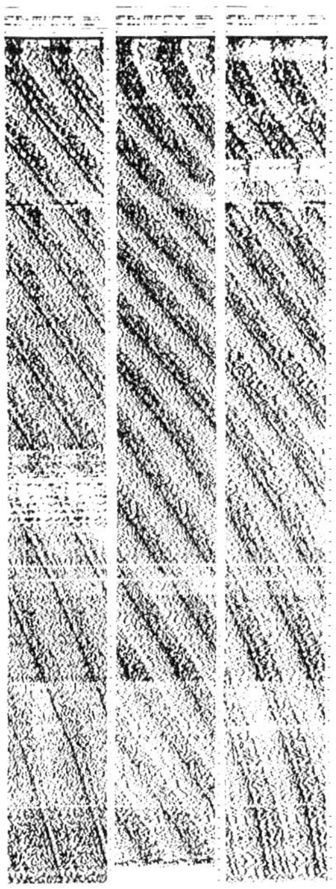

Figure 2. Long term recording of food intake in three individual rats during 700 consecutive days. Note the decrease in period length especially in the animals at the left hand and at the right hand side of the figure.

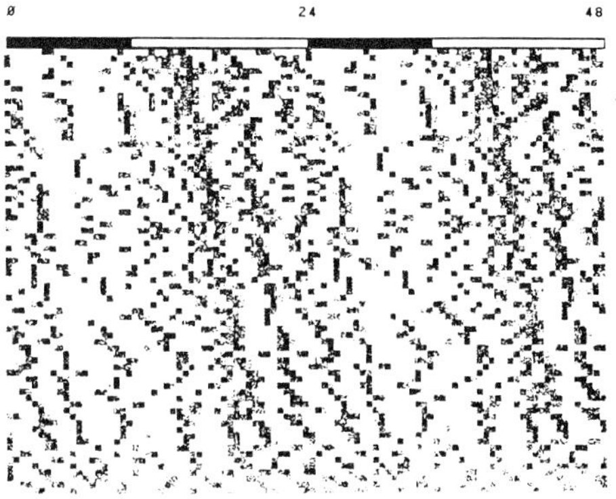

Figure 3. A detail of the last 35 days of the rat at right-hand side of figure 2. Note the appearance of ultradian components.

Another argument in favour of the network hypothesis is the fact that while aging the free running period of locomotor activity and food intake in rats shortens monotonously by about a second a day (9), see figure 2.
This corresponds well with the loss of cells in the SCN as described by Swaab, et al. (10).
A few days before death the circadian pattern is replaced by a number of ultradian components sometimes with different period lengths, see figure 3.

4. PROPERTIES OF THE SYSTEM

4.1 The effect of constant light

Due to the presence of a sustained oscillator, a circadian timing system free runs under constant conditions. This does not exclude an effect of the conditions themselves on the pacemaker structure.
For example, the amount of light during constant illumination is of great importance. As mentioned earlier, rats and hamsters that have been blinded by enucleation of the eyes free run for years with a rather stable period length (9). Sighted animals, however, under conditions of constant light show highly variable behaviour (11). Some of them free run, the activity rhythm of others splits into two or more components, all of which maintain the same frequency. A complete loss of circadian organization also might occur, especially in the rat. Spectral analysis of the activity reveals a persistence of ultradian components in some cases.
Such a breakdown under constant illumination has been recognized a long time, but neither the effects of this breakdown on the organism nor the mechanism responsible for it are fully understood. The fact that it occurs rather fast under conditions of dim light suggests some critical threshold of light intensity. The effect is not

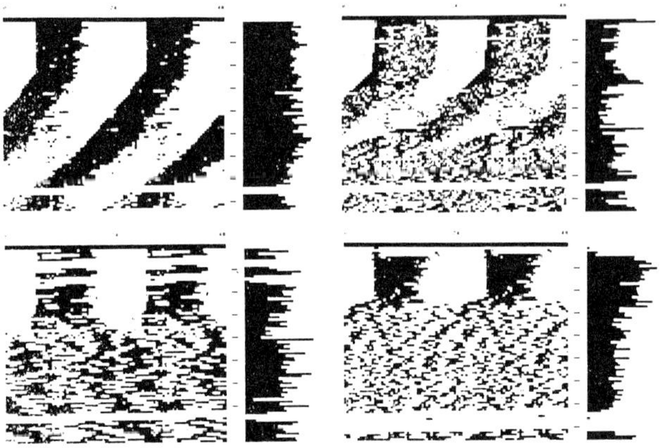

Figure 4. Recordings of locomotor activity (wheel running) of four different chipmunks. Legend as in figure 1. During the first 25 days the animals were under conditions of L/D, thereafter at LL. Light intensity: 100 lux. Note the different behaviour ranging from free running to complete breakdown.

exclusively restricted to night time active animals as the same breakdown can be seen in the chipmunk, a day-active animal (figure 4).
The persistence of ultradians suggests that the underlying periodicity of elements comprising the rat circadian system is ultradian. But it also may be the result of a change in phase relationship between a number of basically circadian oscillators.

4.2 A multi-oscillator pacemaker

Several other properties of a circadian control system can be explained in terms of a multi-oscillator pacemaker system.
Hamsters that are placed under constant light conditions show a phenomenon that is known as splitting. The activity/rest pattern splits up in different components, often with different period lengths. Interaction between two or more oscillators may account for this and several other properties of circadian rhythms, especially in rodents. Constant light or special entraining cycles can compress the duration of the activity as compared to the period length. A single phase-shifting light or dark pulse often induces transient changes in period length. Pittendrigh and Daan (12) propose a two oscillator pacemaker model in which two oscillators or populations of oscillators interact. Each oscillator is coupled to either the dark-to-light transition (morning) or to the light-to-dark (evening) change. In this model the periods of these oscillators are oppositely dependent on the light intensity. This means that in constant light their phase relationship changes, inducing a compression of the activity duration. The concrete anatomical localization of such separate but interacting oscillators has not yet been achieved.
It has been suggested that the SCN lying at both sides of the midline of the hypothalamus not only contribute to the control of the circadian rhythmicity but are also the two oscillators proposed in the model. This is supported by the fact that some authors describe that unilateral lesions of the SCN disrupt splitting of the activity rhythm in hamsters (13). Others claim that there is no evidence that the two SCN have different oscillator properties (14,15).

4.3 A multi-oscillator circadian system

In a multi-oscillator circadian system a pacemaker structure, whether or not dual, could also be responsible for maintaining the synchronization or the phase relationship between itself and lower-order oscillators, which may exist for example in other neural structures or endocrine glands. In vitro circadian rhythmicity has been demonstrated in the adrenal glands and in the pituitary (16,17). It has been shown that rats with a lesion of the SCN show entrained rhythms of corticosteron and body temperature when placed on a restricted feeding schedule (18). However this might be due to passive driving of the rhythmicity, a phenomenon known as masking. On the other hand there is experimental evidence that in animals with a bilateral lesion of the SCN meal timing induces an activity rhythm that shows anticipatory activity before the time of feeding (19,20,21). After reinstitution of ad libitum feeding this anticipatory activity disappears within a few days. If, even after 60 days or more the animals are placed in a fasting condition this anticipatory locomotory activity reappears at exactly the same time point. Experiments with rats under free running conditions demonstrate the real circadian pattern of this anticipatory rhythm. Although the exact location for the oscillator has not yet been demonstrated, preliminary experiments by Ruis (22) suggest an important role of the dorsomedial hypothalamic nucleus (DMH) as in animals with a bilateral lesion of the DMH no anticipatory activity can be seen, neither in controls nor in SCN lesioned DMH rats.

5. MANIPULATION BY DRUGS

In addition to lesion studies many neuropsychopharmacological experiments have been done in order to elucidate the possible role in circadian time keeping of the various neuropeptides present in the SCN neurones (23). Drugs affecting these peptides were given either by adding them to the food or water or by implantation of osmotic minipumps subcutaneously. Direct application into the SCN was done iontophoretically or by the use of implanted canules. The results of these experiments are sometimes contradictory, depending on the kind of animal used, and not easy to understand. Neither acetylcholine nor vasopressin seems to play a role in the rhythm generation mechanism. Local injection of alpha-bungarotoxin, an irreversible cholinergic antagonist, into the SCN does not affect circadian rhythmicity in pineal activity. Brattleboro rats that lack vasopressin in the SCN show undisturbed circadian rhythms. Injection of vasopressin in the rat SCN does not change the period of free running activity rhythms.

Serotonin (5-HT) in the SCN is located in terminals, the perikarya of which are situated in the midbrain raphe nuclei. 5-HT may act as a transmitter between these nuclei and the SCN. Electrophysiological studies reveal a response of SCN neurones to iontophoretically applied 5-HT as well as to clorgyline, a MAO inhibitor. In spite of this there is no effect on the free running period of food intake in the rat after local application of 5-HT into the SCN. However, in case of local implantation of clorgyline there is some evidence of an increase in period length. Wheel running activity of hamsters slows down after implantation of osmotic mini pumps filled with clorgyline or imipramine another anti-depressant drug.

This effect is absent in the rat.

When lithium is added to the food the rest/activity rhythm as well as food intake slows down in both rat and hamster.

Another interesting effect is seen after application of meth-amphetamine into the drinking water of rats (24). Food intake decreases with a concomitant increase in locomotor activity. In addition, the drug induces a shift of the activity (locomotor, food intake as well as water intake) towards the subjective day. Control, untreated animals usually have three bouts of activity during the subjective night. The shift towards the subjective day is mainly due to a shift of the middle and late activity bouts. In addition to the shift in activity, an internal desynchronization occurs as well as the appearence of circabidian (double length) days (figure 5).

Firstly, it is not clear whether this is an effect related to the psychotomimetic action of the drug or due to the central stimulant action. It is noteworthy that after administration of haloperidol an abrupt return of the original circadian of all forms of activity takes place, suggesting a dopaminergic effect.
Secondly, the question arises whether this is an effect on the pacemaker itself or an effect on a more peripheral level. If one tries to describe these phenomena according to a similar model as given by Daan et al. (25) for the control of sleep, these effects can be simulated in three ways. First by lengthening the period of the circadian pacemaker, second by decreasing the amplitude of the circadian oscillator and third by increasing the threshold to food intake behaviour or to locomotor activity (24). Up to now there is not enough experimental evidence to exclude one of these possible explanations.

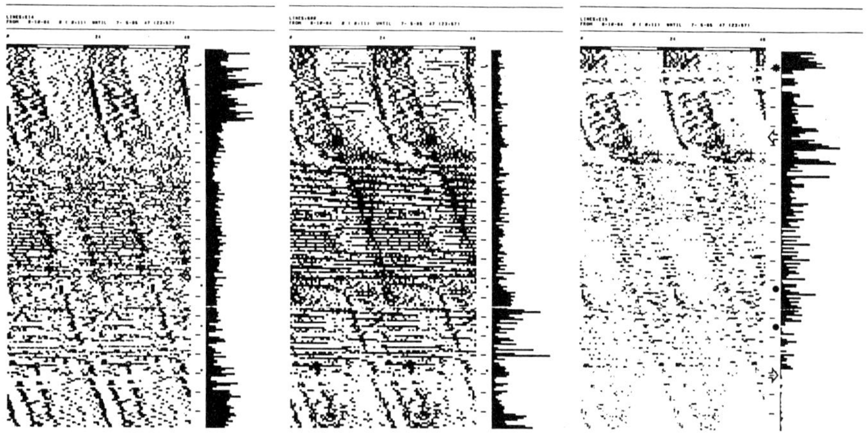

Figure 5. Food intake (left), drinking activity (middle) and wheel running activity (right) of one rat under free running conditions (after blinding:). Inward and outward arrows indicate application and withdrawal of meth-amphetamine in the drinking water. The two black dots indicate administration of haloperidol. Note the shift towards the resting phase of the middle bout of activity. The pattern is similar in all three forms of activity. Administration of haloperidol blocks the effect, indicating a possible role of dopamine.*

More promising seems to be the fact that application of the GABA-ergic, anti-epileptic drug sodium valproate into the drinking water of rats results in a reversible shortening of the period length of free running activity, figure 6.
So although the SCN have been definitively established as the main driving oscillators for a large number of circadian rhythms, several functions still remain to be elucidated. By what mechanisms the endogenous activity is generated, how entrainment is achieved as well as the existence and localisation of secondary oscillators. More experiments will be needed not only on cellular level in one particu-

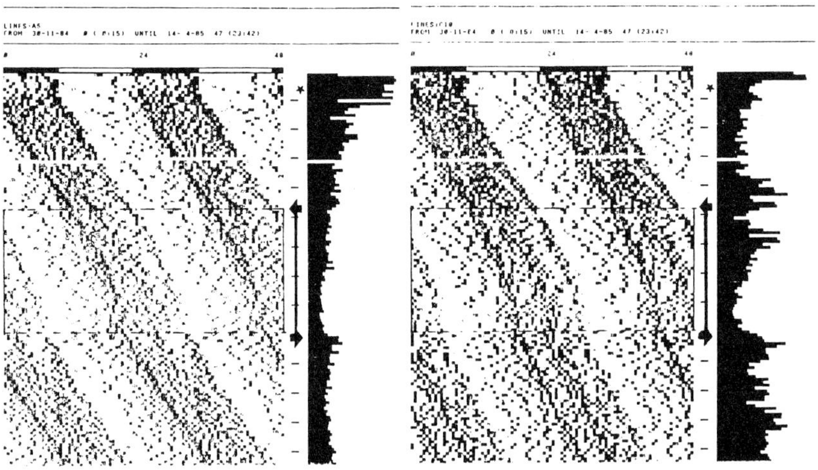

Figure 6. Legend as in figure 1. Valproate is given in the drinking water starting from 50 mg per kg per day up to 1000 mg per kg per day. Days of administration are marked at the right hand side of the actograms by a vertical line. Note the changes in pattern as well as in period length.

lar species (rat or hamster) but also comparing the properties of circadian systems in different species.

Literature

1. B. Rusak, and G.A. Groos: Science 215, 1407-1409 (1982)
2 R.Y. Moore: Brain Res., 49, 403-409 (1973)
3. B. Rusak, I. Zucker: Physiol Rev., 59, 449-526 (1979)
4. B. Rusak, G.A. Groos: Science, 215, 1407-1409 (1982)
5. W.J. Schwartz, L.C. Davidson and C.B. Smith: J. Comp. Neurol., 189, 157-167 (1980)
6. S.I. Inouye and H. Kawamura: Proc Natl. Acad. Sci. USA, 76, 5962-5966 (1979)
7. A.N. van den Pol and K.L. Tsujimoto: Neuroscience, 15, 1049-1086 (1985)
8. W.J. Rietveld: In Annual review of chronopharmacology, ed. by A. Reinberg, M. Smolensky, and A. Labreque, 1-5 (Pergamon Press, Oxford, 1984)
9. W.J. Rietveld, M.E. Boon, J. Korving and K. van Schravendijk: Neuroscience Lett Suppl., 22, 449-450 (1985)
10. D.F. Swaab, E. Fliers, and T.S. Partiman: Brain Research, 342, 37-44 (1985)
11. H.E. Albers, A.A. Gerall and J.F. Axelson: Neuroscience Letters, 25, 89-94, (1981)
12. C.S. Pittendrigh and S. Daan: J. Comp.Physiol., 106, 223-252 (1976)
13. G.E. Pickard and F.W. Turek: J. Comp. Physiol. A., 165, 803-815 (1985)
14. J.A. Donaldson and F.K. Stephan: Physiology and Behavior, 29, 11611169 (1982)
15. F.C. Davis and R.A. Gorski: J. Comp. Physiol. A., 154, 221-232, (1984)
16. F. Ungar and F. Halberg: Science, 137, 1058-1060 (1962)
17. F. Ungar and F. Halberg: Experientia, 19, 158-160 (1963)
18. D.T. Krieger, H. Hauser and L.C. Krey: Science, 197, 398-399 (1977)
19. F.K. Stephan, J.M. Swann and C.L. Sisk: Behavioral and Neural Biology, 25, 340-365 (1979)
20. F.K. Stephan: Physiol Behav., 32, 663-671 (1984)
21. C. Boulos, A.M. Rosenwasser and M. Terman: Behav. Br. Res., 1, 39-65 (1980)
22. J. Ruis: J. Interdiscipl. Cycle Res., 16, 321-322 (1985)

23. W.J. Rietveld: In Circadian rhythms in the central nervous system, ed. by P.H. Redfern, C. Campbell and J.A. Davies, 45-47 (The Macmillan Press Ltd., Basingstoke, 1985)

24. A. Wirz Justice, K. Krauchi, T. Morimasa and W.J. Rietveld: In Circadian rhythms in the central nervous system, ed. by P.H. Redfern, C. Campbell and J.A. Davies, 123-135 (The Macmillan Press Ltd., Basingstoke, 1985)

25. S. Daan, D.G.M. Beersma, and A.A. Borbély : Am. J. Physiol., 246, R161-R178, (1984)

Perturbations of Cellular Circadian Rhythms by Light and Temperature

L. Rensing and W. Schill

Biology/Mathematics Department, University of Bremen,
D-2800 Bremen, Fed. Rep. of Germany

1. Introduction

The main natural "Zeitgeber"-periodicities for circadian rhythms are the cycles of light and temperature in the course of a solar day. They entrain the endogenous circadian oscillation of organisms to exactly 24 h, or perturb (phase shift) the oscillation in cases of transmeridian flights or shift work. The entrained state itself is a dynamic state of repetitive changes of phase, amplitude and period of the endogenous oscillation caused by the Zeitgeber periodicity. Two classes of effects of the Zeitgeber can be distinguished especially in the rectangular form of light and temperature cycles in the laboratory: a) differential (phasic) effects of the different directions (up and down) of change, and b) proportional (tonic) effects of longer exposures to higher or lower intensities. Differential and proportional effects, can to some extent, be tested separately either 1) by applying steps or pulses of light, dark or different temperatures and by analysing the resulting phase shifts ($\Delta\varphi$) of the circadian oscillator, or 2) by exposing the oscillator to different constant light intensities or temperatures and by analysing the resulting changes of τ and amplitude (A). A third approach is to abolish ("hold") the circadian oscillation by long exposures to light or high temperature and then initiate the oscillation by a single transfer to darkness or lower temperature and then to analyse the subsequent phasing of the rhythm (1,2).

We would like to address the following 5 questions: 1) Are the effects of light and elevated temperature on the circadian rhythm identical or similar? If they have similar effects, what is the common cellular mechanism of their effects? Special attention shall be given to the possibility of common changes in Ca^{++} concentration, protein phosphorylation and protein synthesis. 2) Is there a way to draw a conclusion about the oscillatory mechanism from phase response curves (PRCs) to light, temperature and various drugs? The possibilities and limits of this approach are discussed on the basis of simulations and experimental results. 3) What are the effects of long-term (constant) exposure of the circadian oscillator to different light intensities or temperatures? Again, we shall compare the responses of the model oscillator with the experimental data. We were especially interested in the effects of changed synthesis or degradation rates of an oscillatory compound on the period and amplitude of the oscillator. 4) Which cellular mechanism may be responsible for the comparatively small effects of long-term exposures of the oscillator to different light intensities or temperatures (temperature compensation), and finally 5) How can exogenously induced changes in the synthesis and/or degradation rates entrain the circadian oscillation?

2. Are the effects of light and elevated temperatures on the circadian rhythm similar or identical?

A preliminary answer to this question may be derived from a look at a) the phase relation to either of both Zeitgeber periodicities, b) the phase shifting effect of pulses of light or temperature, c) the effects of longer exposures to different temperatures or light intensities on the free-running period length and d) the "holding" and subsequent initiation of the endogenous oscillation by a stepwise change in either of the two Zeitgeber intensities.

Data on the entrained state in different organisms (reviewed by Bünning (3)) consistently reveal that the phase of the circadian oscillator (for example expressed by the rhythm of conidiation in Neurospora) is locked to light in the same way as to elevated temperature. Furthermore, in Neurospora high light intensity pulses phase-shift the rhythm very similarly to the phase shifts elicited by high temperature pulses (Fig. 1). The phase positions of the PRCs are identical within the limits of measurements in different laboratories. The same is true in several well analysed organisms such as Phaseolus, Kalanchoe and Gonyaulax (reviewed by Cornelius and Rensing (4)). Light- and temperature-PRCs are apparently also rather similar in multicellular animal organisms (5,6) revealing generally lesser phase shifts during the "subjective" day phase compared to the stronger shifts during the "subjective" night phase.

The effects of different constant light and temperatures on amplitude and period of the circadian oscillation appears to be similar in most cases as discussed below. When Neurospora is exposed to a higher light intensity for more than 12 h and then transferred to darkness, the rhythm of conidiation appears with the same phase as compared to a transition from high temperature to lower temperature (2). Altogether, these similarities in the effects of high light

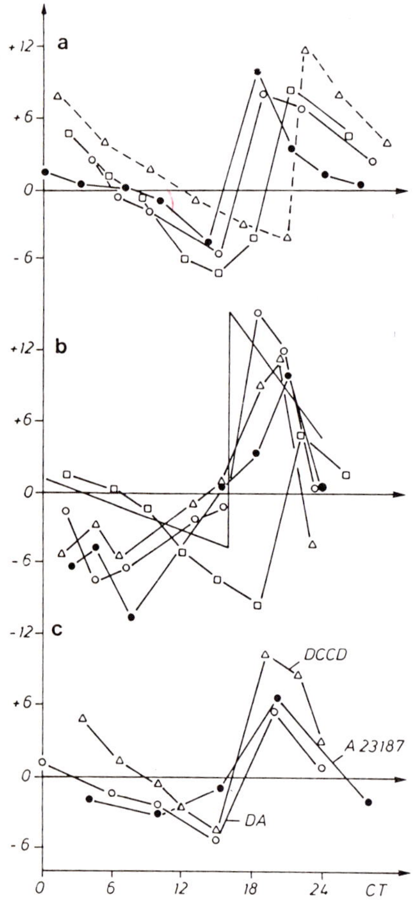

Fig. 1 Phase response curves of Neurospora conidiation rhythm to a) light, b) elevated temperatures and c) drugs affecting Ca^{++} transport. a) Δ - Δ 45 min light pulses of 1430 ftc (65), ● - ● 5 min, 50 ftc (66), o - o 5 min (22), □ - □ 5 min (67), b) —— 6 h 35°C (63), Δ - Δ - 3h 30°C (38), ● - ● 3h 35°C (38), o - o 3h 40°C (38), c) Δ - Δ 3h 200 µM dicyclohexylcarbodiimide (DCCD (22)), o - o 3h 30 µg/ml dantrolene (28), ● - ● 3h 1 µMA 23187 (28). Ordinates: Phase shifts in hours, advances (+) above, delays (-) below the abscissae; abscissa: circadian time (free running period length divided into 24 time units).

intensity and high temperature on the variables of the circadian rhythm led us to conclude that both light and temperature may have a common cellular effect. We shall, therefore, discuss briefly the known effects of these signals on receptor cells and unspecialized cells and search for a possible common target for both stimuli.

3. Intracellular effects of light signals

In animals, light signals reach the circadian oscillator of pacemaker regions in the brain (for example: suprachiasmatic nuclei in vertebrates, optic lobes in insects, eyes of some gastropods) via retinal or extraretinal light receptors. In these cases the light signal is transformed into changes of membrane potentials and transduced to the pacemaker cells by way of neurotransmitters and/or neuropeptides. Apart from this type of signal transmittance light may directly act on a cellular circadian rhythm by way of specialized visual pigments in light receptor cells or by other pigments or receptors (for example in pineal cells of birds and lower vertebrates (6)). The latter may apply to other tissues as well if those tissues maintain a cellular rhythm of their own, which is not yet clear from many tissues and animal species (see (7)). Direct effects of light on cellular oscillators are often mediated by a cellular blue light receptor which exists in Drosophila, Acetabularia, Neurospora and other organisms (review: (8)).

In order to analyse the cellular mechanism of the phase shifting effect of light, it would be interesting to compare the intracellular processes induced by 1) illumninated visual pigments, 2) stimulated optic neurons and their transmitters and 3) illuminated cellular photoreceptors. In vertebrate rods, light causes a decrease in the dark current and thus hyperpolarizes the membrane potential. Recently, evidence has been presented that this is the result of a sequence of events starting from activated rhodopsin molecules, which activate a phosphodiesterase (PDE) via a GTP-binding protein. The activated PDE lowers the cGMP content and closes the sodium (and calcium) channels causing hyperpolarization and a drop in Ca^{++} (reviews: (9,10,11).

The hyperpolarization of the rod cell is transformed into "on" and "off" signals (12,13) which are then transmitted via the retino hypothalamic tract (and perhaps by the primary optic tract) to the pacemaker cells in the suprachiasmatic nuclei (14). These neurons are mainly cholinergic. Apart from effects on sodium channels muscarinic cholinergic receptors as well as receptors for adrenalin, histamine, 5-hydroxytryptamine, substance P, neurotensin, V_1-vasopressin elicit a response via the inositol phospholipid (PiP_2) pathway (15). This pathway ultimately leads to a release of Ca^{++} from intracellular sources (i.e. endoplasmatic reticulum) and to an activation of protein kinase C.

In Neurospora and plants and animals it has been shown that light acts on the circadian rhythm via a blue light receptor in the membranes (16,8). Blue light perception consists of a flavin-mediated cytochrome b reduction (17), as documented also using riboflavin mutants (18) : Flavin deficiency causes a significant decrease in light sensitivity assayed as photosuppression of circadian conidiation and phase shifting. The probable mechanism of the primary blue light action on membrane flavins has been reviewed by SCHMIDT (19). Blue light-reducible cytochromes have been shown to exist in the plasma membrane, the ER and mitochondrial membranes (20). The mitochondrial mutant "poky" is grossly deficient in mitochondrial cytochrome b (21) and is considerably less sensitive to phase by shifting light (22).

The illumination of cells with blue light leads to a hyperpolarization of the cell membrane (20-25 min: 40-60 mV (23, 24)) and is probably due to an activation of the H^+-ATPase and to increased electrogenic H^+-transport. That proton translocation is involved in the transmission of the light signal is further supported by the finding that higher extracellular pH (6,7) diminished the phase shifting by light (25). This pH dependency was abolished by addition of ammonium. Diethylstilbestrol, an inhibitor of plasma membrane ATPase, completely suppressed phase shifting by light (26). Phase shifting by light, furthermore, decreases with increasing temperatures (27). Light may act on the Ca^{++} content of the cytoplasm and/or other compartments of the cell. This is indicated by recent findings of Nakashima and Cornelius (pers. comm.) that mutants defective in Ca^{++} transport were less sensitive to light pulses. Since this mutant can still be phase-shifted by temperature pulses the effects of light and temperature on the Ca^{++} level must be different. Pulses of N,N'-dicyclohexylcarbodiimide, giving rise to a similar phase response curve as light and elevated temperature (Fig.1) have been shown to inhibit Ca^{++} transport into the vacuole (Cornelius and Nakashima, in press). The light-induced transient increase in the activity of the PDE (24) may depend on the Ca^{++} change. It leads to a decrease in the cAMP level during 15-20 min, which, however, does not seem to phase shift the circadian rhythm to the same extent as light does: antagonists of cAMP such as a stereoisomer did not result in a PRC similar to light (28). Ultimately, light seems to act on gene expression on the level of translation and transcription(29,30,31,32). Light acting through neurotransmitters and the direct effects of light on cells may thus have changes of Ca^{++} concentration, and subsequent processes, in common.

4. Intracellular effects of temperature signals

If elevated temperature is perceived by sense organs, it may be transmitted to the circadian pacemaker cells via neurotransmitters and the cellular processes discussed above. The direct reaction sequence in cells to elevated temperature will be discussed using Neurospora as a model organism.

There are numerous effects of temperature on enzyme catalyzed reaction rates in cellular metabolism and membrane-associated processes (reviewed by (33)). More specifically, all cells react to elevated temperatures by synthesizing so-called "heat shock proteins" and often repressing the synthesis of other proteins (34,35,36,37). We will concentrate on the induction of this heat shock response for the following reasons: a) apart from heat shock this response is triggered by many agents that also have a strong phase shifting effect on the circadian rhythm (38) b) The dose dependence of phase shifts and of the induction of HS-proteins by temperature pulses of different amplitudes is almost linear in both cases (38). Apart from this effect on gene expression, elevated temperatures increase the concentration of H^{+} and Ca^{++} as shown in yeast (39) and Drosophila (40) as well as the level of cAMP in Chinese hamster ovary cells (41). Several proteins were shown to increase or decrease their phosphorylation after heat shock in Neurospora as well as in other organisms (42,43). Recently, the degradation of proteins and the transient depletion of ubiquitin has been proposed as an important HSP-inducing process (reviewed by Schlesinger (37)).

When comparing the known effects of light and elevated temperatures, common links may be Ca^{++} changes and associated processes, i.e. changes of phosphorylation or synthesis rates of proteins.

5. Principal relations between phase of perturbed variable and phase of PRC as analyzed by a model oscillator

A theoretical interlude may be appropriate in order to relate the phase response curves of light and temperature pulses and the light and temperature dependent intracellular effects discussed above to the perturbation of rhythmic variables of the oscillator. We have used a model of Goodwin (44) producing limit cycle oscillations to stimulate pulsed perturbances (45, 46). The model assumes that a protein X whose concentration is dependent on the synthesis rate (influenced by an inhibitor Z) and the degradation rate. X is involved in the synthesis of Y, which concentration, in turn, determines the amount of active inhibitor Z. This arrangement of the three variables represents a classical feed-back system:

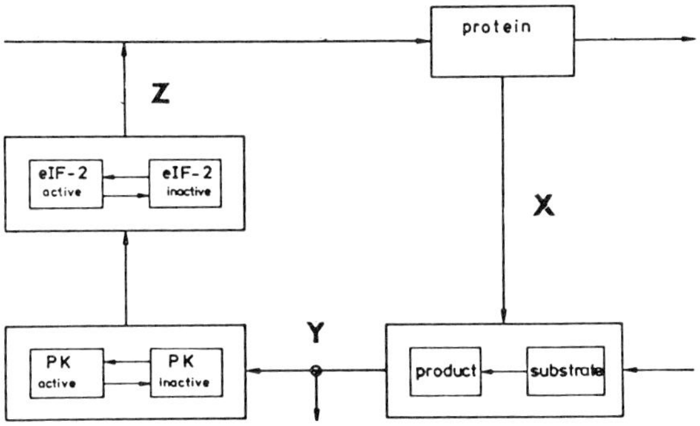

$$dX/dt = Ax/Z^9 + 1) - Bx*X$$

$$dY/dt = Ay*X - By*Y$$

$$dZ/dt = Az*Y - Bz*Z$$

Fig. 2 Model oscillator consisting of three variables: a protein species (X) which catalyses a reaction leading to product Y. Y determines the active form of a protein kinase (PK) which inactivates the initiation factor eIF2 (Z). This, in turn inhibits the synthesis of X.
For computer simulations of phase-shifting experiments the Goodwin model (44) is used (see 45). The parameter values for the unperturbed system were Ax = Ay = Az = 1, Bx = By = Bz = 0.2

The synthesis rates of X (Ax) were lowered for three hours at different phases of the oscillation and the resulting PRCs show delays during the decreasing portion of X and advances during the later increasing portion of X (Fig. 3a). These responses occur because a decreased synthesis rate of X during the decreasing portion of X causes a lower minimum and thus a delay. A decreased synthesis rate during the increase of X, in contrast, causes a lower maximum and thus an advance. The reverse is true for the increase of the synthesis rate (Fig. 3b).

Changes in the degradation rate of X (Bx) for 3 h at different phases also reveal PRCs: a decreased rate leading to phase delays, an increased rate to phase advances during the increasing portion of X (Fig.3c,d). It is interesting to note that the PRCs for increased or decreased decay rates result in either more or less advances or more or less delays, which differ from the PRCs or changes in the synthesis rate. There are some experimental PRCs, for example with cyclic nucleotides in Neurospora (28) which show similarities to the decay-type response curves. The same types of PRCs shown for perturbations of X exist for perturbations of Y and Z. The phasing of those PRCs is, however, different (45).

6. Conclusions from Zeitgeber and other pulses PRCs on the underlying oscillating variables

In an attempt to correlate the experimental data with the simulated PRCs, we summarized the available Neurospora PRCs in the following way (Fig. 4): the maximum advance of a certain treatment is plotted as a square (more than 8 h phase shift between the extreme values) or as a circle (less than 8 h) above the circadian time axis, and the maximum delay below this axis. If the four types of PRCs for each rhythmic variable exist as discussed above, the assignment of a specific PRC to a certain variable (out of an unknown number of variables) appears difficult or impossible. However, when assuming the simplest cases one may arrive at two clusters of PRCs that affect the same variable in

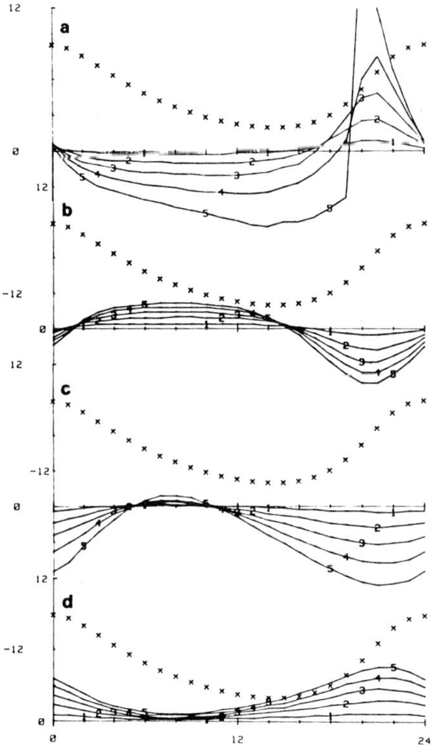

Fig. 3 Computer simulations of the relation between PRCs and perturbed variable (x) with the model oscillator. The rate of synthesis Ax of the protein X is decreased (a) or increased (b) for three hours. Ax was changed in five equal steps from 1 to 0.1 (decrease) or to 1.9 (increase). The degradation rate Bx of X is decreased (c) or increased (d) for three hours (from 0.2 to 0.11 or 0.29). The resulting phase shifts were determined after one transient period. x-x - Concentration changes of X. Ordinates: advance (+) and delay (-) phase shifts in hours. Abscissa: phase of the oscillation at which the 3h perturbation was applied.

different directions, or two variables that are 180° out of phase affected in the same direction. The PRC from protein synthesis-inhibiting pulses (cycloheximide) indicates a rhythm of protein synthesis or concentration of a protein X with a maximum around CT 6 - 12 and a minimum around 18 - 24 hours (see Fig. 3a).

This theoretical maximum coincides approximately with the maximum inducibility of HS-protein synthesis (Fig. 4c). The PRCs of a number of inhibitors of energy metabolism, such as DNP, CCCP, antimycin A, cyanide, azide and oligomycin are similar in principal to that of CHX. These drugs also strongly interfere with protein synthesis; and this may be the more relevant effect on the rhythms, rather than the perturbance of energy metabolism (47). Inhibitors of H^+-ATPase activity such as DES and vanadate show maximal advances at the same time, which might suggest that an ATPase activity changes parallel to the protein concentration changes. Ca^{++}-depletion by means of A23187 without Ca^{++} causes maximum phase advance at about CT 14 (48). This may mean that Ca^{++} (or Ca^{++}-calmodulin) levels or Ca^{++} dependent enzymes oscillate in a cell compartment (cytoplasm, mitochondria, ER) with a maximum at about CT 16 - 20.

Another cluster of PRCs centers around PRCs caused by light and high temperature (maximal advances at CT 18-24). They may be due to changes of Ca^{++} levels which would be in line with a similar PRC of dantrolene and DCCD which probably increase either the cytoplasmic or ER Ca^{++} contents. Ca^{++} may act positively on the synthesis rate of certain polypeptides (HS-proteins; light-activated proteins?).

Chlorophenylthio cAMP and phosphodiesterase inhibitors show maximal advances between CT 0-12 suggesting a positive effect on protein degradation or a negative effect on protein synthesis (see Fig. 2a,c). A negative effect of phos-

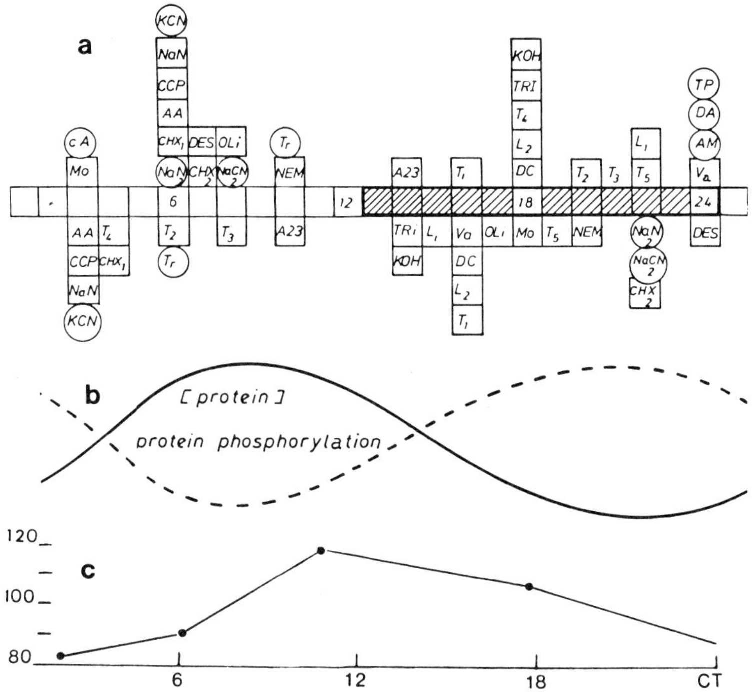

Fig. 4 a) PRCs of Neurospora conidiation rhythms to light, elevated temperature and drugs

Maximal delays and maximal advances of the circadian rhythm of conidiation induced by various signal pulses. Delays are plotted below, advances above the time axis either as squares (maximal shifts more than 8 h) or circles (maximal shifts less than 8 h). Time axis in CT unit, each CT unit is the 1/24 part of the endogeneous period length (21 h); the thick lines indicating the "subjective" dark phase within constant darkness. This "subjective" dark phase corresponds to that phase of the endogeneous oscillator occurring during the dark phase of a 12:12 light to dark cycle.

Pulses are abbreviated as follows:

AA - 3 h 0.7 µg/ml antimycin C (47)
A23 -3 h 1 µM A 23187 without Ca^{++} (48)
AM - 3 h 100 or 250 µM amiloride (28)
CA - 3 h 0.5 mM chlorophenylthio cAMP (28)
CCP - 3 h 30 µM carbonylcyanide m-chlorophenyl hydrazone (CCCP(47))
CHX_1 - 3h 1 mM cycloheximide (49)
CHX_2 - 3h 1 µg/ml cycloheximide (22)
DA - 3 h 30 µg/ml dantrolene (28)
DC - 3 h 200 µM N,N' dicyclohexylcarbodiimide (DCCD (22))
DES - 3 h 50 µM diethylstilbestrol (26)
KCN - 3 h 2 mM KCN (47)
KOH - 3 h KOH (pH 8) (68)
L_1 5 min light (1000 lx) (67)
L_2 5 min light (22)
Mo - 3 h 50 mM molybdate (22)
NaN_1 - 3 h 4 mM NaN_3 (47)
NaN_2 - 3 h 0.5 mM NaN_3 (22)
NaCN - 3 h 0.5 mM NaCN (22)
NEM - 3 h 5 mM N-ethylmaleimide (22)
OLI - 3 h 10 µg/ml oligomycin (22)
T_1 - 6 h 35°C (63)
T_2 - 3 h 30°C (38)
T_3 - 3 h 35°C (38)
T_4 - 3 h 40°C (38)
T_5 - 3 h 35°C (67)
Tr - 3 h 30 µM trifluorperazine (67)
TRi- 3 h Trisbase (pH 8) (38)
TP - 3 h 50-2000 ng/ml tetradecanoyl phorbolacetate (28)
V_a - 3 h 10 mM vanadate (22)

b) Hypothetical variables derived from two clusters of PRCs: concentration changes of a protein and changes of protein phosphorylation.

c) Measurements of the inducibility of heat shock (HS) proteins by a 3h temperature increase to 42°C (49) Ordinate: rate of synthesis of 3 HS proteins, abscissa: circadian time.

phorylating agents can also be found with molybdate pulses. Molybdate inhibits phosphatases and thus enhances protein phosphorylation: Pulses of molybdate cause a PRC very similar to the PRC of cycloheximide (22). In other organisms such as Aplysia a similar 12 h difference between the PRCs of light and protein synthesis inhibitors is observed (50). However, in Gonyaulax and Phaseolus the PRCs coincide (review: (4)) indicating an opposite direction of the effect of light and temperature with respect to CHX in these organisms.

7. The effects of different constant light intensities and temperatures on period length and amplitude

The tonic effect of light and temperature on the period length (τ) and amplitude (A) has been analyzed mainly under different constant values of these parameters. τ and A were shown to change with changes of either parameter in a species specific way (review: (51,52)), but in the same range of a few hours. If the implicated similarity of the effects of light and higher temperature is correct, we might expect in any one species parallel changes of τ and A with increasing light intensities as well as with temperature. This is observed in general (reviewed by Bünning (3)) with at least one exception: in Gonyaulax, τ increases with increasing temperature but decreases with increasing light intensities (53,54,55). This discrepancy, however, may be due to the uncertainty about which temperature change is equivalent to which change in light intensity. In Neurospora, τ and A of the conidiation rhythm decrease with increasing light intensities and temperatures (18,56,57,58).

The limited range of changes of τ in different temperatures, which is observed in all circadian clocks, led to the term "temperature compensation" regarded as a characteristic feature of circadian rhythms.

8. The effect of different synthesis and degration rates on period length and amplitude

If we assume that light and temperature affect synthesis and degradation rates (or activity) of proteins in the oscillatory mechanism, it could be interesting to analyse the effects of changes of these rates on period length and amplitude of the oscillation in more detail. We shall first discuss these effects by using the model oscillator (46) without considering adaptation to changes in the synthesis or degradation rates or activity (Fig. 5). This informal discussion is based on computer simulations, as exact calculations of global parameters like period length seem rather intractable.

As a rule, period length is more sensitive to variations in Bx than to variations in Ax. If we divide the cycle of variable X into a phase of X - degradation and a phase of X-synthesis, changes in Bx influence both phases in the same direction, i.e. prolong or shorten both phases. This differs from changes in Ax.

1. Changes in the rate of synthesis (Ax)

Ax+ lengthens the degradation phase of X, but shortens its synthesis phase: prolongation of the degradation phase seems mainly due to an increased maximal X-concentration, which results in additional time necessary to reach the minimum. Acceleration of the synthesis phase is a direct consequence of the increased rate of synthesis. Since the phase of X-degradation is longer than the time of X-increase (approximately 6:4), a longer period length results.

2. Changes in the rate of decay (Bx)

Bx+ will accelerate both degradation and synthesis-phase of X, and will thus shorten the period length: acceleration of the degradation phase is a direct

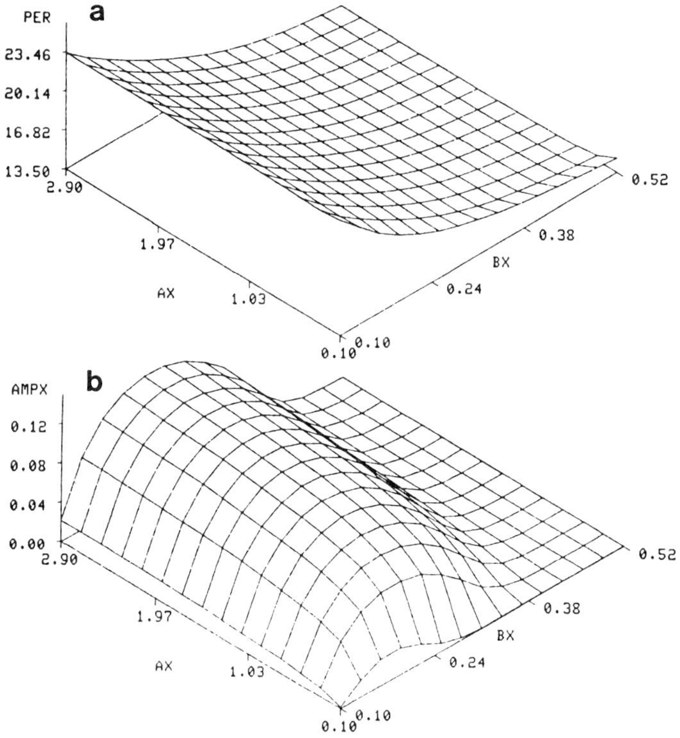

Fig. 5 Computer simulations of the effect of permanent changes of the synthesis rate (Ax) and the degradation rate (Bx) of the variable X on period length (a) and amplitude A (b).

consequence of the increased decay-rate. Acceleration of the synthesis phase is due to the fact that Bx+ diminishes the amount of X available for synthesis of the intermediary Y and thus leading to lower concentration of the inhibitor Z. Thus the velocity is increased. This behaviour can be related to the effects of pulsed changes as expressed in the PRCs (Fig. 3a-d): higher Ax led to delays as well as advances whereas changes of Bx led to only delays or advances.

The experimental data on the effects of various inhibitors of protein synthesis (on 80-S ribosomes) on τ and A were summarized by Hastings et al. (59): The effects on τ were either small (Gonyaulax) or τ was lengthened and A decreased. There is little known, however, how these treatments affected protein synthesis and degradation. Because of these open questions, it is difficult to compare the results of the simulations with the experiments cited above. Since there is evidence at least for elevated temperatures to affect synthesis and degradation rates of proteins, including an adaptation to elevated temperatures, we will focus on these processes in the following section.

In Neurospora total protein decreases 4.5 h after heat shock (40°C) to less than 20% of the untreated controls and then slowly recovers. Similar kinetics can be observed with single protein species (Rensing, unpubl.). When testing the rate of total protein synthesis after 48 h at different temperatures (30°, 35°C) there is little difference to the controls at 22°C whereas a considerable decrease is observed at 40°C. The temperature dependence of the conidiation rhythm appears to be rather similar: it remains constant between 20-30°C and then decreases (above 30°C). In Gonyaulax, total protein synthesis also decreases with increasing temperatures (Fig. 6, (54)). The same, perhaps to a different extent, is true for protein degradation. In this case, however, τ increases in contrast to Neurospora. Possibly, the ratio between synthesis and degradation is decisive for this increase of τ. In many other organisms an adaptation of protein synthesis to higher temperatures is described (reviewed by (49,36). A controversial point is the role of heat shock proteins in the stabilization of the translational machinery and thermotolerance (see for example (60)).

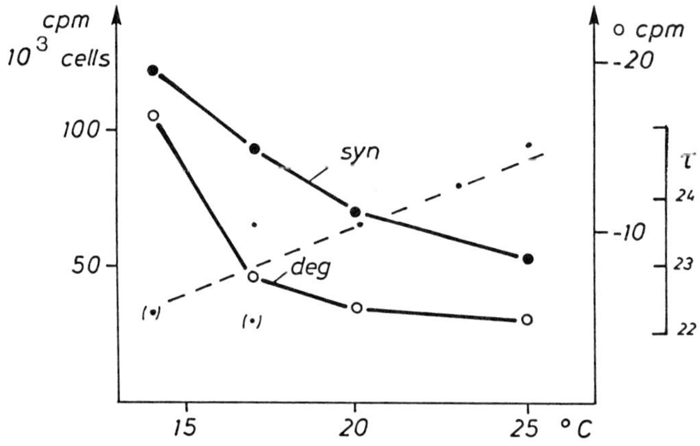

Fig. 6 Possible correlations between protein synthesis and degradation rates and period length in Gonyaulax. Inverse changes of synthesis and degradation rates of total protein (measured at different growth temperatures) and τ(54). Ordinates cpm/10^3 cells and the changes of activity during a time interval (Δcpm). Abscissa: temperature in °C.

In Tetrahymena, Hallberg (61) presented evidence that protein synthesis is not required to stabilize the translational machinery until about 43°C. Above 43°C the cells need previously synthesized HS-proteins for their survival. It is interesting that adaptation to cycloheximide, i.e. to a protein synthesis inhibitor, conveys the same thermotolerance to the cells (62). However, the mechanism of this adaptation is still unknown.

As an alternative to the adaptation of normal protein synthesis, one may consider the adaptation of heat shock protein synthesis (or the possibly coupled degradation rate, see below) decisive for the temperature compensation of the circadian period length. This may even be more likely because τ in most organisms decreases with the temperature, indicating an enhanced process. Neurospora crassa shows an increased rate of HSP-synthesis mainly in the first 3 h after heat shock and then a decrease to a new steady state which is somewhat higher than that of the controls (38). Similar kinetics were observed also in other organisms such as Drosophila (review: (68)). The mechanism of this adaptation is not well understood. The amount of HSPs synthesized seems to feed back to the synthesis rate probably acting on transcriptional as well as on translational control mechanisms. Recently, the following feed back mechanism has been proposed (37) : heat (or other inducing agents) cause alterations of protein conformations leading to higher concentration of "abnormal" proteins. These proteins bind to ubiquitin, labelling them for proteases. Since the amount of ubiquitin is limited, heat shock causes a depletion of ubiquitin, which in turn leads to activation of HS-genes (and HS-mRNA-translation?). Among the HS proteins, ubiquitin is then synthesized at a higher rate, thus leading to higher concentration of ubiquitin and a higher degradation rate of the "abnormal proteins". At the same time the synthesis rate of HS-proteins is slowed down.

9. Long exposures to high light intensities and temperatures

Long constant exposures to high light intensities and temperatures often exceed the adaptive capacity of the oscillatory system and lead to an apparent abolition of the rhythm. However, it is often not possible to distinguish between abolition of the rhythm of a driven function from abolition of the basic oscillator itself. Even if variables of the basic oscillator were known, it would be hard to distinguish between a very low amplitude or absence of a rhythm. The apparent induction of a rhythm or coupling of a driven function to the basic oscillator by a single light-dark, or high temperature-low temperature transition (1,2) gives no definite clues for a decision between complete absence and low amplitude of the circadian rhythmicity.

10. The entrained state of the circadian oscillator

The differential and proportional effects of a rectangular temperature cycle on the circadian rhythm mediated by a series of intracellular processes can, thus, be summarized and based on some data in Neurospora. The change from lower to higher temperature causes transient changes in Ca^{++}, and, after about 1 h, in the HS-synthesis rates (and a decrease of normal protein synthesis). The differential changes are followed by adaptive reactions that lead to new steady states, which are proportional to the temperature amplitude. After the temperature is switched back to 25°C it is probable, but not yet documented, that opposite differential and adaptional changes occur at the cellular level.

The change from lower to higher τ causes an immediate phase shift ($\Delta\Phi$) of the endogenous oscillation (see Fig. 1). is dependent on the phase of the oscillation (63) and on the amplitude of the temperature difference (38). Furthermore, there is a shortening of τ during the subsequent high temperature period. Concomitantly the phase response to the step-down signal of the temperature after 12 h is shifted. The step-down signal causes an immediate phase shift followed by a relative lengthening of τ during the low temperature; a corresponding lengthening of the PRC is the response to the following step-up signal etc. These phase shifts and alterations of τ during the entrained state are characterized by a steady state of daily changes of the endogenous oscillator in different direction (66).

In the model oscillator we simulated the tonic effects of a Zeitgeber cycle by imposing regular changes of synthesis (Ax) and degradation (Bx) rate on the oscillation of X. The oscillator was entrained better when Bx was changed compared to corresponding changes of Ax, i.e. the range of entrainment by changes of Bx was larger and the needed Zeitgeber amplitude smaller than with Ax. These results show that entrainment in the model can be achieved by using tonic effects of the Zeitgeber cycle alone. However, we need to know more about the processes affected by light and elevated temperatures in the pacemaker cells of man or in Neurospora before we can trace deviations from the normal entrainment in man to the cellular processes responsible for it.

11. References

1. D. Njus, L. McMurry, J.W. Hastings: J. Comp. Physiol. 117, 335 (1977)
2. V. Gooch: In Temporal Order, ed. By. L. Rensing, N. Jaeger (Springer, Heidelberg 1985)
3. J. Bünning: In The Physiological Clock (Springer, Heidelberg 1977)
4. G. Cornelius, L. Rensing: BioSystems 15, 35 (1982)
5. J. Aschoff: In Circadian Clocks", ed. by J. Aschoff (North-Holland, Amsterdam 1965)
6. C.S. Pittendrigh: In Handbook of Behavioral Neurobiology V, Chap.7, Plenum Press, New York (1981)
7. C. Kasal, J.R. Perez-Polo: TIBS, 59 (Febr. 1982)
8. H. Senger (ed): In Blue Light Effects in Biological Systems (Springer, Heidelberg 1984)

9. T.D. Lamb: Trends in Neurosci. 9, 224 (1986)
10. W. Baehr, M.L. Applebury: Trends in Neurosci. 9, 198 (1986)
11. L. Stryer: Ann. Rev. Neurosci. 9, 87 (1986)
12. P. Sterling, M. Freed, R.G. Smith: Trends in Neurosci. 9, 186 (1986)
13. R.F. Miller, M.M. Slaughter: Trends in Neurosci. 9, 211 (1986)
14. B. Rusack: In Vertebrate Circadian Systems, Structure and Physiology, ed. by J. Aschoff, S. Daan, G. Gross (Springer, Heidelberg 1982) p. 62
15. C.P. Downes: Trends in Neurosci. 6, 313 (1983)
16. V. Munoz, W.L. Butler: Plant Physiol. 55, 421 (1975)
17. R.D. Brain, J.A. Freeberg, C.V. Weiss, W.R. Briggs: Plant Physiol. 59, 948 (1977)
18. J. Paietta, M.L. Sargent: Proc. Natl. Acad. Sci. USA 78, 5573 (1981)
19. W. Schmidt: In Blue Light Effects in Biological Systems ed. by H. Senger (Springer, Heidelberg 1984)
20. C.E. Borgson, B.J. Bowman: Plant Physiol. 78, 433 (1985)
21. A.W. Lambowitz, C.W. Slayman, C.L. Slayman, W.D. Bonner: J. Biol. Chem. 247, 1536 (1972)
22. R. Schulz, U. Pilatus, L. Rensing: Chronobiol. Intern. 2, 223 (1985)
23. T.V. Potapova, N.N. Levina, T.A. Belozerskaya, L.M. Chailakhian, M.S. Kritsky: Arch. Microbiol. 137, 262 (1984)
24. M.S. Kritsky, T.P. Afanasieva, T.A. Belozerskaya, L.M. Chailakhian, E.K. Chernysheva, S.Yu Filippowich, N.N. Levina, T.V. Potapova, V. Yu Sokolovsky: In Blue Light Effect in Biological Systems" ed. by H. Senger (Springer, Heidelberg 1984)
25. H. Nakashima, Y. Fujimura: Planta 155, 431 (1982)
26. H. Nakashima: Plant Phyisol. 70, 982 (1982)
27. H. Nakashima, F. Feldman: Photochem. Photobiol. 32, 247 (1980)
28. D. Techel, L. Rensing: unpubl. experiments
29. R.W. Harding, R.V. Turner: Plant Physiol. 68, 745 (1981)
30. M.S. Kritsky, V. Yu. Sokolevsky, T.A. Belozerskays, E.K. Shernysheva: Arch. Microbiol. 133, 208 (1982)
31. U. Mitzka-Schnabel, E. Warm, W. Rau: In Blue Light Effects in Biological Systems ed. by H. Senger (Springer, Heidelberg 1984)
32. J.A.A. Chambers, K. Hinkelammert, V.E.A. Russo: The EMBO Journal 4, 3649 (1985)
33. V.Y.A. Alexandrov: In Cells, Molecules and Temperature (Springer, Heidelberg 1977)
34. M. Ashburner, J.J. Bonner: Cell 17, 241 (1979)
35. M.J. Schlesinger, M. Ashburner, A. Tissières: In Heat Shock From Bacteria to Man (Cold Spring Harbor Laboratory 1982)
36. L. Nover: In Heat Shock Response in Eukaryotic Cells (Springer, Heidelberg 1984)
37. M.J. Schlesinger: J. Cell Biol. 103, 321 (1986)
38. L. Rensing, A. Bos, J. Kröger, G. Cornelius, unpubl.
39. G. Weitzel, U. Pilatus, L. Rensing: Exp. Cell Res. 159, 252 (1985)
40. J.A.S. Drummond, S.A. McClure, M. Poenie, R.S. Tsien, R. Steinhardt: Mol. Cell Biol. 6, 1767 (1986)
41. S.K. Calderwood, M.S. Stevenson, G.M. Hahn: Biochem. Biophys. Res. Comm. 126, 911 (1985)
42. V. Ernst, E. Baum, Reddy, P.: In Heat Shock From Bacteria to Man Cold Spring Harbor Laboratory 1982
43. J.M. Kennedy, R.H. Burdon, D.P. Leader: FEBS 169, 267 (1984)
44. B.C. Goodwin: Adv. Enzyme Regul. 3, 425 (1965)
45. K. Drescher, G. Cornelius, L. Rensing: J. theor. Biol. 94, 345 (1982)
46. L. Rensing, W. Schill: In Temporal Order, ed. L. Rensing, N. Jaeger (Springer, Heidelberg 1985)
47. H. Nakashima: Plant Physiol. 76, 612 (1984)
48. H. Nakashima: Plant Physiol. 74, 268 (1984)
49. G. Cornelius, L. Rensing: Europ. J. Cell Biol. 40, 130 (1986)
50. J. Jacklet: Biol. Bull. 160, 199 (1981)
51. J. Aschoff: In Cold Spring Harb. Symp. quant. Biol. 25, 11 (1960)

52. B. Sweeney, J.W. Hastings: In Cold Spring Harb. Symp. quant. Biol. 25, 87 (1960)
53. G. Scholübbers, W. Taylor, L. Rensing: Am.J. Physiol. 247, R250 (1984)
54. A. Schroeder-Lorenz, L. Rensing: Comp. Biochem. Physiol. 85B, 315 (1986)
55. B.M. Sweeney: Plant Physiol. 64, 341 (1979)
56. G.F. Gardner, J.F. Feldman: Plant Physiol. 68, 1244 (1981)
57. M.L. Sargent, W.R. Briggs, D.W. Woodward: Plant Physiol. 41, 1343 (1966)
58. C.S. Pittendrigh, V.G. Bruce, N.S. Rosenzweig, M.L. Rubin: Nature 184, 169 (1959)
59. J.W. Hastings, J.C. Dunlap, W.R. Taylor: In Current Topics in Cell Regul. 18, (Academic Press, New York 1981) p. 519
60. B.G. Hall: J. Bacteriol. 156, 1363 (1983)
61. R.L. Hallberg: Mol. Cell Biol.6, 2267 (1986)
62. R.L. Hallberg, K.W. Kraus, E.M. Hallberg: Mol. Cell Biol.5, 2061 (1985)
63. C.D. Francis, M.L. Sargent: Plant Physiol. 64, 1000 (1979)
64. C.S. Pittendrigh: In Cold Spring Harbor Symp. quant. Biol. 25, 159 (1960)
65. M.L. Sargent, W.R. Briggs: Plant Physiol. 42, 1304 (1967)
66. J. Perlman, H. Nakashima, J.F. Feldman: Plant Physiol. 67, 404 (1981)
67. H.Nakashima: In Circadian Clocks and Zeitgebers, ed. by T. Hiroshyge and and K. Honma (Hokkaido Univ. Press, Sapporo 1985) p. 35
68. L. Rensing, R.Olomski, K.Drescher: BioSystems 15, 341 (1982)
69. H. Nakashima, J. Perlman, J.F. Feldman: Amer. J. Physiol. 241, 31 (1981)

Part V

Ovarian Cycles

Temporal Order and Disorder in a Model That Regulates Ovulation Number

H.M. Lacker

Courant Institute of Mathematical Sciences, New York University, New York, NY 10012, USA

1. INTRODUCTION

The overwhelming majority of follicles that initiate growth in the mammalian ovary atrophy before reaching full ovulatory maturity. However, the number of follicles that emerge fully mature in each cycle, the *ovulation number*, is a controlled and characteristic number of the species or breed. For example, in many mammals removing an ovary does not cut the ovulation number in half. Instead, the number of follicles per cycle that reach full maturity doubles in the remaining ovary to compensate for the removal of its partner [1].

The temporal disorders that we will consider arise in a mathematical model that is proposed to explain the physiological mechanism regulating ovulation number [2,3,4]. Disturbances in the timing of maturation will therefore often be associated with a loss of control in ovulation number as well. We consider disturbances where there are sudden transitions from cyclic to non-cyclic states and also where there is a more gradual loss of temporal control that occurs in the normally aging reproductive system.

2. THE MODEL

Our model takes the form of a many-body problem where the interaction between bodies, follicles in this case, occurs through circulatory feedback involving estradiol and pituitary gonadotropic hormones. As a follicle matures its estradiol secretion rate increases [5]. In many species a follicle's secretion rate is directly proportional to the concentration that it supports in the circulation. This is because estradiol is removed from the circulation by a first order process that is fast on the time scale of follicle development [6]. In the model, we measure follicle maturity by the circulating estradiol concentration that a follicle supports.

Let us denote the maturity of the ith follicle as a function of time by $x_i(t)$. Follicles are activated into the interacting population from a non-secreting reserve pool at random times. In the model these activation times are generated from a given probability distribution. Let $\{T_i$ $i=1,2,...\}$ denote a sequence of follicle activation times on $t > 0$. Let the initial activation maturity of follicles be a given (small) constant x^*. Then,

$$x_i(T_i) = x^* \quad . \tag{1}$$

At any time the estradiol concentration in the circulation is the sum of the contributions made by the activated follicle population. If we denote the estradiol concentration as a function of time by $X(t)$ then,

$$X(t) = \sum_{\{i:\, t > T_i\}} x_i(t) \quad . \tag{2}$$

Through the mediation of pituitary hormones, the circulating estradiol concentration, X, feeds back upon each developing follicle influencing its maturation rate. Since the response of a follicle to pituitary hormones depends on its maturity, the maturation rate of the ith follicle is a function of both x_i and X. Therefore,

$$\frac{dx_i}{dt} = f\,(x_i,X) \qquad t > T_i \quad . \tag{3}$$

In the model every active follicle influences the maturation rate of every other active follicle through its contribution to X.

Note that there is a great deal of symmetry in the model. Since f(,) is the same function for all follicles, they are all assumed to inherit the same program of development. All follicles start growing at the same maturity x* and all follicles interact through X which at any time is the same value for all.. To regulate ovulation number the symmetry must be broken. More precisely, the developing follicle population must split into two groups: those that ovulate and those that undergo atresia (atrophy). In addition,physiological observations suggest that the ovulation number should be nearly independent of the number of follicles in the interacting population, the mean activation rate, and the specific sequence of activation times.

In principle,the maturation function f(x,X) could be determined directly from experiments, but the techniques for generating this data are not yet available. It is possible, however, to generate examples of maturation functions that account for features of follicle development over a wide range of experimental conditions.

Consider the example illustrated in Fig.1. The maturation surface takes the form

$$f(x,X) = C\,x\,\{1 - D(X - M_1x)(X - M_2x)\} \tag{4}$$

where $M_1 = 3.85$, $M_2 = 15.15$, $C = 1.0$ and $D = 0.0025$. If follicles are activated at random times generated from a Poisson process, the following numerical solution of the system (1-4) is obtained (Fig. 2).

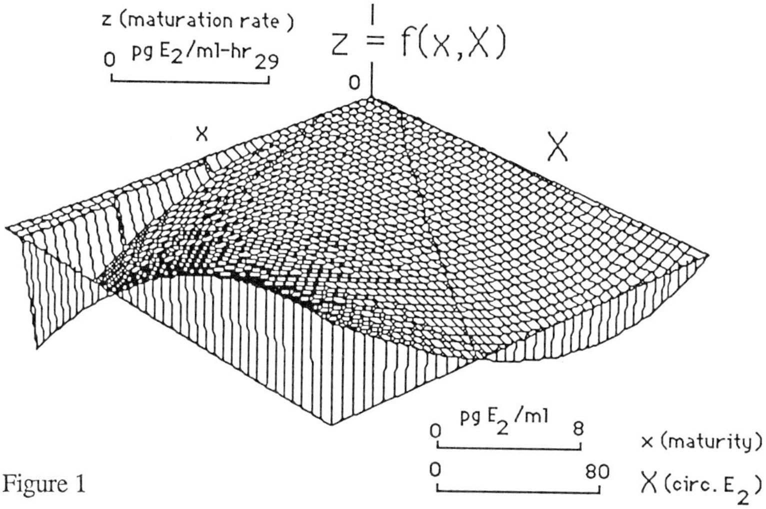

Figure 1

Figure 2

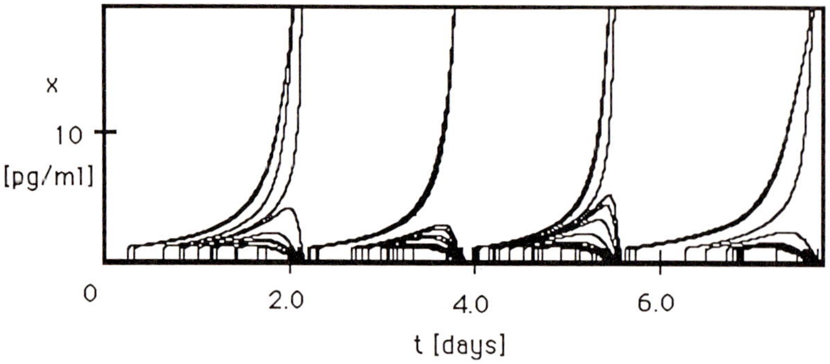

Ovulation Time (Days)	Ovulation Number
2.145	5
3.905	4
5.575	4
7.785	4

In this example $x^* = 2$ pg/ml, and the mean activation rate is 12 follicles per day. Even though all follicles obey the same growth law, f(,), interact through a common feedback signal, X, and start growing at the same maturity, x^*, 4 or 5 follicles are repeatedly selected for ovulation. When $X=X^\dagger$ (a sufficiently large constant) these follicles are assumed to ovulate, that is, they are removed from the interacting population and their contribution to X is set to 0. Physiologically, this corresponds to the triggering of the ovulatory surge mechanism when the circulating estradiol concentrations become sufficiently high [7].

Note the temporal synchronization of the ovulatory follicles in the model and the full repression of the non-ovulatory follicles by the time of ovulation. The temporal order that emerges from the chaotic activation mechanism is a well-known physiological property of the system regulating follicle development.

3. Symmetric Solutions

What is it about the follicle maturation program illustrated in Fig. 1 that allows it to repeatedly select 4 or 5 follicles for ovulation? Figure 3 shows that the maturation function separates the (x,X)-plane into regions of growth ($f > 0$) and atresia ($f < 0$).

Consider the special case where M follicles start growing with identical maturity and the remaining follicles remain dormant. Since $X=Mx$, the M identical follicles mature along the line with integer slope M in the (x,X) plane. When M is in the interval (M_1, M_2), the line of integer slope M remains in the growth zone and all M follicles ovulate. Substituting Mx for X in f(x,X) shows that the M follicles satisfy the differential equation

$$\frac{dx}{dt} = C\,(x + \mu x^3) \tag{5}$$

where $\mu = -D(M-M_1)(M-M_2)$. The sign of μ is positive when $M \in (M_1, M_2)$ and x approaches infinity in a finite time (idealized ovulation time). This follows from $dx/dt \sim x^3$ for sufficiently large x. In the example above, the interval $(M_1,M_2) = (3.85,15.15)$ includes the integers 4 and 5. Although ovulatory solutions also exist for larger numbers (6-15), these ovulation numbers have never been observed numerically for reasons that will be explained shortly. When $M \notin (M_1, M_2)$, then the line with integer slope M in Fig. 3 crosses into the atretic

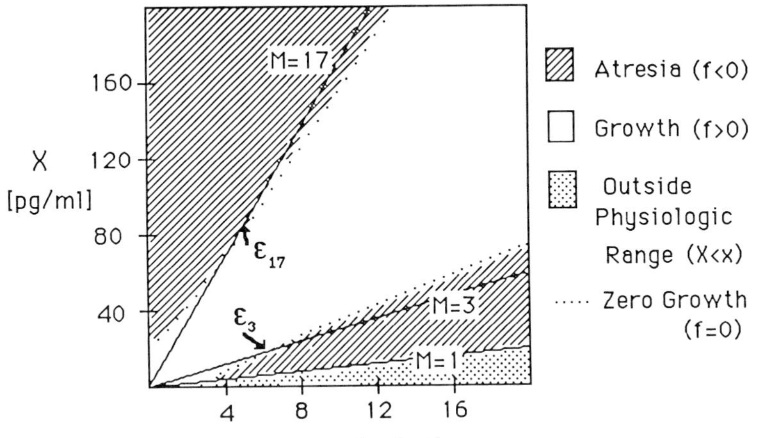

Figure 3

zone. This prevents the follicles from fully maturing. At the point of crossover f = 0 ($x=\mu x^3$) and an equilibrium, ξ_M, occurs. Two equilibrium points for 3 and 17 identical follicles are labelled in Fig. 3.

4. Stability of Symmetric Solutions for the N-Follicle Initial Value Problem

The reason why the higher ovulation numbers and the ξ_M equilibria are not seen in numerical solutions is that they are usually unstable and therefore occur with probability zero. Factors that stabilize the equilibria, produce pathology in the model. We postulate that these factors may also cause pathology in some mammals including humans.

Although we do not yet have a method for directly analyzing the system with random entry into interacting follicle population, we can analyze the initial value problem

$$\frac{dx_i}{dt} = f(x_i, X) \quad i = 1,\ldots,N$$

$$X = \sum_{j=1}^{N} x_j \tag{6}$$

$$f(x,X) = C\,x\{1 - D(X - M_1 x)(X - M_2 x)\} \quad \left(x_1(0), x_2(0), \ldots, x_N(0)\right)$$

when there is a fixed number N of interacting follicles. Consider the following change of variables

$$y_i = \sqrt{\frac{x_i}{X}} \quad , \quad i = 1,\ldots,N \quad ,$$

$$\tau(t) = \int_0^t C X^2(s)\, ds \quad , \tag{7}$$

which transforms the system above into the following gradient system on the unit sphere S in N-dimensions

$$\frac{dY}{d\tau} = \nabla_S V \; ,$$
$$V(Y) = \frac{1}{2}\sum_{i=1}^{N} \int^{y_i} s\,\xi(s^2)\,ds \; , \qquad (8)$$
$$\xi(s) = D\,s(M_1 + M_2 - M_1 M_2 s) \; .$$

The symbol ∇_S is the gradient projected onto S, and $Y(\tau) = (y_1(t(\tau)),..., y_N(t(\tau)))$ is a solution on S. If M of the N follicles are non-zero, and have the same maturity x, then x/X= 1/M. Therefore, each line of integer slope in Fig. 3 corresponds to a point on S with coordinates

$$y_i = \begin{cases} \sqrt{\dfrac{1}{M}} & i = 1, \ldots, M \\ 0 & i = M+1, \ldots, N \end{cases} \; . \qquad (9)$$

It can be checked that these points (and points whose coordinates are permutations of the above coordinates) are critical points of V restricted to S (V/S) and therefore represent equilibria for the gradient system. Because of the gradient property, it can be shown that all solutions of the system on S asymptotically approach a critical point of V/S. (Actually, there may be other critical points of V/S besides the symmetric equilibria described above, but these are not local maxima and therefore are not stable [4].) The stability properties of the M-fold symmetric equilibria are summarized in Fig. 4.

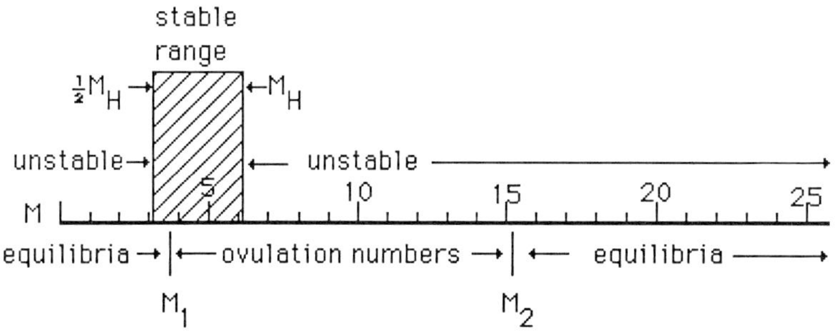

Figure 4

The interval of ovulatory solutions (M_1,M_2) is broken into two intervals by M_H, the harmonic mean of M_1 and M_2,

$$1/M_H = 1/2 \cdot (1/M_1 + 1/M_2) \; . \qquad (10)$$

Only ovulation numbers in the stable interval (M_1,M_H) will be observed for the N follicle system. For the example above, $M_H = 6.12$ and so ovulation numbers larger than 6 are unstable. Since the stability properties are independent of N, the range of observed ovulation numbers would not change, for example, if N were reduced by 1/2 (something like removing an ovary). The number of interacting follicles in a cycle is also a decreasing function of age. (The reserve pool of follicles decreases exponentially and the mean number of follicles activated per unit time declines gradually with age.)

5. A Functional Role for Atretic Follicles

Although the eigenvalues are independent of N, the geometry of the phase space on S and the domain of attraction of each stable equilibria does change with N. This results in a change in the frequency with which a stable ovulation number is observed. This is illustrated in Fig. 5. As the size of the interacting follicle population decreases, there is a shift towards the higher ovulation numbers in the stable range. This is consistent with the steady statistical increase in the dizygotic twinning rates with age in humans [8]. (The identical twinning rate does not change with age.)

The model results suggest that the mechanism activating large numbers of follicles from the reserve pool during each cycle actually helps to keep the ovulation number down. This may represent an evolutionary adaptation of a mechanism that was originally designed to release large numbers of eggs into the external environment. This could represent yet another example where an older scheme is not discarded when the demands of the environment change but rather is adapted to different (and in this case opposite) purposes by newly superimposed regulatory mechanisms.

Figure 5 also shows that the timing of maturation is much less regular when N is small. This loss of control in the timing of ovulation is a well-known feature of the human reproductive

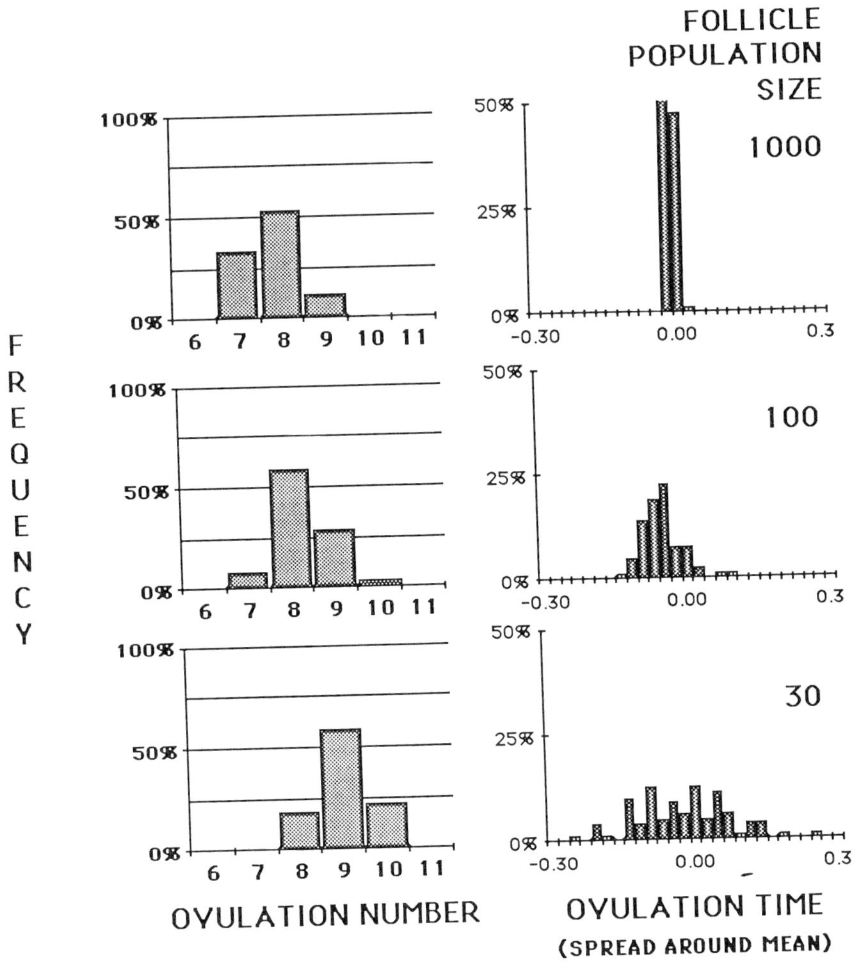

Figure 5

system as menopause is approached [9]. The model therefore suggests important functional roles for what might first appear simply as follicle wastage: The large numbers of follicles that are activated and atrophy in each cycle may actually be helping to control the timing of ovulation and number of follicles that ovulate.

6. Anovulation

The stability analysis summarized in Fig. 4 suggests another possibility. If integers exist in the interval between $M_{H/2}$ and M_1 then they should correspond to stable non-ovulatory equilibria. Since there are no integers in the interval $(M_{H/2}, M_1) = (3.06, 3.85)$ for our particular example, none of the equilibria ξ_M are stable in the N-follicle system. Nevertheless, for special choice of the parameters M_1 and M_2, some of the non-ovulatory equilibria could become stable. This is illustrated in Fig. 6. In this case the stable interval $(M_{H/2}, M_1)$ includes the integers 5 and 6.

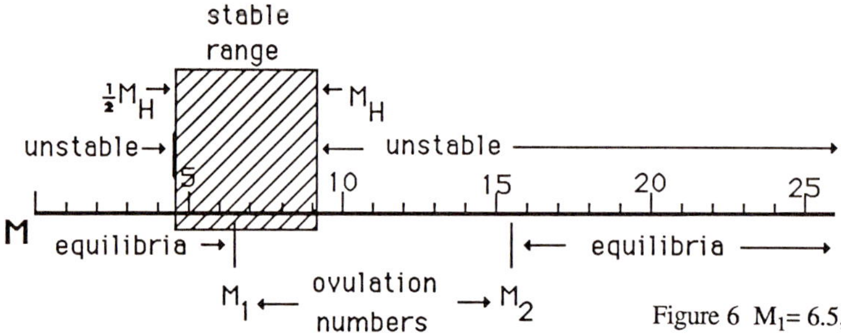

Figure 6 $M_1= 6.5, M_2=15.5, M_H=9.16$

Figure 7 shows two numerical solutions of the initial value problem. In each case the number of interacting follicles N=10. The initial maturities are chosen independently from a uniform distribution in the interval (0.00,0.05). In Fig. 7a, a number of follicles (7) mature to ovulation, but in Fig. 7b, several follicles (6) get "stuck" at an intermediate maturity. (The equilibrium corresponding to 5 "stuck" follicles was observed in 2 out of 1000 trials similar to Fig. 7).

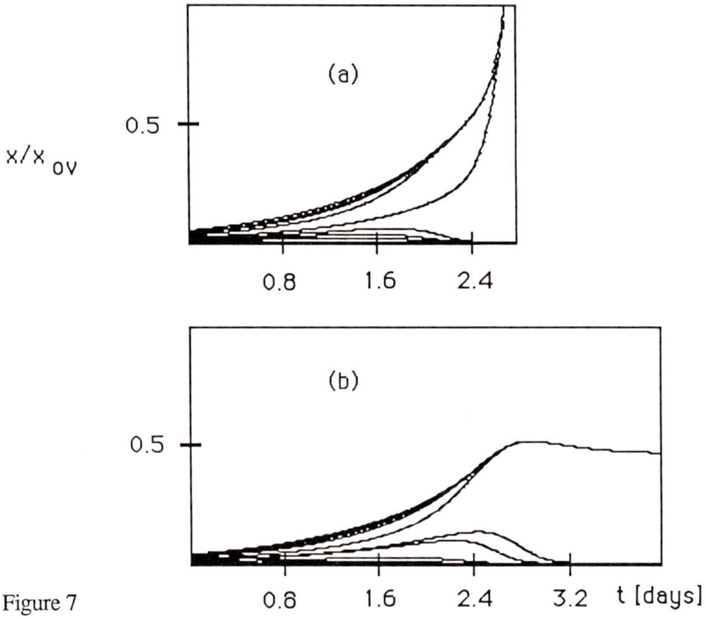

Figure 7

Figure 8 shows that when follicles are activated at random times, spontaneous transitions from cyclic to non-cyclic states can occur. Similar transitions have been observed in some members of some species including humans [10]. It is important to understand how such transitions occur because long-term exposure to steady concentrations of estradiol can produce pathology in estrogen-sensitive tissues in the breast and uterus including endometrial carcinoma.

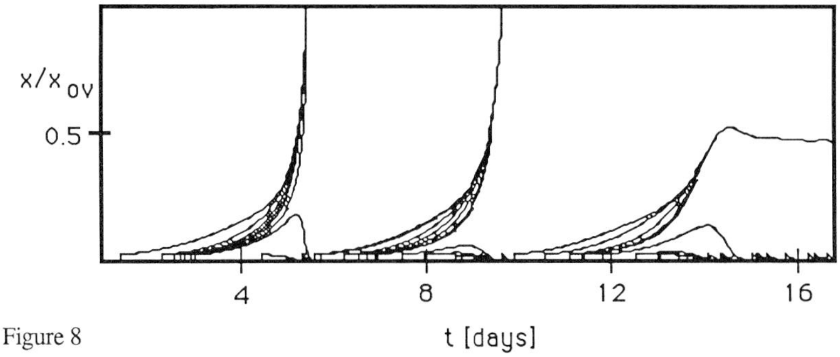

Figure 8

During the non-cyclic state, the estradiol concentrations produced by the "stuck" follicles (there are 5 such follicles in Fig. 8) are sufficient to repress the growth of newly activated follicles. With each new activation the phase space of the interacting system increases by one dimension. This changes the position of the equilibrium point as well as the geometry of its capturing region, and produces the fluctuations that are observed in Fig. 8. Escape from anovulation and return to cyclic activity could occur if the system were perturbed outside of the domain of attraction of the stable ξ_M equilibrium. This might occur spontaneously or it might be "forced" by the exogenous administration of estradiol or its antagonist.

Although the stability analysis of the N-follicle system appears to explain many numerical observations of the system with random follicle entry, there are some unexpected numerical results. The first of these is illustrated in Figure 9a. The parameters M_1 and M_2 are the same as those chosen originally (3.85 and 15.15). Three follicles approach an equilibrium maturity although there are not supposed to be any integers in the stable range $(1/2\ M_H, M_1)$, (Fig. 4). It appears as if the random entry of follicles has stabilized ξ_3. This is supported by the numerical experiment shown in Figure 9b. This is the same run as Fig. 9a, except that at $t = 3$ (arrow), the random entry of follicles is stopped. From this point on, the system is an N-follicle system. As predicted ξ_3 becomes unstable. Another follicle joins the three and all four (a stable number) ovulate. As a first approximation, one could consider the repressed follicle population as sustaining a constant estradiol concentration $\lambda = \nu\ x^*$, where ν is the mean poisson activation rate. A stability analysis of the N-follicle system with

$$X = \sum_{j=1}^{N} x_j + \lambda(\nu) \quad . \tag{11}$$

shows that when the bifurcation parameter ν increases past a critical value ν_c, ξ_3 becomes stable.

This suggests that the anovulatory state could be broken by removing estradiol from the circulation or by giving an estradiol antagonist. (Some types of anovulation in humans have been treated with the estrogen antagonist clomiphene citrate). Figure 10 illustrates an example in which cycling activity is restored in the model when the circulating estradiol concentration is

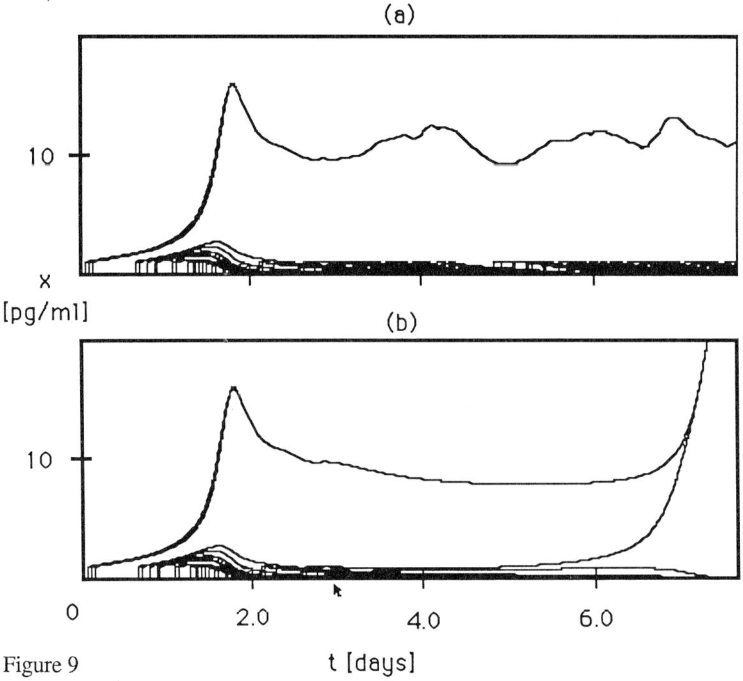

Figure 9

lowered by 10 pg/ml during the time indicated between the arrows. The system of equations (1)-(4) is solved numerically, except that during the time between the arrows (2) has been changed to

$$X(t) = \sum_{\{i:\, t > T\}} x_i(t) - 10 . \tag{12}$$

In the model, escape from steady anovulation to cyclic follicle maturation can also occur as a result of gradual changes in the mean entry rate of follicles into the estradiol secreting population. This is illustrated in Fig. 11. The maturation surface in Fig. 11a is obtained from a generalization of the two parameter (M1,M2)-model [4]. When follicles enter the dynamically interacting population at times generated by a poisson process (mean rate 1/day), one follicle emerges with ovulatory maturity approximately every 12 days (Fig. 11b). Figure 11c shows the circulating estradiol concentration as a function of time when follicles are activated at times generated by an exponential distribution. At the beginning of the simulation, the activation rate is sufficiently high to prevent any follicle from maturing to ovulation. A steady non-ovulatory state is achieved. (This steady state does not exist in the initial value formulation of the model.) As the mean rate gradually declines towards 1 per day a spontaneous and sudden transition to cyclic activity occurs where one follicle periodically escapes from the remaining population and reaches ovulatory maturity.

Figure 10

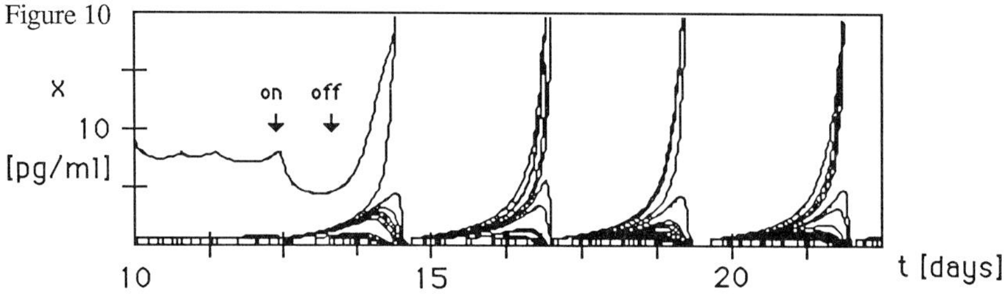

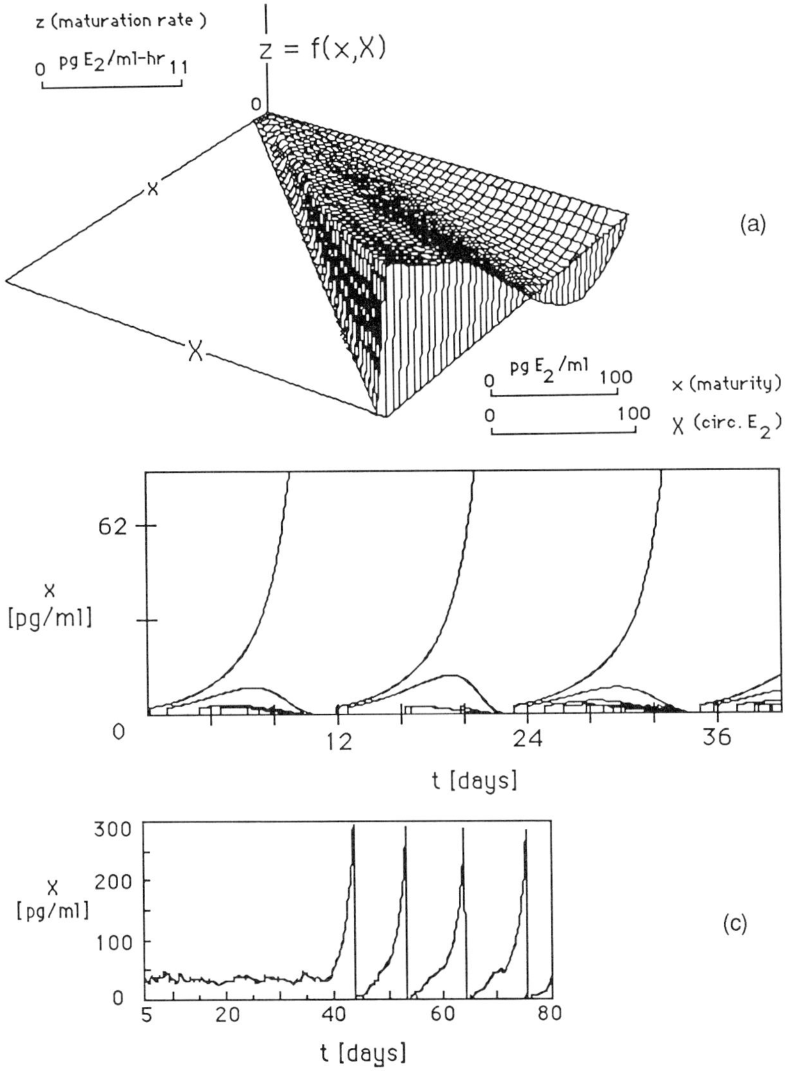

Figure 11

1. A. Lipschütz: Br. J. Exp. Biol. 5, 283 (1928)
2. H. M. Lacker: Biophys. J. 35, 433 (1981)
3. H. M. Lacker, C. S. Peskin: In Lect. Math. Life Sci. 14, 21 ed. by S. Childress (The Amer. Math. Soc.,Providence 1981)
4. E. Akin, H. M. Lacker: J. Math. Biol. 20, 113 (1984)
5. L. Speroff, R.L. VandeWiele: Am. J. Obstet. Gynecol. 109, 234 (1971)
6. D. T. Baird, R. Horton, C. Longcope, J. F. Tait: Recent Prog. Horm. Res. 25, 611 (1969)
7. E. Knobil: Recent Prog. Horm. Res. 30, 1 (1974)
8. N, McArthur: Ann. Eugen. 17, 249 (1954)
9. S. G. Korenman, B. M. Sherman, J. C. Korenman: Clin. Endocrinol. Metab. 7, 625 (1978)
10. L. Speroff, R. H. Glass, N. G. Kase: In Clinical Gynecologic Endocrinology and Infertility (The Williams & Wilkins Co., Baltimore 1973)

Index of Contributors